American Public Health Association
VITAL AND HEALTH STATISTICS MONOGRAPHS

Marriage and Divorce: A Social and Economic Study

Marriage and Divorce: A Social and Economic Study

Revised Edition

HUGH CARTER and PAUL C. GLICK

HARVARD UNIVERSITY PRESS

Cambridge, Massachusetts, and London, England

Library of Congress Catalog Card Number 76–3977
ISBN 0–674–55076–5
Printed in the United States of America

PREFACE TO SECOND EDITION

The nature and extent of recent changes in marriage, divorce, and living arrangements have been so sweeping that a new concluding Chapter 13 has been prepared for the second edition of *Marriage and Divorce*. This chapter describes also some measures of the parameters of marriage and divorce that have become available during the 6 years since the first edition was published.

The sections of Chapter 13 treat the subject matter in the same sequence as Chapters 1 to 12, obviously in selective detail. Besides updating key statistics in the original edition, Chapter 13 features such entirely new material as the following: first-marriage, divorce, and remarriage rates for the United States during the last 50 years; projection of the proportion of first marriages that eventually end in divorce; distributions by marital status for persons in consistently high and consistently low socioeconomic groups; quartiles of age at marriage by previous marital status of bride and groom; classification by race for children with parents of unlike race; proportion of white children and black children living with both parents who are in their first marriage; number of adults living with unmarried partners of the opposite sex; proportion of wives with more income than their husbands; number and characteristics of persons ever divorced; socioeconomic level of widowed and divorced persons who have not remarried; reasons for low incomes, on the average, of single and separated men but high incomes of single and divorced women; new indicators of the relation between health and marital status; and evidence of extensive changes in the legal and administrative aspects of marriage and divorce during the last decade, including a discussion of the pros and cons of no-fault divorce.

Although Chapter 13 highlights extensive recent changes in lifestyles relating to marriage, it also documents the continuing preference of a vast majority of postadolescent adults for life as married (or remarried) persons. Many of the changes may be properly interpreted as reflections of a deep desire for greater satisfaction from married life, even if delayed marriage or divorce is required to realize it.

We express our gratitude to the Population Division of the Bureau of the Census for its support in preparation of the manuscript for this new edition; to those who reviewed the manuscript and offered many helpful suggestions; to Arthur J. Norton and his staff in the Census

Bureau's Marriage and Family Statistics Branch, who were responsible for preparation of many of the reports from which data were drawn for use in the new chapter; and to Joyce K. Balch for her able assistance in typing the text and tables. We thank the United States National Center for Health Statistics and the United Nations for providing statistics in advance of publication, and Isabel Gordon Carter for aid in compiling and analyzing large quantities of data.

Hugh Carter
Sociologist and Consultant
2039 New Hampshire Avenue, N.W.
Washington, D.C. 20009

Paul C. Glick
Senior Demographer
Population Division
Bureau of the Census
U.S. Department of Commerce
Washington, D.C. 20233

February 1976

PREFACE TO FIRST EDITION

The upward trend in divorce during most of the twentieth century has attracted far more attention than the concurrent upward trend in marriage. Probably few people realize that for every unit of increase since 1940 in the proportion divorced among adults in the United States there have been five units of increase in the proportion married. This is one of many developments that can be found in the analysis presented in this monograph.

This study presents a systematic documentation of important trends and variations in demographic aspects of marital behavior in the United States during recent decades. Many "obvious facts" are substantiated and many others are shown to be "nonfacts." Emphasis is placed on selective factors in marriage; that is, information about who does and who does not follow the norm of mature adulthood by becoming married and remaining married through middle age.

The material documented here is limited largely to such biological characteristics as age, sex, and race and to such social and economic characteristics as national origin, residence, education, occupation, and income, though attention is also given to legal and administrative aspects of marriage and divorce. These variables set limits within which other important forces — including psychological variables and marriage counseling — can take place. They do not reveal how many people are happily married nor how many unmarried persons are happier because they are still single or are "single again." Nonetheless, the subject matter covered is of primary importance to those who wish to learn more about the situation within which steps can be taken to improve the quality of life as it relates to marriage.

This monograph is one of a series that has been sponsored by the American Public Health Association. One chapter deals specifically with the relationship between marital status and health. In that chapter, the findings from other chapters on the association between marital status and socioeconomic status are used to develop hypotheses about the interaction among all three phenomena: marital status, socioeconomic status, and health.

This book is an introduction to the growing body of demographic and socioeconomic facts concerning marriage. The limitations of these data are set forth in the publications cited. Little attention is devoted to marriage patterns as a factor in fertility, because that subject is covered in another monograph in this series by Kiser, Grabill, and Campbell, *Trends and Variations in Fertility in the United States.*

Because of the nationwide concern about problems among families in the black community, a conscious attempt is made to compare white and nonwhite groups with regard to as many facets of marriage as possible. Marriage patterns among persons at all social and economic levels are analyzed, and information bearing on the marital behavior of numerous groups with distinct social problems is provided: persons with early marriage, late marriage, or no marriage; children of separated, unwed, or divorced persons; orphans; persons from different social groups who intermarry; couples who double up with relatives after marriage; working wives and mothers; school dropouts; and highly educated women.

After the first three chapters, several chapters are organized around the successive ages at which marriage, separation and divorce, and widowhood tend to occur, with a special chapter on those who marry late or never. Primary responsibility was assumed by Hugh Carter for the preparation of chapters 1 to 4, 8, and 12; by Paul C. Glick for chapters 5 to 7 and 9 to 11; and by both authors for chapter 13.

Working for several years on the preparation of this book was a complex undertaking and involved the cooperative efforts of many more persons than those named below. The late Mortimer Spiegelman, however, deserves to be singled out for a special tribute for the constant encouragement he gave the authors and for his unstinting effort to improve the substance and form of the manuscript through all of the drafts. Conrad Taeuber likewise provided valuable counsel at all stages of the preparation of the manuscript and made a number of valid criticisms. Robert D. Grove was helpful in obtaining funds for special tabulations used in this study. David M. Heer and Robert Parke, Jr., made important contributions in the designing of tables for census reports that are cited extensively. Carl E. Ortmeyer and Alexander Plateris similarly made important contributions to the preparation of relevant vital statistics reports.

Hugh Carter expresses gratitude to Sylvia Goldstein for statistical assistance, including the preparation of numerous tables, and to Ruth Ritchey, his former secretary, for typing and editorial assistance.

Paul C. Glick gratefully acknowledges the valuable technical assistance he has received from Wilson H. Grabill through many years of close collaboration, particularly on the analysis of the cycle of married life. He wishes to thank Leone M. Forgo, his secretary, for her devotion to the project and for the skilled editorial assistance she cheerfully rendered.

Any errors in the book that have gone undetected are, of course, the responsibility of the authors.

Finally, the authors express their deep appreciation to their wives, Isabel Carter and Joy Glick, for their patience and sustained interest while this study of other husbands and wives was being undertaken.

H.C.
P.C.G.

October 1969

CONTENTS

TABLES

FIGURES

FOREWORD

Rapid advances in medical and allied sciences, changing patterns in medical care and public health programs, an increasingly health-conscious public, and the rising concern of voluntary agencies and government at all levels in meeting the health needs of the people necessitate constant evaluation of the country's health status. Such an evaluation, which is required not only for an appraisal of the current situation, but also to refine present goals and to gauge our progress toward them, depends largely upon a study of vital and health statistics records.

Opportunity to study mortality in depth emerges when a national census furnishes the requisite population data for the computation of death rates in demographic and geographic detail. Prior to the 1960 census of population there had been no comprehensive analysis of this kind. It therefore seemed appropriate to build up for intensive study a substantial body of death statistics for a three-year period centered around that census year.

A detailed examination of the country's health status must go beyond an examination of mortality statistics. Many conditions such as arthritis, rheumatism, and mental diseases are much more important as causes of morbidity than of mortality. Also, an examination of health status should not be based solely upon current findings, but should take into account trends and whatever pertinent evidence has been assembled through local surveys and from clinical experience.

The proposal for such an evaluation, to consist of a series of monographs, was made to the Statistics Section of the American Public Health Association in October 1958 by Mortimer Spiegelman, and a Committee on Vital and Health Statistics Monographs was authorized with Mr. Spiegelman as Chairman, a position he held until his death on March 25, 1969. The members of this committee and of the Editorial Advisory Subcommittee created later are:

Committee on Vital and Health Statistics Monographs

Carl L. Erhardt, Sc.D., Chairman
Paul M. Densen, D.Sc.
Robert D. Grove, Ph.D.
Clyde V. Kiser, Ph.D.
Felix Moore

George Rosen, M.D., Ph.D.
William H. Stewart, M.D. (withdrew June 1964)
Conrad Taeuber, Ph.D.
Paul Webbink
Donald Young, Ph.D.

Editorial Advisory Subcommittee

Carl L. Erhardt, Sc.D., Chairman
Duncan Clark, M.D.
E. Gurney Clark, M.D.
Jack Elinson, Ph.D.

Eliot Freidson, Ph.D. (withdrew February 1964)
Brian MacMahon, M.D., Ph.D.
Colin White, Ph.D.

The early history of this undertaking is described in a paper presented at the 1962 Annual Conference of the Milbank Memorial Fund.[1] The Committee on Vital and Health Statistics Monographs selected the topics to be included in the series and also suggested candidates for authorship. The frame of reference was extended by the committee to include other topics in vital and health statistics than mortality and morbidity, namely fertility, marriage, and divorce. Conferences were held with authors to establish general guidelines for the preparation of the manuscripts.

Support for this undertaking in its preliminary stages was received from the Rockefeller Foundation, the Milbank Memorial Fund, and the Health Information Foundation. Major support for the required tabulations, for writing and editorial work, and for the related research of the monograph authors was provided by the United States Public Health Service (Research Grant HS 00572, formerly CH 00075 and originally GM 08262). Acknowledgment should also be made to the Metropolitan Life Insurance Company for the facilities and time that were made available to Mr. Spiegelman before his retirement in December 1966, after which he devoted his major time to administer the undertaking and to serve as general editor. Without his abiding concern over each monograph in the series and his close work with the authors, the completion of the series might have been in grave doubt. These sixteen volumes are a fitting memorial to Mr. Spiegelman's resolute efforts.

The New York City Department of Health allowed Dr. Carl L. Erhardt to allocate part of his time to administrative details for the series from April to December 1969, when he retired to assume a more active role. The National Center for Health Statistics, under the

---

[1] Mortimer Spiegelman, "The Organization of the Vital and Health Statistics Monograph Program," *Emerging Techniques in Population Research* (*Proceedings of the 1962 Annual Conference of the Milbank Memorial Fund*; New York: Milbank Memorial Fund, 1963), p. 230. See also Mortimer Spiegelman, "The Demographic Viewpoint in the Vital and Health Statistics Monographs Project of the American Public Health Association," *Demography*, 3:574 (1966).

supervision of Dr. Grove and Miss Alice M. Hetzel, undertook the sizable tasks of planning and carrying out the extensive mortality tabulations for the 1959–61 period. Dr. Taeuber arranged for the cooperation of the Bureau of the Census at all stages of the project in many ways, principally by furnishing the required population data used in computing death rates and by undertaking a large number of varied special tabulations. As the sponsor of the project, the American Public Health Association furnished assistance through Dr. Thomas R. Hood, its Deputy Executive Director.

Because of the great variety of topics selected for monograph treatment, authors were given an essentially free hand to develop their manuscripts as they desired. Accordingly, the authors of the individual monographs bear the full responsibility for their manuscripts, and their opinions and statements do not necessarily represent the viewpoints of the American Public Health Association or of the agencies with which they may be affiliated.

William H. McBeath, M.D., M.P.H.
Executive Director
American Public Health Association

Marriage and Divorce

1 / DEVELOPMENT OF STATISTICS ON MARRIAGE AND DIVORCE

Policy concerning official records of the registration of marriages in the United States has followed a slow course toward centralization in each state capital. In order to prevent fraudulent marriages in the early days, as well as to keep a permanent record, essential information about each wedding became the responsibility of local magistrates. Gradually, as a matter of convenience in referring to them, copies of all marriage records for an entire state were concentrated in one place. At the present time, there are central files in nearly all the states.

The evolution with respect to divorce registration has been more complex. In the early days of the republic, opinion about divorce varied considerably. There were those who opposed divorce under any circumstances. Among those who would allow divorce, there was a question as to whether a legislative or a judicial body should grant individual divorces. In time, state legislatures discontinued acting on individual divorce petitions, and the granting of divorces became a judicial function. The custody of records of divorce then reposed in the court that had heard the case.

However, many practical questions arose in using these court records. For example, if rival heirs claimed the estate of a deceased man, his alleged divorce sometimes became an important question. Court records could settle the matter, but if the decedent had lived in many places the urgent problem might be in which court the records would be found. Much time, money, and unnecessary delay were involved in attempting to locate such records. Some states, in the interest of efficiency, accordingly established a statewide index of their divorce records. Other states followed suit, and very slowly the practice became more common. At the present time, nearly all states maintain central files of their divorce records.

As a by-product of the state files of marriage and divorce records — and of great interest to social scientists — certain demographic information becomes available. The first successful effort to prepare national statistics from marriage and divorce records occurred about 90 years ago, and was stimulated by reports of the rising number of divorces. Following that first survey of marriages and divorces, the federal government has followed a strange start-and-stop program in

1

this important field of social statistics. Not until the 1920's did it initiate the annual publication of marriage and divorce data, but it discontinued this program within a dozen years; and not until 1960 did it begin the preparation of national data from microfilm copies of the state marriage and divorce records, the method long used in preparing statistics of births and deaths.

History of Marriage and Divorce Registration in the United States

Early years. Marriage customs in early America were carried over, to some extent, from Old World customs but differed markedly from area to area. The early Puritans of the Massachusetts Bay Colony, holding strongly that marriage was a civil contract rather than a sacrament, ruled that marriage ceremonies should be performed by magistrates rather than clergymen. The *registration* of marriages also was made a civil function. All of early New England tended to follow the same pattern. In due time, church marriages were permitted and most weddings came to be conducted by ministers, although magistrates continued to perform some.

By contrast, in early Virginia the clergy of the Church of England had the exclusive right to solemnize marriages. However, since an increasing majority of the settlers were adherents of other faiths, this exclusive right was not enforced; many weddings were conducted by ministers of other churches and by magistrates. Moreover, *custody* of the records of marriage became a lay rather than a clerical function.

Other southern colonies tended to follow the Virginia pattern, but in the middle colonies practices differed widely. Pennsylvania, under the influence of the Quakers, permitted variation in marriage customs by the different groups within the colony. New York felt the influence first of Dutch and later of English marriage customs. In all of the colonies, however, keeping the official records of marriages became a civil rather than a church function.[1]

In Colonial America there was also a lack of uniformity in official actions regarding divorce. In New England, divorce from the bonds of matrimony was allowed. In Massachusetts during the seventeenth century, the Court of Assistants, meeting periodically, heard petitions for divorce and related matrimonial matters. There was also legislative divorce in the New England colonies. The General Court of Massachusetts, which was both a judicial tribunal and a legislative body, received such petitions but normally referred them to the Court of Assistants (later referred to as Court of Assizes) for disposition.[2]

In the southern colonies, the situation was radically different. The English law provided means for dealing with proposed divorces, beginning with hearings in the ecclesiastical courts, but in the colonies these courts were not established and this route to divorce, or more properly to separation (divorce "from bed and board"), was not available. According to George Elliott Howard, prior to the Revolution the records of southern colonies reveal no instance of divorce by legislative action or otherwise.[3] In the middle colonies, the situation regarding divorce was different from both New England and the South. In New Netherland, for example, the civil courts had jurisdiction in matrimonial matters and could grant divorce but rarely did so. The Dutch civil authorities frequently attempted to arbitrate difficulties that arose between husband and wife. In Pennsylvania, divorces were granted by legislative authority.[4]

Growth of state files of marriage and divorce records. One of the important motives for the early marriage regulations was to assure that parties who wished to marry were in fact eligible to do so. Banns were published, frequently on three different occasions; parental consent was obtained; a license was issued; and after the marriage a careful record was made of the date and names of bride and groom. Despite these efforts, innocent persons continued to be victimized by the unscrupulous who did not report an existing marriage contracted in another community. The population was highly migratory and communications were slow and uncertain. Thus, after the American Revolution it became apparent that files of marriage records should not be limited to a single community but should include all marriages occurring within an entire state. Such files, of course, would remove much of the uncertainty regarding the eligibility of an individual to marry, since a state file could be searched to verify needed information more easily than could numerous local files. (There would also be added security against loss of records from fires or floods through having a copy of each marriage certificate in both a local office and a state file.) Before 1900, 12 states had established central files of marriage records. During the next 50 years the number of such states increased by 25, so that in 1950 the list included 37 states.[5] By 1968 only 3 states lacked such files of marriage records.

After the granting of divorces was recognized as a function of the civil courts of the various states, the records of divorces granted became part of the official records of the numerous local courts throughout the country having jurisdiction in these matters. But consulting these court records, particularly if one did not know the exact court in which a decree had been granted, was a time-consuming and expensive matter. Frequently, important questions — such as rights of inheritance, alleged bigamy, and legitimacy of children — could not be resolved without official records establishing that a divorce had been granted. The advantage of having one central file of the records of divorce granted within a state soon became evident. In 5 states such files were established before 1900. During the next 50 years 23 additional state files were set up, so that in 1950 a total of 28 states had files of the divorces granted within their boundaries. There were also central files in the District of Columbia and in the Commonwealth of Puerto Rico.[6] In 1968 only 5 states lacked central files of divorce records.

Early National Surveys of Marriage and Divorce

The United States has lagged behind a number of European countries in developing adequate statistics of marriage and divorce. Since the registration of these events is a state rather than a federal function in this country, each of the 50 states passes such laws and keeps such records as seem appropriate to it. Another important reason for our poor statistics may be traced back more than a century to circumstances surrounding the first two national surveys of marriage and divorce. A strong desire for divorce reform was evident in the early agitation for these surveys. The resultant statistics were to be used to persuade the states to adopt uniform laws and to curb easy divorce. Such action immediately placed marriage and divorce statistics in an area of controversy. Unlike the decennial censuses of population, originally authorized for the purpose of determining each state's representation in Congress, the proposed statistics of marriages and divorces were intended to bring about changes in laws relating to marital conflict; it is easy to understand why so many legislators avoided this emotionally charged subject.

First national survey, 1867–1886. The motivation for the first national survey is well summarized in the final publication[7] issued in

1889. The New England Divorce Reform League began operations in 1881 and included in its membership numerous clergymen and others concerned with the confusion and maladministration of the many marriage laws and with divorce reform. Members of the League expressed the desire to bring about greater uniformity in divorce laws through legislation by the several states. Numerous petitions were presented to the Congress requesting a survey of marriage and divorce, but several years passed before authorization was granted in the spring of 1887.

The survey, based on data available in the records of numerous courts and local officials, was far more modest in scope than had been envisioned by Reverend Samuel W. Dike, secretary of the National Divorce Reform League (formerly known as the New England Divorce Reform League), and more limited than had been desired by the Commissioner of Labor, Carroll D. Wright, who directed the survey. Regarding divorces, information was secured on date of marriage, cause for which divorce was granted, whether absolute or limited divorce, number of children, and whether petitioner was husband or wife. Regarding marriages, there was an incomplete count of events; in many areas the records were inadequate. Special agents of the government visited the offices of local officials and recorded most of the data, but in more remote areas attempts to secure information by correspondence were not always successful. Since the survey covered events occurring during 20 years, extending back to the period immediately following the Civil War, there are probably serious gaps in the data, especially for the early years. In 160 listed counties some of the needed records had been destroyed, mostly by fire, but the survey of existing records was evidently done with care.

Second national survey, 1887–1906. Twenty years passed before another survey of marriage and divorce was undertaken. Although the first report was widely circulated and petitions for another survey began to reach Congress in 1902, the enabling legislation was not enacted until 1905. The purpose of the second survey was set forth by President Theodore Roosevelt in a message to Congress containing the following statement: "The hope is entertained that cooperation amongst the several states can be secured to the end that there may be enacted upon the subject of marriage and divorce uniform laws, containing all possible safeguards for the security of the family. Intelligent and prudent action in that direction will be greatly promoted by securing reliable and trustworthy statistics upon marriage and divorce." [8]

The survey was initiated in the summer of 1906. Although this survey, like the first one, placed the primary emphasis on divorce, the results were to improve on the earlier marriage data by securing for the first time, in addition to a count of the number of marriages, a count of marriage licenses. Since two states had no laws for licensing marriages, data on marriage licenses were obtained only as a check on the accuracy of the count of marriages. By contrast, the divorce schedule was expanded from the first survey to a total of 18 items. (The first survey had included much supplementary data from 45 so-called representative counties.) Of special interest were the following items: "Occupation of parties," "Was case contested?" "Was decree granted?" and, as an echo of the times, "If not direct, was intemperance an indirect cause?" There were also two questions on alimony.

Reporting was more nearly complete than on the first national survey, although again much information from the smaller counties — more than one-fourth of all counties — was secured by correspondence. A summary volume published in 1909 (see reference 8) combined data from both the first and second national surveys.

Survey of 1916. Plans were initiated to conduct a third survey covering the period 1907 to 1916, but the United States was preoccupied with its approaching entry into World War I. Coverage of the survey[9] was limited to the one year 1916 and there was no further significant action until 1922.

Reporting of Marriage and Divorce, 1922–1956

The 35-year period beginning with 1922 witnessed great variation in the adequacy of reporting of marriage and divorce. During the first 11 years, the reporting was good. Beginning with the year 1922 and continuing through 1932, the Bureau of the Census made annual comprehensive surveys of marriage and divorce through mail surveys.[10] This was a noteworthy series, and the report for 1926 contained estimates for 1907–1915 and 1917–1921, the missing years in the earlier surveys. The volume for 1932 was somewhat truncated and the program was terminated in 1933. During the next several years, official national data were not available and private efforts were made to fill the gap.[11]

The next important governmental effort was made in connection with the 1940 Census of Population. Copies (transcripts) of the original state records of marriage and divorce were collected from a few states that could provide usable data. The entrance of the United States into World War II brought an end to this promising program. Thereafter, through 1956, the data published by the federal government on marriages and divorces based on the original records were derived from pretabulated material provided by state and local agencies. There were also useful publications by several states.

Beginning in 1948, under a cooperative arrangement between appropriate state agencies and the federal government, detailed table plans calling for the number and characteristics of persons at the time of marriage or divorce were distributed to the states annually. State officials wherever possible completed the forms. In the other states, more limited data, including as a minimum the estimated numbers of marriages and divorces, were prepared in cooperation with state officials. Frequently questionnaires were sent to local officials.

This system of using state tables had obvious weaknesses. There was no consistent group of reporting states from year to year, because some dropped out and others were added, and this made the interpretation of national trends difficult; only limited quality checks for accuracy were possible, because each state office operated independently. Moreover, the chief financial burden of this federal statistical program fell on the states rather than on the federal government.

Establishment of Marriage and Divorce Registration Areas, 1957 and 1958

Recent efforts to improve statistics of marriage and divorce have stressed (1) the need for statewide central files of these records in all states, with (2) the record of each case providing the same essential statistical information and with (3) modern and reliable methods of compiling the data. As a promotion device, reporting areas were established similar to the birth and death registration areas completed in 1933. Before this came about, however, it was necessary to get over several hurdles.

In 1952 the staff of the National Office of Vital Statistics (later identified as the Division of Vital Statistics of the National Center for Health Statistics) gave approval to a plan to establish officially recognized registration areas for marriage and divorce. The first step envisioned for this plan involved securing broad agreement, from state registrars of vital statistics and representatives of serious users of the data, on standards that should be established for participation by states in these areas. After numerous meetings a special committee of state registrars and technical consultants reached general agreement in 1954. However, when their plan was submitted for ratification to a representative group of state registrars, it was voted down on the grounds that the standards were unreasonably high. Thus it was necessary to retreat, regroup, and try again.

The nub of the controversy concerned the statistical report form to be used by the states. A special committee (the Working Group on Marriage and Divorce) agreed on a minimum list of items. One such item, "race or color," would have made possible the analysis of marriage and divorce data for the white and nonwhite population. Many of the state forms contained the race item, but it was missing from several others. Some registrars indicated that the item was controversial in their states and that it would not be feasible to add it to their report forms. Another controversial item on the proposed form was "occupation and industry." There was general agreement in the working group that an indicator of socioeconomic status was essential. Again, some registrars indicated that because of local conditions it would not be possible to add this item to their report forms. As a compromise, the Marriage Registration Area (MRA) was established, recommending but not requiring the inclusion of these items.[12]

Another hurdle concerned approval by the next layer of officialdom. Before the MRA could be launched it was necessary to obtain approval by the Association of State and Territorial Health Officers, made up of the heads of state health departments. This approval was given in 1956, and on January 1, 1957 the Marriage Registration Area was officially launched. A press release from the Surgeon General of the Public Health Service (January 4, 1957) pointed out that more than one-half of the marriages in the country took place within the original registration states. "The 29 states have also agreed to cooperate in making periodic tests of the completeness and accuracy of their marriage registrations," the press release indicated and added, "The states will use most of the items on a recommended Standard Record of Marriage."

The Divorce Registration Area, established one year later, began with a much smaller geographic coverage. "Under the new system, uniform data will be collected . . . in cooperation with 14 states and 3 territories. . . . The new registration area is a start toward obtaining figures on divorces and annulments comparable in reliability and comprehensiveness with data now available on births and deaths," stated a Public Health Service press release of December 23, 1957. Again, there was agreement with the states for testing of registration completeness and accuracy and a *recommended* statistical report form, the Standard Record of Divorce or Annulment.

The MRA and DRA served to dramatize the importance of marriage and divorce registration. The maps of the areas, which changed from time to time as new states were added, served to highlight the states that were lagging and to quicken interest in the program. Sociologists officially moved to help by establishing a committee on marriage and divorce statistics; a sociologist residing in each state not included in both areas was appointed to help with moving the program forward in his state.[13] Influential groups endorsed the program and urged their members to support it.[14] In the American Bar Association consideration of the program began in the Section of Family Law at its 1961 annual meeting, which recommended endorsement by the Board of Governors of ABA. This endorsement was given some weeks later.[15]

The registration areas have grown but are considerably short of national coverage. In 1968 the MRA included 42 states and the DRA 26 states, which are shown in Figure 1.1.

Reporting of Marriage and Divorce, 1959–1967

National Survey of 1960. Long before the establishment of the Marriage and Divorce Registration Areas, there was general agreement among many users of the data and the federal professional staff that the method of collecting the data for national statistics was inadequate; the "pretabulated program" of special tables prepared by state offices could be defended only because of its low cost to the federal government. In the mid-1950's professional staff discussion began, concerning the possible collection of sample statistical records (transcripts) from the states for tabulation of data by the

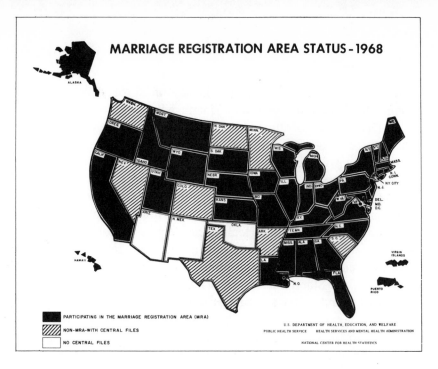

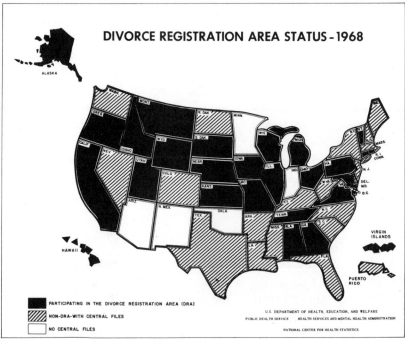

Fig. 1.1. Marriage and divorce registration areas: United States, December 1968

Source: National Center for Health Statistics.

10

federal government in the same way that mortality data were prepared. A small sample of the 1960 transcripts, representative of the entire country, was collected for the preparation of benchmark data.

The first national sample consisted of 41,000 marriage and 16,000 divorce records. In addition to national tabulations, these records permitted simple state tabulations for the registration states and regional tabulations for the remainder of the country. Even with such a small sample, difficulties were encountered in collecting the information from areas outside the registration states. Many social scientists and others residing in these areas aided in the collection process.[16]

Publication of the 1960 data marked an important advance in the collection of national marriage and divorce data; it also underlined some weaknesses in the program.[17] Analysis of the sample transcripts indicated that the sampling errors were less serious than errors of other types. Even in a few of the registration states such essential variables as age, color, and number of this marriage were seriously underreported. For divorce, there was severe underreporting of several important variables.[18]

Later developments. This situation raised the serious question of how to maintain high standards for the MRA and DRA. In the developmental stages of the earlier birth and death registration areas, states were dropped for failing to meet established minimum standards.[19] This action served the double purpose of keeping registration-area statistics at established standards and making each state continually aware that it might be dropped for incomplete reporting. The same procedure was not invoked with the MRA and DRA, however; at the end of 1967 no state had been dropped from either area for any cause.

Reporting for the years 1961–1967 was of two types. A sample of marriage and divorce transcripts was obtained from the states in the MRA and DRA, and detailed reports were prepared from tabulations based on these transcripts. From the remaining states only information on the number of marriages and divorces by county of occurrence was collected and published.

In 1967 plans were far advanced for the development of revised statistical report forms to be titled "Standard Certificate of Marriage" and "Standard Certificate of Divorce and Annulment." These forms were drafted after extensive consultation with the state registrars and with users of the data. The new forms, shown in figures 1.2 and 1.3,

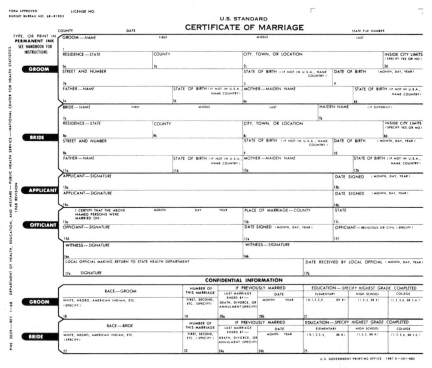

Fig. 1.2. United States standard certificate of marriage: 1968

Source: National Center for Health Statistics.

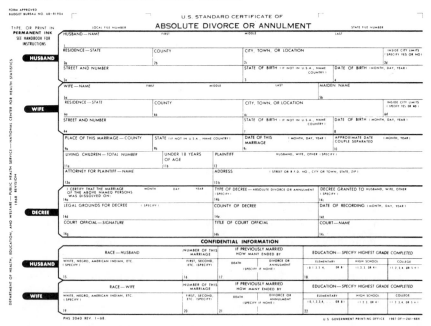

Fig. 1.3. United States standard certificate of divorce or annulment: 1968

Source: National Center for Health Statistics.

were adopted in 1966 and were recommended for use by all states in 1968.

Census Data on Marital Status

In recognition of the revealing insights into family life that can be attained from information on marital status of the population by age and sex, decennial census reports in the United States since 1890 have included tables on this subject.[20] At first the age detail terminated with 65 years and over, but as larger proportions of the population reached the older ages the final age group was advanced to 75 and over in 1930, and to 85 and over in 1940. Because of the rapid change in marital-status distribution of the younger ages, statistics on marital status by single years of age have been provided for ages 14 (or "under 15") to 29 since 1910.

Very few persons living in family groups fail to have marital status reported for them. However, the situation is less satisfactory for persons living in rooming houses, institutions, and other places where census information is difficult to collect. A category for "not reported" was shown in the marital-status distribution through the 1930 census. Simple methods of eliminating this category were used in the 1940 and 1950 censuses, with the result that some persons were incorrectly assigned to the category "single" and none to the category "divorced." An improved method was used in 1960, whereby for persons with no report on marital status the electronic computer allocated the entry on marital status for the most recently processed person of similar characteristics whose status had been reported.[21]

Married persons were first coded and tabulated as "spouse present" or "spouse absent" in connection with the preparation of tables on marital status of family heads for the 1930 census. This improvement was extended in the 1940 census to the marital-status classification of persons and has been continued in later censuses and surveys.

"Married persons with spouse absent" were subdivided in the enumeration for the 1950 and 1960 censuses into two categories, "separated" (because of marital discord) and "other." This subdivision was made originally to provide a more meaningful response category on marital status for persons who were in the process of obtaining a divorce or whose spouse had deserted them. Incidentally, a small pretest of the 1950 census held in Wilmington, North Carolina, showed that about one-third of the persons reported as "separated" had obtained legal separations.

The category "separated" is admittedly imperfect, as attested by the fact that half again as many women as men use the term to describe themselves (the two numbers obviously should be the same); this observation is taken as evidence that separated men are probably underreported and, perhaps more importantly, that unwed mothers often use the term to avoid admitting that they have children born out of wedlock. Yet the statistics on demographic and social characteristics of separated persons throw valuable light on the subject of marital instability. The same statement can be made of divorced persons and remarried persons, for whom the counts also have weaknesses.[22]

A further subcategory of "married persons with spouse absent" has been recognized by the Bureau of the Census each year since 1951 in its Current Population Reports. This subcategory is married women with husband absent in the armed forces.

Most of the basic decennial census reports since 1940, and many of the special reports, have contained tables on marital status classified by other demographic and social characteristics. Full citations for those reports which are most relevant to readers of this monograph can be found in the source notes on the tables in subsequent chapters.

2 / COMPARATIVE INTERNATIONAL TRENDS IN MARRIAGE AND DIVORCE

In this chapter trends in marriage and divorce in selected countries throughout the world are reviewed. This presentation will serve as background for a more detailed analysis in later chapters of such trends in the United States. Inevitably, making meaningful comparisons of rates and trends in the United States and in other countries involves a great many hazards. In a general way, the statistics show that both marriage and divorce rates are higher in the United States than in other countries. The divorce rate, however, has serious limitations as an index of marital discord in the several countries, since the number of divorces granted varies more with the legal and administrative obstacles placed in their way than with the general level of discontent between spouses. These obstacles vary sharply between countries and within the same country over time as new laws and regulations come into effect.

Despite these limitations, comparisons of divorce rates among the countries over time serve to demonstrate how much the rate of marital disruption through the process of divorce is changing. For as the divorce rate increases, the number of persons eligible for remarriage increases, and the marriage rate therefore tends to rise also.

Marriage Trends

Crude marriage rate. There are various ways of measuring the rate of marriage; the simplest is the crude marriage rate, which records the number of marriages per 1,000 population during one year. It is easy to compute but does not take into account the age, sex, and marital distribution of the population. Table 2.1 gives the crude marriage rate for 15 countries and the United States for selected years between 1932 and 1965.

During this relatively brief span of years, encompassing the trough of the Great Depression, World War II, and the postwar era, noteworthy fluctuations in the crude marriage rate were recorded. In 1932, about the low point of the depression, low rates prevailed in all of these

Table 2.1. Crude marriage rates: Selected countries, 1932 to 1965

Country	Year[a]											
	1965	1964	1963	1962	1961	1960	1955	1950	1945	1940	1935	1932
Australia[b,c]	8.3	7.7	7.4	7.4	7.3	7.3	7.8	9.2	8.5	11.1	8.4	6.6
Canada	7.4	7.2	6.9	7.0	7.0	7.3	8.2	9.1	9.0	10.8	7.1	5.9
Chile[b,c]	7.6	7.2	6.9	6.8	7.2	7.2	8.9	7.6	7.7	8.3	6.9	6.4
Denmark[c]	8.8	8.4	8.2	8.1	7.9	7.8	7.9	9.1	9.0	9.2	9.3	7.8
France[c]	7.1	7.2	7.1	6.7	6.8	7.0	7.2	7.9	10.1	4.4	6.9	7.6
Germany (Fed. Rep.)	8.3	8.6[c]	8.8	9.2	9.4	9.4	8.8	10.8	--	--	--	--
Ireland	5.9	5.7	5.5	5.5	5.4	5.5	5.6	5.4	5.9	5.1	4.8	4.4
Italy[c]	7.7	8.2	8.3	8.1	8.0	7.8	7.6	7.7	6.9	7.1	6.7	6.4
Japan[b,c]	9.7	9.9	9.8	9.8	9.5	9.3	8.0	8.6	--	9.2	8.0	7.8
Mexico[b]	6.9	6.8	6.5	6.6	6.3	6.8	7.1	6.9	6.7	7.9	6.6	5.6
Netherlands[c]	8.8	8.5	8.0	7.9	8.0	7.8	8.3	8.2	7.8	7.6	7.2	6.9
Spain	7.2	7.4	7.6	7.7	7.8	7.2	8.1	7.5	7.2	8.4	6.1	6.6
Sweden	7.8	7.6	7.0	7.1	7.0	6.7	7.2	7.7	9.7	9.3	8.2	6.7
Switzerland	7.6	7.5	7.6	7.8	7.7	7.8	8.0	7.9	8.1	7.7	7.3	7.8
United Kingdom (England & Wales)[b,c]	7.8	7.6	7.5	7.4	7.5	7.5	8.1	8.2	9.3	11.2	8.2	7.6
United States[d]	9.2	9.0	8.8	8.5	8.5	8.5	9.3	11.1	12.2	12.1	10.4	7.9

Source: United Nations, Demographic Yearbook, Vols. 10, 14, 15, 16, and 19.

[a]Rates are number of legal (recognized) marriages performed and registered; i.e., excluding unions established by mutual consent or by tribal or native custom, per 1,000 population.

[b]Tabulated by year of registration rather than occurrence.

[c]For population and territorial inclusions and exclusions, see source.

[d]Official publications of National Center for Health Statistics.

countries, and for a majority of them this year marked the lowest point for the period examined. It is evident that when economic conditions are extremely bad, the number of marriages tends to be drastically reduced. In 1935, when business conditions in most countries had improved, almost all the rates were higher, the exceptions being France, Spain, and Switzerland. In the war year 1940, marriage rates were generally still higher. There were two exceptions: in Denmark the rate was fractionally lower, while in France — its armies defeated and Paris occupied — the rate was down more than one-third. In the latter country during this period, the reporting may have been incomplete. During the next five years, up to 1945, the trends are contradictory. In six countries there were higher marriage rates than in 1940 (France, Ireland, Netherlands, Sweden, Switzerland, and the United States), whereas in eight countries (Australia, Canada, Chile, Denmark, Italy, Mexico, Spain, and the United Kingdom) the rate was lower. The changes in marriage rates between 1945 and 1950 reflected the impact of war and its aftermath and the extent to which economic conditions recovered.

Table 2.1 also illustrates the relationship between varying characteristics of the several countries and the level of their marriage rates. Ireland, with a rate near 5.5, was usually 10 to 50 percent below the other countries listed. The rate for the United States was usually the highest recorded. Italy, with a gradual upward trend, illustrates a country in which year-to-year changes were slight, even though somewhat larger variations would appear if the rate were examined for each of the thirty years covered. Italy may be compared with Australia, where the rate rose from 6.6 to 11.1 in the eight years from 1932 to 1940, thereafter moving irregularly downward to stabilize near 7.4.

Rate for the marriageable population. As pointed out above, the the crude marriage rate is based on the entire population. The more refined rates in Table 2.2 relate only to persons 15 years of age and over who are eligible to be married (that is, single, widowed, divorced) or of unknown marital status. By eliminating persons under 15 years of age, as well as those currently married, the rate — in theory — is based on the population at risk. Although a few marriages do occur at ages below 15, these very young marriages probably do not greatly affect the rate. (In general, the marital-status statistics compiled by the U.S. Bureau of the Census relate to persons 14 years old and

Table 2.2. Marriage rates by sex: Selected countries, 1935 to 1963

Country and year	Marriage rates[a] Male	Female	Country and year	Marriage rates[a] Male	Female
Australia[b]			Japan[b,f]		
1963[c]	64.6	66.2	1962[c]	75.1	63.7
1960-62[c]	61.9	63.1	1959-61[c]	70.2	59.6
1953-55	63.9	66.3	1955	38.2	32.4
1946-48	71.4	70.2	1950	33.7	28.4
Canada			Mexico[b]		
1963[c]	64.5	65.9	1962[c]	57.2	45.9
1960-62[c]	63.6	65.1	1959-61[c]	54.5	43.8
1950-52	71.6	74.1	1949-51	50.7	39.2
1940-42	66.1	73.5	1939-41	51.7	39.8
Chile[b]			Netherlands		
1962[c]	52.9	46.5	1962[c]	66.9	61.3
1959-61[c]	54.1	47.5	1959-61[c]	64.6	59.2
1951-53	54.4	49.9	1952	64.1	59.3
1939-41	52.4	49.8	1946-48	72.5	67.3
Denmark			Spain		
1962[c]	63.5	57.4	1962[c,g]	57.7	45.4
1959-61[c]	60.2	54.4	1959-61[c,g]	58.3	45.9
1944-46	66.5	60.6	1949-51	46.1	36.4
1939-41	59.9	54.8	1939-41[h]	46.0	36.3
France			Sweden		
1961-63[c]	55.0	43.7	1962[c]	48.5	46.0
1953-55[d]	57.0	42.2	1959-61[c]	45.9	43.5
1945-47	81.7	59.3	1949-51	52.6	49.5
1935-37	54.4	41.2	1939-41	51.0	48.0
Germany			Switzerland		
(Fed. Rep.)			1949-51	54.1	42.1
1963[c]	78.1	51.3	1940-42	49.7	40.6
1960-62[c]	81.1	53.3	United Kingdom[b]		
1949-51	83.5	56.0	(England		
1946-47[e]	83.1	49.5	and Wales)		
Ireland[b]			1963[c,d]	69.2	52.6
1963[c]	30.3	30.8	1960-62[c,i]	68.2	51.9
1960-62[c]	30.1	30.6	1945	72.1	54.7
1945-47	26.2	28.2	1940	80.5	63.4
1940-42	23.2	24.7	United States		
Italy			1963	87.2	73.4
1950-52	49.9	42.2	1960	88.2	73.5
1935-37	55.0	46.2	1950[j]	82.6	74.7

over.) However, the inclusion of persons in the upper age groups and those of unknown marital status tends to obscure the real differences between countries, because the percentage in these groups is considerably higher in some countries than in others.

The great majority of the marriage rates for the 16 countries shown in Table 2.2 are averages of the rates for three years. This smoothing

Table 2.2 (continued)

Source: United Nations, Demographic Yearbook, Vols. 6, 10, 14, 15, and 16; for population and territorial inclusions and exclusions refer to these volumes: Unpublished data from the Statistical Office of the United Nations; Yearbook of the Commonwealth of Australia, No. 49 (1963); Vital Statistics of the United States, 1959, Vol. 1, and 1962, Vol. 3; unpublished data from the National Center for Health Statistics; Statistical Review of England and Wales for the years 1960, 1961, and 1962, Part II.

[a]Average annual number of marriages per 1,000 marriageable (single, consensually married, widowed, divorced, or of unknown marital status) male or female population 15 years or over or of unknown age; Mexico, male population 16 years or over, female 14 years or over.

[b]Tabulated by year of registration rather than occurrence.

[c]Rates computed from latest data available in the sources listed. When population figures were not available for the data year, populations for the nearest year were used: Australia, Canada, Federal Republic of Germany, Ireland, and United Kingdom, 1963 data and 1961 population; Chile, Denmark, Japan, Mexico, Netherlands, Spain, and Sweden, 1962 data and 1960 population; France, 1964 data and 1962 population. Denmark, 1955 population base, was unpublished estimate from the United Nations.

[d]Provisional.

[e]Average for years 1946 and 1947. Population base in French and United States zones of occupation includes persons "separated."

[f]Population includes persons "separated" but excludes "consensually married."

[g]Based on one-percent sample of census returns and includes persons "separated" because classified with "divorced," a category considered unreliable because of sampling errors.

[h]Population excludes persons "consensually married."

[i]Rates based on estimated 1961 population rounded to the nearest thousand.

[j]Rates represent a total of 17 states: calculated from unpublished data in the files of the National Center for Health Statistics for 15 states (Connecticut, Delaware, Florida, Idaho, Iowa, Kansas, Maine, Michigan, New Hampshire, Oregon, South Dakota, Tennessee, Vermont, Virginia, and Wyoming); from Vital Statistics of the United States, 1950, Vol. II, and Population Census, 1950, Vol. II, Parts 21 and 32 for Massachusetts and New York. New York excludes New York City, with estimates made for age groups 45-49 and 50-54 in the city in the same proportion these age groups were in the state.

process tends to minimize exceptional rates which arise from unusual circumstances prevailing in one year. Single-year rates are also shown where it was not feasible to prepare three-year averages.

Marriage rates for males are higher than the corresponding rates for females in nearly all countries. Several factors may be involved in this situation. Because of greater longevity of females, the age distribution of the two sexes differs. There is usually a much larger number of females over age 60, an age bracket in which few marriages occur. Differences in number between the sexes are increased by the higher war losses and accidental deaths among males than females. Differential migration rates may also be an important, though temporary, factor. In some instances, the male marriage rate is lower, as in Ireland and Canada for all years shown and in Australia for the most recent years shown. In general, rates for the United States are higher than those for the other countries.

Marriage rate by age. A more meaningful view of what has been happening to marriages in recent years is afforded by making an examination of the rates by age. This type of examination provides a more detailed analysis of the impact of marriage on different segments of the eligible population. Unfortunately, the basic data are not available to compute these rates for many countries; and for others, rates are available only for selected years. In Table 2.3, comparative data for 13 countries are shown. Three areas of special interest in this table are: (1) the youngest marriages (ages 15 through 19 years); (2) the oldest marriages (persons over 60); and (3) the most active marriage years (20 through 29 for women and 20 through 34 for men).

(1) Marriage under 20. For women, the proportion marrying under 20 years of age has varied markedly among countries. In the earlier years shown in Table 2.3, around 1940, rates of less than 20 per 1,000 persons were reported for Spain, Sweden, and Switzerland. In contrast to these low rates, there were three countries besides the United States (Australia, Canada, and Chile) with high rates of over 40 per 1,000 females 15 to 19 years of age. Probably several additional countries belong in this group, but their data are unavailable. The other countries fell in an intermediate position. Twenty-five years later, around 1960–1962, these national rates for females under 20 were generally higher, in some cases dramatically so. For France, rates were lower; but in Canada, Denmark, and the United Kingdom, increases were marked. At both the earlier and later dates, the United States had the highest rate.

Grooms under 20 years of age were relatively rare in the years 1935–1941. Rates of less than 2.5 per 1,000 eligible males were recorded for Denmark, France, Spain, Sweden, and Switzerland. For the three countries besides the United States with the highest rates (Canada, 5.4; Chile, 8.0; and the United Kingdom, 5.8) the rates were moderate. But 25 years later a great increase in teenaged grooms was recorded; the rates rose in the United States and eight other countries (Canada, Chile, Denmark, France, Netherlands, Spain, Sweden, and the United Kingdom). For the United States, rates were higher in 1960 than in 1950 and were above those for the other countries shown.

(2) *Marriage over age 60.* Marriages of persons over 60 were infrequent in the 13 countries shown in Table 2.3. For women, rates during the years around 1940 were highest in the United States, Australia, Canada, and the United Kingdom; especially low rates were recorded for France, Italy, Spain, Sweden, and Switzerland. Around 1960, rates for women were highest for the United States, the United Kingdom, and Canada, while the lowest rates were recorded for Denmark, Spain, Sweden, and the Federal Republic of Germany. More of the rates moved up than moved down.

At ages over 60, rates were substantially higher for men than for women. This was notably true of Chile, the United Kingdom, the United States, and Canada in the early years; around 1960, rates were relatively high for Germany, Canada, the United States, and the United Kingdom.

(3) *Marriage for women aged 20 to 29 and for men aged 20 to 34.* The highest concentration of marriages in these economically developed countries was for persons aged 20 to 29 years, although some of the rates for men were notably high at ages 30 to 34 years.

Marriage rates for women of 20 to 24 years around 1940 were especially high in the United States, United Kingdom, Canada, and Denmark, with the range between 142 and 285 per 1,000 eligibles. By contrast, low rates were recorded for Chile (76.2), Spain (91.4), and Switzerland (98.4). Twenty-five years later most of the rates were higher; in the United States, United Kingdom, and Denmark rates were above 250 (more than 1 eligible female in 4), while in Canada, France, Germany, and the Netherlands more than 1 eligible in 5 was married within a year.

In the majority of countries, marriage rates were somewhat lower among women in the next age group, 25 to 29 years. For the earlier

Table 2.3. Marriage rates of women and of men, by age: Selected countries, 1936 to 1963

Country and year	All ages	15-19	20-24	25-29	30-34	35-39	40-44	45-49	50-54	55-59	60-64	65 & over
	Age (years)[a]											
Women												
Australia[b]												
1954	66.1	57.8	266.9	194.5	111.5	71.3	45.3	28.9	16.2	9.0	4.9	1.5
1947	69.8	49.6	225.0	190.2	114.3	70.9	42.9	25.6	13.3	7.5	4.5	1.2
Canada												
1963[c]	65.9	62.7	243.8	142.7	75.8	44.9	32.5	23.4	17.2	11.7	3.6	
1941	72.1	45.1	166.2	167.8	102.1	57.9	33.2	21.9	13.7	8.4	6.1	1.7
Chile[b]												
1962[c]	46.5	48.9	92.7		40.8			6.2				
1940	48.7	43.6	76.2	94.7	74.7	52.7	37.3	25.5	12.2		2.6	
Denmark												
1962[c]	57.4	51.4	266.1	199.0	87.4	50.1	32.1	18.2	11.1	4.8	0.7	
1940	55.3	30.2	167.1	164.0	80.1	40.5	21.2	11.9	5.6	2.5	2.2	0.7
France												
1962[c]	42.8	33.7	211.0	172.7	81.7	45.8	29.0	17.8	11.6	6.7	1.1	
1936	41.2	39.4	157.9		51.2		15.9		5.1		0.7	
Germany (Fed. Rep.)												
1963[c]	51.3	37.1	205.1	240.4	82.1	39.5	30.5	10.6	8.9	5.0	1.0	
1950	57.5	25.2	154.4	192.6	127.5	71.9	28.0	18.4	8.9	3.9	0.5	
Italy												
1951	40.8	23.8	109.1	124.7	66.1	31.0	16.0	8.6	4.3	2.5	1.3	0.4
1936	44.7	65.7		115.8	59.5	29.6	15.8	8.4	4.7	2.7	1.9	0.6
Netherlands												
1963[c]	62.8	32.4	204.2	224.7	87.7	43.1	28.4	16.9	10.4	7.2	1.7	
1947	67.9	20.2	141.2	226.8	136.8	74.6	44.1	28.7	17.0	10.2	5.2	0.9
Spain												
1963[c]	45.5	16.8	126.5	166.9	86.9	37.4	14.2		3.7		0.6	
1940	42.8	11.3	91.4	146.4	75.8	34.3	13.3		3.2		0.5	

Sweden												
1962[c]	46.0	35.5	195.4	179.2	92.1	51.8	31.7	18.3	9.7	4.5	0.6	
1940	47.7	19.9	123.5	155.9	95.2	48.0	23.5	12.0	5.2	2.1	1.0	0.1
Switzerland												
1950	41.9	13.7	116.0	145.7	86.5	48.2	28.3	16.4	9.4	4.8	2.2	0.3
1941	41.7	9.6	98.4	150.4	89.6	45.8	23.6	15.0	8.5	3.7	1.7	0.2
United Kingdom (England & Wales)[b]												
1962[c]	52.1	63.3	269.2	186.1	104.7	55.6	38.0	23.3	14.2	8.1	2.1	
1940	63.4	38.4	221.6	197.8	87.2	44.0	26.9	16.3	9.4	5.3	3.7	1.1
United States												
1960[c]	73.5	100.3	284.7	196.7	119.1	89.5	58.7	39.4	23.4	13.2	4.0	
1950[d]	74.7	92.3	260.8	180.8	114.7	75.1	48.4	32.1	19.2	4.4		
Men												
Australia[b]												
1954	63.8	7.8	126.9	148.0	97.9	68.3	50.4	39.8	31.4	23.5	18.8	7.9
1947	70.9	6.6	129.8	187.0	137.2	91.8	64.2	43.1	30.6	23.8	16.4	6.4
Canada												
1963[c]	64.4	11.8	159.8	166.1	94.3	58.0	41.6	30.7	27.5	23.0	11.6	
1941	64.9	5.4	95.5	168.8	140.7	89.5	56.8	38.3	28.1	20.3	15.2	6.4
Chile[b]												
1962[c]	52.9	12.2	105.6		66.7			20.4				
1940	51.3	8.0	56.1	112.2	99.6	79.0	64.3	56.8	43.3		18.2	
Denmark												
1962[c]	63.5	7.4	146.2	220.1	121.0	73.5	54.0	37.0	24.3	20.8	4.8	
1940	60.5	1.3	80.1	172.8	137.1	89.5	60.5	45.0	31.4	23.3	10.9	2.4
France												
1962[c]	53.9	5.8	108.5	171.7	83.4	50.4	38.2	28.3	21.9	16.2	7.0	
1936	54.4	2.4	110.7		80.1		39.2		20.3		4.9	

Table 2.3 (continued)

Men (con.)

Country and year	All ages	Age (years)[a]										
		15-19	20-24	25-29	30-34	35-39	40-44	45-49	50-54	55-59	60-64	65 & over
Germany (Fed.Rep.of)												
1963[c]	78.1	2.4	102.6	246.4	169.5	136.6	117.0	47.5	50.8	40.3	13.7 ————	
1950	85.9	3.1	97.6	217.0	255.7	241.6	134.4	106.1	74.8	54.3	9.8 ————	
Italy												
1951	48.3	2.7	42.9	129.5	153.5	102.1	55.9	32.8	23.5	17.9	11.1	3.8
1936	53.2	26.0 ————		152.8	130.4	86.7	54.9	35.3	22.1	15.4	10.9	4.1
Netherlands												
1963[c]	68.5	6.7	107.1	232.5	145.1	78.3	57.0	36.1	28.8	24.9	8.3 ————	
1947	73.1	3.7	69.2	214.9	217.2	149.1	103.0	74.5	56.6	41.5	26.8	5.8
Spain												
1963[c]	57.9	2.0	39.9	190.4	157.5	87.3	46.5 ————		17.3 ————		4.5 ————	
1940	54.2	1.4	32.7	169.9	173.6	100.3	49.0 ————		18.7 ————		4.3 ————	
Sweden												
1962[c]	48.5	5.3	108.9	172.8	100.7	59.1	41.4	23.7	16.1	12.3	3.0 ————	
1940	50.7	0.8	53.3	134.6	122.4	82.0	53.7	33.8	20.1	13.9	7.3	1.3
Switzerland												
1950	53.8	1.2	57.0	149.8	131.7	88.9	56.9	42.1	30.9	25.9	16.5	4.2
1941	51.1	0.6	41.8	134.5	133.9	88.1	54.8	41.2	27.7	21.2	14.0	3.8
United Kingdom (England & Wales)[b]												
1962[c]	68.6	14.0	159.1	192.6	114.9	69.9	47.3	36.7	32.9	25.9	12.4 ————	
1940	80.5	5.8	128.4	236.9	161.5	94.1	60.6	48.8	34.9	26.1	17.0	6.8
United States												
1960	88.2	31.3	218.3	210.7	145.3	112.0	94.7	65.0	52.2	40.4	20.2 ————	
1950[d]	82.6	19.3	180.3	198.9	147.5	103.7	76.4	57.9	43.6		16.9 ————	

Source: United Nations, _Demographic Yearbook_, Vols. 2, 6, 10, 14, 15, and 16. For population and territorial inclusions and exclusions refer to these volumes. Unpublished data from files of the Statistical Office of the United Nations. _Vital Statistics of the United States_, 1950, Vol. II, and 1960, Vol. III, Section 2; unpublished data from files of the National Center for Health Statistics. _Statistical Review of England and Wales_ for the year 1961, Part II.

aRates are the number of women and men of the specified age per 1,000 marriageable (single, consensually married, widowed, divorced, unknown) population of the same age and sex, with the exception of the 15-19 rate, which includes marriages of those under 15 computed on marriageable population 15-19; total rates based on marriages at all ages but computed on marriageable population aged 15 years and over and unknown.

bData by year of registration rather than occurrence.

cRates computed from latest data available in the sources listed. When population figures were not available for the data year, populations for the nearest year were used.

dRates represent a total of 17 states (see note j, Table 2.2).

25

period all the rates were below 200, with many of them under 155. Changes in rates over the course of time were mixed, with about an equal number of countries recording higher and lower rates. The modal age group for marriage shifted downward (from 25 to 29 years to 20 to 24 years) in Canada, Denmark, France, and Sweden. However, at the end of the period under study the modal age was in the upper twenties in the Netherlands, Spain, and Germany.

The highest marriage rates for males occurred in the ages from 20 to 34 years, with greatest concentration usually at 25 to 29 years. There were some exceptions to this prior to 1960, with the peak occurring at 30 to 34 years of age in Germany, Italy, and Spain. However, for 1960–1963 all countries had the highest rates at 25 to 29 years of age, except the United States where the peak came at 20 to 24 years. There was a fairly general tendency for rates to rise at the younger ages, while changes were mixed at the older ages. Overall, during the 25 years ending in the early 1960's, the trend was toward marriage at younger ages.

Divorce Trends

Meaningful international comparisons are more difficult for divorce rates than for marriage rates. Official statistics are available, but interpreting them is not simple.

To begin with, there are varying uses of the term "divorce." A *final decree of absolute divorce* terminates the legal status of husband and wife, formalizes financial and parental obligations between spouses, and permits each of them to remarry. In addition, there are *limited decrees of divorce* (also referred to as legal separations) which do not permit the parties to remarry but otherwise legally terminate the marriage, and there are *annulments of marriage* in which the court indicates that a valid marriage has not taken place. In the divorce statistics of different countries, there is some variation in definition of terms and in coverage. The official statistics of the United States, for example, include both absolute decrees of divorce and annulments of marriage; also included, inadvertently, are some limited decrees of divorce, or legal separations.

There are important differences in the laws of various countries concerning divorce. In several, divorces are not granted; the *Demographic Yearbook* (1963) lists countries from which divorce statistics were not collected, including Argentina, Brazil, Chile, Colombia, Ireland, Italy, Paraguay, Philippines, and Spain. These nine countries — all predominantly of Roman Catholic culture — do not grant legal divorce.

Although a country does not permit divorce and there are no legal provisions under which a decree of divorce may be granted, serious marital discord — the subject of greatest interest to analysts of divorce statistics — may nevertheless exist. Again, if one country has extremely restrictive divorce laws while another country has broadly permissive laws, then a substantially lower divorce rate in the first country would be expected, although obviously this evidence would not prove that the amount of marital discord there was substantially less.

A further complication of analyzing trends in the divorce rates results from major changes in divorce laws that occur within a country. In England, for example, during the 80 years prior to 1938, absolute divorce was granted solely on grounds of adultery, but thereafter other grounds were added, including (with various restrictions) desertion, cruelty, and insanity. Part of the increase in divorce rates after 1938 must be attributed to these changes in the laws.[1]

In general, marital discord is not easily measured in statistical terms. It manifests itself in certain observable ways, such as desertions and separations (for which statistics are generally unreliable), but it may also be present when no objective and measurable event takes place. Furthermore, a consensual union, or common-law marriage, may continue until the death of one of the marital partners, or it may be disrupted after a brief period, but there are no comprehensive data on the number of such unions nor on the rate of their disruption. Perhaps because divorce figures are available, they are used as an index of marital discord, but in fact they constitute such an index in a very limited sense. Divorce is only one of the ways in which societies deal with serious marital discord.

Crude divorce rate. In Table 2.4 divorce rates for the selected years 1932–1965 are presented for 12 countries. Like crude marriage rates, they measure events per 1,000 population without regard to age, sex, or marital status. Data are not available for all these countries for each year. The Federal Republic of Germany is first represented in 1950; hence, it is omitted from the following tabulation of rates in 1932 and in 1965:

Divorce rate per 1,000 population	Number of countries with specified divorce rates in —	
	1932	1965
0.1–0.3	6	0
0.4–0.6	3	2
0.7–0.9	1	5
1.0 and over	1	4

Figure 2.1 shows this tabulation graphically.

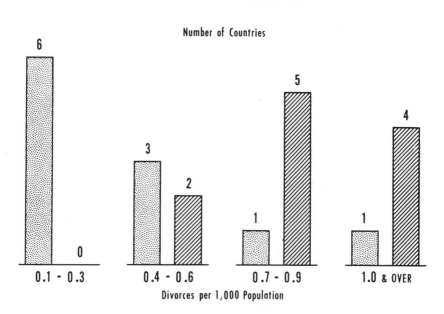

Fig. 2.1. Number of countries with specified divorce rates: 1932 and 1965
Source: Table 2.4.

The generally upward trend of the divorce rates is apparent, except in Japan where the rate was 0.8 in both 1932 and 1965. For Japan, rates were based on the date of reporting and not the date of occurrence; consequently, the true trend may be obscured by eccentric reporting practices. In the other ten countries the rate advanced — in most cases substantially. For seven countries, the rate more than doubled between 1932 and 1965, including three where the increase

Country	Year[a]											
	1965	1964	1963	1962	1961	1960	1955	1950	1945	1940	1935	1932
Australia[b]	0.8	0.7	0.7	0.7	0.6	0.7	0.7	0.9	1.0	0.5	0.4	0.3
Austria[b]	1.2	1.2	1.1	1.1	1.1	1.1	1.3	1.5	0.7	0.9	0.1	0.1
Canada[b]	0.5	0.5	0.4	0.4	0.4	0.4	0.4	0.4	0.4	0.2	0.1	0.1
Finland[b]	1.0	1.0	0.9	0.9	0.9	0.8	0.9	0.9	1.5	0.4	0.4	0.3
France[b]	0.7	0.7	0.6	0.7	0.7	0.7	0.7	0.9	0.6	0.3	0.5	0.5
Germany[b] (Fed. Rep.)	0.9	1.0	0.9	0.8	0.8	0.8	0.9	1.6	--	--	--	--
Japan[b],[c]	0.8	0.8	0.7	0.8	0.7	0.7	0.9	1.0	--	0.7	0.7	0.8
Netherlands[b]	0.5	0.5	0.5	0.5	0.5	0.5	0.5	0.6	0.5	0.3	0.4	0.4
Norway	0.7	0.7	0.7	0.7	0.7	0.7	0.6	0.7	0.6	0.3	0.3	0.3
Sweden	1.2	1.2	1.1	0.8	0.9	0.9	1.2	1.1	1.0	0.6	0.4	0.4
United Kingdom[b] (England and Wales)	0.8	0.7	0.7	0.6	0.5	0.5	0.6	0.7	0.4	0.2	0.1	--
United States[d],[e]	2.5	2.3	2.3	2.2	2.3	2.2	2.3	2.6	3.5	2.0	1.7	1.3

Source: United Nations, Demographic Yearbook, Vols. 10, 14, 15, 16, and 19.

[a]Rates are the number of final divorce decrees granted under civil law, per 1,000 population. Annulments and legal separations are excluded, unless otherwise specified.

[b]For population and territorial inclusions and exclusions, see source.

[c]Tabulated by year of registration rather than occurrence.

[d]Data include annulments.

[e]Official publications of National Center for Health Statistics.

29

was fivefold or greater. The greatest relative increases occurred in countries with the lowest initial rates (Austria, Canada, Finland, Sweden, United Kingdom), while the smallest relative change occurred in countries with the highest initial rates (United States, Japan, France, Netherlands). As a result, there was less relative spread between rates in 1965 than in 1932; in 1932 the highest rate was 13 times the lowest, whereas in 1965 the highest rate was five times the lowest rate.

A relatively high divorce rate in these 12 countries was usually recorded for the immediate postwar period. In a majority of the countries the highest rates occurred in 1945 or 1950, or the rate did not move higher in the years after 1950. If rates for every year had been shown in the table, the pattern would have been modified. For example, the highest rate for the United States was recorded in 1946.

After the postwar peak the trend was generally downward, followed by a temporary leveling, then by a further rise in the rate. Incomplete data on these countries for 1966 picture a rising trend in the divorce rate in four countries (Australia, Germany, Netherlands, and Sweden) and an unchanging rate for the remaining reporting countries (Austria, Canada, Finland, Japan, Norway, and the United States). In 1967 and 1968 the provisional rate for the United States was up, with 2.7 and 2.9 reported for these years. It is also noteworthy that a rate of 2.8 for both 1966 and 1967 was reported for the U.S.S.R. — more than double the 1963 rate of 1.3. Such an abrupt rise may well have been associated with changes in divorce laws and regulations. There is no evidence of a declining divorce rate in any of these countries from the data available for years subsequent to 1965.

Divorces per 1,000 married couples. In divorce statistics the population at risk consists of all married persons. Since the proportion of the total population that is married varies markedly from country to country, a comparison of the crude divorce rates of two countries may be misleading; the divorce rate per 1,000 married couples should give a more meaningful picture. Such data are given in Table 2.5 for the same 12 countries as the preceding table. The rates are shown, in most instances, for three years combined.

The general trend between 1935 and 1945 for all available rates was upward. The peak rate was usually reached within a few years after the close of World War II. The highest rates were recorded dur-

Table 2.5. Divorce rate per 1,000 married couples: Selected countries, 1935 to 1964

Country and year	Rate	Country and year	Rate	Country and year	Rate
Australia		Germany		Sweden	
1963[a]	3.1	(Fed. Rep. of)		1962[a]	5.0
1960-62[a]	2.8	1963[a]	3.5	1959-61[a]	4.9
1953-55	3.3	1960-62[a]	3.4	1949-51	4.9
1946-48	4.4	1949-51	6.4	1944-46	4.2
Austria		1946-47	6.3	1939-41	2.7
1950-52	6.7	Japan		1934-36	2.3
1938-40	3.8	1962[a]	3.7	United Kingdom	
Canada		1959-61[a]	3.7	(England and	
1963[a,b]	1.9	1954-56	4.4	Wales)	
1960-62[a]	1.7	1949-51	5.3	1960-62[c]	2.1
1955-57	1.7	Netherlands		1950-52	2.8
1950-52	1.7	1962[a]	2.2	1944-46	1.8
1940-42	1.1	1959-61[a]	2.2	1939-41	0.7
Finland		1951-53	2.6	United States	
1962[a]	4.4	1946-48	4.5	1964	10.7
1959-61[a]	4.1	Norway		1963	10.3
1955[a]	4.2	1962[a]	2.9	1962	9.4
1949-51	4.6	1959-61[a]	2.8	1960	9.2
1939-41	2.2	1949-51	3.2	1955	9.3
France		1945-47	3.2	1950	10.3
1961-63[a]	2.9			1945	14.4
1953-55	2.9			1940	8.8
1945-47	4.9			1935	7.8
1935-37	2.3				

Source: United Nations, Demographic Yearbook, Vols. 6, 10, 14, 15, and 16. For population and territorial exclusions and inclusions refer to these volumes. Unpublished data from the United Nations Statistical Office; unpublished data from the Division of Vital Statistics and the Bureau of the Census; Vital Statistics of the United States, Vol. 1, 1959, and Vol. 3, 1962; Yearbook of the Commonwealth of Australia, No. 49 (1963); Statistical Review of England and Wales for the year 1961, Part II.

[a]Rates computed from latest data available in the sources listed. When population figures were not available for the data year, populations for the nearest year were used.

[b]Provisional.

[c]Rate based on estimated 1961 population rounded to the nearest thousand.

ing the years 1945–1948 for Australia, France, Netherlands, Norway, and the United States. For four other countries (Finland, Germany, Japan, and the United Kingdom), the peak came between 1949 and 1952. The exceptions to this general pattern of divorce were Sweden, for which the rate rose to its highest point in 1962, and Canada, with a peak in 1963. Between 1960 and 1962 the rate declined in a majority of the countries but moved upward in some (Australia, Finland, Germany, Norway, and the United States).

Age-specific divorce rate. Divorce records may also be considered in relation to the age of the marital partners at the time of the decree. Age-specific rates provide important information on the divorce patterns, but such data are readily available for only a few countries. In Table 2.6 the divorce rates for husbands and wives (per 1,000 married persons of the specified sex and age) are given for six selected countries plus limited data for the United States covering four states. Although divorce may occur to married couples of any age, the table indicates a concentration in the early age brackets.

Considering first the divorced wives, the highest rate of divorce in four of the six countries was for women 20 to 24 years of age. This was the case in Germany, the Netherlands, Norway, and Sweden. However, the peak rate in France and the United Kingdom was at ages 25 to 29 years. Limited data for the United States indicate peak rates at 15 to 19 years of age. After rising to a peak, the rates declined steadily with advancing age, but the rise and fall of the age-specific rates were different in these countries. The Netherlands had the lowest peak rate, 4.3, at ages 20 to 24 years, and a relatively high rate (3.6) at ages 15 to 19; the rate declined slowly with ages above 24 years. Both France and the United Kingdom had about the same peak rates at ages 25 to 29, but since the rate declined more rapidly with age in the United Kingdom, France had higher rates at ages 30 and above. In the United States, limited data indicate that the rate declined steadily with advancing age.

The divorce rates for husbands showed greater diversity in the age at which the rates were highest. Two countries (the Netherlands and Norway) reached the peak at ages 20 to 24; two reached their highest point in the next age group, 25 to 29 (Sweden and Germany); and two countries (France and the United Kingdom) reached their peak at ages 30 to 34. For four states in the United States, the highest rates were recorded at ages 15 to 19 years, with only slightly lower rates at ages 20 to 24 years. After reaching the highest level, the rates moved downward with advancing age of husbands, and at age 50 and above the rates fell between 0.8 for the United Kingdom and 2.0 for Sweden.

For both husbands and wives, some consistencies in rates may be noted:

Table 2.6. Divorce rates by age of husband and of wife: Selected
countries, 1959 to 1962

Country and year	Age (years)[a]								
	All ages	15-19	20-24	25-29	30-34	35-39	40-44	45-49	50 & over
Husband									
France[b] 1961	2.6	0.2	3.0	3.8	4.6	4.3	3.4	3.3	1.1
Germany (Fed. Rep. of) 1961	3.4	0.4	6.3	7.5	5.6	4.8	4.5	3.0	1.3
Netherlands[c] 1959-61	2.2	1.7	4.1	3.4	3.2	3.0	2.5	2.1	0.9
Norway[c] 1959-61	2.8	3.5	5.5	3.8	4.7	3.9	3.1	2.8	1.3
Sweden[c] 1959-61	4.9	1.6	9.4	10.3	9.0	7.4	6.0	4.9	2.0
United Kingdom[c] (England & Wales) 1960-62	2.2	0.1	1.5	3.9	4.1	3.4	2.8	2.1	0.8
United States[d] 1960-61	7.5	24.8	22.0	15.5	10.2	7.5	6.9	5.6	2.5
Wife									
France[b] 1961	2.7	1.3	3.4	4.7	4.5	3.9	2.8	2.7	0.9
Germany (Fed. Rep. of) 1961	3.4	3.8	7.6	6.7	4.9	4.2	3.9	2.5	0.9
Netherlands[c] 1959-61	2.2	3.6	4.3	3.4	3.0	2.7	2.3	1.9	0.7
Norway[c] 1959-61	2.8	2.3	5.9	5.1	3.9	3.5	3.0	2.5	1.0
Sweden[c] 1959-61	4.9	3.7	10.1	9.8	7.9	6.7	5.4	4.2	1.6
United Kingdom[c] (England & Wales) 1960-62	2.2	0.1	2.7	4.6	3.8	3.1	2.4	1.8	0.6
United States[d] 1960-61	7.5	29.0	18.9	11.1	9.0	7.1	5.9	4.2	1.8

Source: United Nations, Demographic Yearbook, Vols. 10, 14, and 15.
For population and territorial inclusions and exclusions, refer to these volumes.
Unpublished data from the United Nations Statistical Office; Statistical Review
of England and Wales, 1960, 1961, and 1962, Part II; Divorce Statistics Analysis:
United States, 1962, National Center for Health Statistics, 1965, table 4.

[a]Rates are the number of divorces within a given age group per 1,000
married (including the consensually married) and separated male and female
population.

[b]The divorces were of year 1961, the population base 1962.

[c]Divorces are an average of three years centered on a census year which
is the base for computing rates. The married population of Sweden excludes those
consensually married. The population base for United Kingdom is estimated.

[d]Data are for four States (Hawaii, Iowa, Tennessee, Wisconsin). Rates
for United States unavailable.

(1) France and the United Kingdom had their highest rates at older ages than the other countries — 25 to 29 years for wives and 30 to 34 years for husbands.

(2) After the United States, Sweden had the highest rates, whereas the Netherlands and the United Kingdom had the lowest rates.

(3) In the Netherlands both husbands and wives had their highest divorce rates at ages 20 to 24 years.

(4) Quite generally, the peak divorce rates fell in the same age groups for husbands and wives (three countries) or within an age group for wives five years younger than for husbands (four countries).

A marked concentration in the age at which divorce occurs, in most countries among marital partners who were relatively young, is evident from Table 2.7. For wives, the modal age group at divorce appearing in the largest number of countries was 25 to 29 years, followed by 30 to 34 years, and this followed by 20 to 24 years. For husbands, the modal age group at divorce in the largest number of countries during the earliest years shown was 30 to 34 years, followed by 25 to 29 years; in the latest years shown, however, about the same number of countries fall in these two age brackets. In a substantial majority of these countries the modal age for men at divorce was between 25 to 34 years. The most frequent changes were in the direction of divorce at an earlier age.

Divorce rate by other characteristics. Divorce patterns for various countries are clarified by data on the duration of marriage for divorced couples. In some countries divorces usually take place after one or two years of marriage, but in others divorces normally take place after six or eight years of married life. In Table 2.7 the modal duration of marriage in years (the most frequent interval between marriage and divorce) is shown for 17 countries plus limited data for the United States. The most frequent duration of marriage prior to divorce was three or four years, and in recent years marriages have tended to end sooner than in earlier years. The detailed tabulations on which this summary table is based show that some of the marriages end at every duration of marriage from less than one year to 20 years or more.

A number of factors may help account for the differences in average duration of marriage prior to divorce. Important differences between countries include: the usual age at marriage; public opinion concerning divorce, including attitudes toward divorced persons; the

Table 2.7. Divorces by modal years duration of marriage and modal age group of husband and of wife: Selected countries, 1950 to 1964.

Country and year	Modal years duration of marriage	Modal age group Wife	Modal age group Husband
Australia			
1963	7	30-34	35-39
Austria			
1964	2	20-24	25-29
1957	3	30-34	30-34
Denmark			
1962	3	25-29	25-29
1955	4	25-29	30-34
Finland[a]			
1963	3	25-29	30-34
1950	4	25-29	35-39
France			
1963	5	30-34	35-39
1954	7	30-34	30-34
Germany (Fed.Rep.)			
1961[b]	3	25-29	25-29
1957	3	25-29	30-34
Hungary[a]			
1963	4	25-29	30-34
1956	3	25-29	25-29
Israel[c]			
1956	Under 1	20-24	25-29
Japan			
1962	Under 1	25-29	25-29
1957	Under 1	25-29	25-29
Netherlands			
1963	3	25-29	30-34
1958	3	30-34	30-34
New Zealand			
1964	7	20-24	20-24
1958	8	20-24	20-24
Norway			
1963	4	25-29	25-29
1956	6	30-34	30-34
Poland			
1953	Under 1	20-24	25-29
Portugal			
1957	6	40-44	40-44
Sweden			
1962	3	25-29	30-34
1956	4	30-34	30-34
Switzerland			
1961	3	25-29	30-34
1956	4	30-34	30-34
United Arab Republic			
1962	Under 1	20-24	25-29
United States[d]			
1963	1 or 2	20-24	25-29

Source: United Nations, Demographic Yearbook, Vol. 10. For population and territorial exclusions and inclusions, refer to this volume. Unpublished data from National Center for Health Statistics and the United Nations Statistical Office; Yearbook of the Commonwealth of Australia, No. 49 (1963).

[a] Data include annulments. [b] Includes West Berlin. [c] Jewish population.
[d] Data for six states: Hawaii, Iowa, Missouri, Rhode Island, Tennessee, and Wisconsin.

Table 2.8. Children in divorce cases: Selected
countries, 1948 to 1963

Country and year	Average number of children[a],[b]		Percent of divorces with children
	Per 100 divorces	Per 100 divorces with children	
Australia[c]			
1963	118.7	194.6	61.0
1948	117.1	191.8	61.1
Austria[c]			
1957	94.1	163.0	57.7
1951	89.9	161.5	55.6
Finland			
1957	133.6	198.7	67.2
1950	112.0	176.3	63.5
France[e]			
1951	59.8	120.2	49.7
Germany, Fed. Rep. of[c],[e]			
1957	92.7	160.1	57.9
1950	100.0	171.1	58.4
Japan[c],[d]			
1962	99.7	171.2	58.3
1951	99.6	169.5	58.8
Netherlands[c]			
1957	122.5	200.2	61.2
1950	118.0	195.5	60.3
Norway[c]			
1957	89.1	156.5	56.9
1950	124.5	180.9	68.8
Sweden			
1950	116.8	173.6	67.3
United Kingdom[c],[e] (England and Wales)			
1962	139.2	201.6	69.1
1951	121.5	185.2	65.6
United States[f]			
1962	130.0	214.0	60.2
1953	84.9	186.6	45.5

Table 2.8 (continued)

Source: <u>United Nations Demographic Yearbook</u>, Vol. 10; <u>Vital Statistics of the United States</u>, 1953, Vol. 1; unpublished data in the Division of Vital Statistics from reporting States and for 1960 from a sample of vital records from all of the United States. Unpublished data from the United Nations Statistical Office; Commonwealth Bureau of Census and Statistics, Social Statistics: Australia, No. 23, Divorce.

[a]Definition of "children" varies as listed: <u>Australia</u>--varied from State to State; since 1961 uniform for the entire country (all living children under 21); <u>Austria</u>--total number of children (living and deceased) born of the marriage, irrespective of dependency status; <u>Finland, France, Norway, United Kingdom</u> (1951)--all surviving children of dissolved marriage irrespective of age or dependency status; <u>United Kingdom</u> (1962)--those alive at the date of petition, irrespective of age, including children legitimized by the marriage and adopted children; <u>Japan</u>--children of dissolved marriage under 20 years of age; <u>Federal Republic of Germany, Netherlands, Sweden</u> (1950)--those under 21 years of age irrespective of dependency status; <u>United States</u>--all under 18, including adopted and those from previous marriages (most of the 50 States). Some States use varying definitions: Alabama and Virginia--number of minor children affected; Alaska--number of children under 21 affected; Hawaii--number of minor children; Idaho and Nebraska--number of children affected by decree; Kansas--number of children; Tennessee--number of children under 18 of this marriage.

[b]Rates were computed from divorces with known number of children except for France and United States, where nonreports were comparatively numerous and were distributed in proportion to those reporting.

[c]For territorial and population inclusions and exclusions, and for inclusions of annulments, see <u>United Nations Demographic Yearbook</u>, Vol. 10.

[d]Data by year of registration rather than occurrence.

[e]Total number of children estimated; method used by United Nations for France, Federal Republic of Germany, United Kingdom (1951), and Japan (1962), unlike that of the United States for its calculations, results in a figure slightly lower.

[f]For 1960, based on sample of vital records from each State. For other years, children per 100 divorces based on estimate for entire country; children per 100 divorces with children and percent of divorces with children based on data from reporting States (22 in 1953 and 21 in 1962).

legal and financial considerations in obtaining a divorce, including the time interval between application and decree; the options open to divorced persons, including employment opportunities for women. In connection with the last point, it may be noted that in an agricultural society opportunities for employment of women outside the home are far more restricted than in an industrial society.

The number of children involved in divorce cases in 11 countries is summarized in Table 2.8. These data have some limitations, especially in the definitions of children, as indicated in notes accompanying the table; nonetheless, certain patterns emerge. From one-half to two-thirds of the divorces involved children, and in recent years there has been a tendency for the proportion of divorcing couples with children to increase. The average number of children per 100 divorces ranged from 60 to 140, with most of the cases falling between 90 and 130 children per 100 divorces. In most countries, the number of children per 100 divorces increased during the period covered. Considering only those divorce cases with children, the average was one or two children per divorce, or about 120 to 214 children per 100 divorces.

Duration of marriage prior to divorce, as well as the varying definition of children, affects the ratio of children to divorces. The longer the average duration of marriage, the greater the number of children. However, where the count of children is limited to those under 18 years of age, as in most American states, the number declines for marriages that continue for more than 20 years. Thus a couple who had been married for 20 years and whose only child was born a year after marriage would have a 19-year-old child at the time of divorce and yet would be reported as having no children (under 18). But since a large proportion of young couples have children within one to three years after marriage and since most divorces take place in less than 15 years after marriage, it is not surprising that so many divorcing couples have one or two minor children.

Discussion

It is clear that the marriage rate in the advanced countries discussed above was responsive to war and other changing social and economic conditions. The changing marriage rates by age indicated that people were marrying younger. Although the most popular ages to marry were between 20 and 34 years old, in recent years there has been a tendency for women, especially, to marry in the early twenties rather than the late twenties and for men to marry either in the late twenties or the early twenties. There has also been an increase in marriages of persons under 20 years of age.[2]

In recent years the divorce rate has moved emphatically upward. An abnormally high peak was reached immediately after the close of World War II, when many hasty wartime marriages were ended.

Since then the rate tended temporarily to stabilize at a level below the peak and later to resume an upward trend. Children are involved in a majority of these divorces, with most couples having one child or two. There is great difference between countries in the usual number of years of marriage before divorce. In a few countries, as in Poland, the modal duration of marriage prior to divorce was less than one year, while in others it was much longer, as in Australia, where it was seven years. There was an evident tendency for this modal duration of marriage to shorten. Recently, it would appear, persons in unsatisfactory marriages are in greater haste to end them.

3 / TRENDS AND VARIATIONS IN MARRIAGE RATES, DIVORCE RATES, AND MARITAL STATUS

The marital status of the population may be viewed as the end product of previous vital trends and net migration of the populace. The past history of variations in the numbers of births, marriages, divorces, and deaths is reflected in the distribution of the total population into the categories single, married, divorced, and widowed. In the present chapter, the first concern is with trends in marriage rates and how these rates vary by age, marital status, educational level, and other characteristics. There is a brief discussion on trends of divorce rates and on variations in these rates by age and residence. The very substantial changes in the marital status of the population in recent decades are described, and the extent and implications of variations in marital status among racial, residence, and educational groups are discussed. Finally, a brief analysis is presented of the interplay of changing trends in marriages and divorces and changes in marital status.

Marriage Rates

Long-term trend of rates. In Chapter 2, marriage rates are compared for various countries. The annual changes in these rates per 1,000 population for the United States from 1920 to 1965 appear in Table 3.1; the rate per 1,000 unmarried females 15 years of age and over is shown in Table 3.2. Figure 3.1 compares the two rates graphically.

Important year-to-year fluctuations in these rates are evident. At the low point of the Great Depression, 1932, the low point of the marriage rate was also reached. The threat of war and later the impact of war are clear. Immediately prior to the entry of the United States into World War II, employment opportunities were greatly enhanced for both men and women. Possible deferments from military service for married men further increased the number of weddings. The marriage rates were also unusually high in 1946, the year immediately following the close of hostilities and the return of men to civilian life; thereafter the rate fell to more moderate levels.

Table 3.1. Marriage rates per 1,000 population: United States, 1920 to 1965

Year	Marriage rate	Year	Marriage rate	Year	Marriage rate
1965	9.2	1949	10.6	1933	8.7
1964	9.0	1948	12.4	1932	7.9
1963	8.8	1947	13.9	1931	8.6
1962	8.5	1946	16.4	1930	9.2
1961	8.5	1945	12.2	1929	10.1
1960	8.5	1944	10.9	1928	9.8
1959	8.5	1943	11.7	1927	10.1
1958	8.4	1942	13.2	1926	10.2
1957	8.9	1941	12.1	1925	10.3
1956	9.5	1940	12.1	1924	10.4
1955	9.3	1939	10.7	1923	11.0
1954	9.2	1938	10.3	1922	10.3
1953	9.8	1937	11.3	1921	10.7
1952	9.9	1936	10.7	1920	12.0
1951	10.4	1935	10.4		
1950	11.1	1934	10.3		

Source: National Center for Health Statistics, Vital Statistics of the United States, 1963, Vol. 3, Marriage and Divorce, table 1-A; and unpublished data from the National Center for Health Statistics and the U.S. Bureau of the Census.

Table 3.2. Marriage rates per 1,000 unmarried women 15 years of age and over: United States, 1920 and 1930 to 1965

Year	Marriage rate	Year	Marriage rate	Year	Marriage rate
1965	75.0	1952	83.2	1939	73.0
1964	74.6	1951	86.6	1938	69.9
1963	73.4	1950	90.2	1937	78.0
1962	71.2	1949	86.7	1936	74.0
1961	72.2	1948	98.5	1935	72.5
1960	73.5	1947	106.2	1934	71.8
1959	73.6	1946	118.1	1933	61.3
1958	72.0	1945	83.6	1932	56.0
1957	78.0	1944	76.5	1931	61.9
1956	82.4	1943	83.0	1930	67.6
1955	80.9	1942	93.0	1920	92.0
1954	79.8	1941	88.5		
1953	83.7	1940	82.8		

Source: National Center for Health Statistics, Vital Statistics of the United States, 1959, Section 2, Marriage and Divorce Statistics, table 2-B, and 1963, Vol. 3, table 1-B; and unpublished data from the National Center for Health Statistics and the U.S. Bureau of the Census.

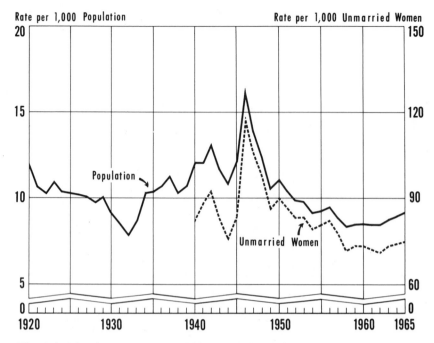

Fig. 3.1. Marriage rates per 1,000 population, 1920 to 1965, and per 1,000 unmarried women 15 years old and over, 1940 to 1965: United States

Source: Tables 3.1 and 3.2.

Another view of the relationship between marriage and such external events as war and the cycle of business prosperity and depression is afforded through an examination of the first-marriage rates of persons who felt the full impact of these events. Table 3.3 features persons who were 30, 35, 40, and 50 years old in 1960 for the following reasons. Those 50 years old in 1960 were 20 years old in 1930 and therefore lived through the depression of the 1930's at the height of their marriageable years; those 40 years old were similarly exposed to the effects of World War II; those 35 were at the height of marriageability during the early postwar marriage boom; and those 30 years old were 20 to 30 years of age during the relatively prosperous 1950's.

The dramatic effects of these variable conditions on the pattern of first-marriage rates are apparent in Figure 3.2. The approximately normal curve of ages at first marriage for those 30 years old in 1960 stands in sharp contrast to the three ensuing curves: the pointed distribution for those 35 years old — many of whom rushed into marriage after World War II; the "hollow-top profile" of the distribution for those 40 years old (who were hit hardest by the war); and the "flat-top profile" of the distribution for persons 50 years old (who tended to postpone marriage until the late 1930's or early 1940's).

Table 3.3. First-marriage rates per 1,000 persons single at beginning of year of age, for white persons 30, 35, 40, and 50 years old at census date, by age at first marriage and sex: United States, 1960

Age at first marriage	First-marriage rates per 1,000 persons single at beginning of year of age							
	White men by age at census (years)				White women by age at census (years)			
	30	35	40	50	30	35	40	50
14 years	3	2	3	2	10	9	11	14
15 years	4	4	4	4	24	24	24	28
16 years	9	7	6	6	58	49	44	46
17 years	20	19	12	14	105	84	69	71
18 years	42	38	26	28	161	118	93	99
19 years	72	52	47	48	181	126	117	114
20 years	117	82	78	65	208	156	153	124
21 years	161	153	122	76	231	230	189	115
22 years	156	184	143	85	220	245	201	109
23 years	173	187	139	98	211	222	166	112
24 years	197	185	123	120	187	192	137	128
25 years	201	175	151	132	171	172	145	125
26 years	188	171	218	136	152	151	200	126
27 years	175	155	210	134	139	134	170	123
28 years	149	148	192	126	127	116	143	108
29 years	141	137	156	120	114	111	115	96
30 years	...	118	153	126	...	93	105	99
31 years	...	107	130	130	...	86	89	90
32 years	...	92	119	120	...	75	73	86
33 years	...	87	114	89	...	62	76	66
34 years	...	74	86	76	...	55	59	57
35-39	...	...	72	44	...	...	40	27
40-44	...	...	...	24	...	...	...	15
45-49	...	...	...	18	...	...	...	9

Source: U.S. Bureau of the Census, U.S. Census of Population: 1960, Detailed Characteristics, U.S. Summary, Final Report PC(1)-1D, table 157; and Subject Reports, Age at First Marriage, Final Report PC(2)-4D, table 2.

The figure reveals the absence of any period with a "normal" marriage pattern for the older persons, but indicates that one is developing for those of marriageable age after World War II whose marriage experience was still incomplete in 1960.

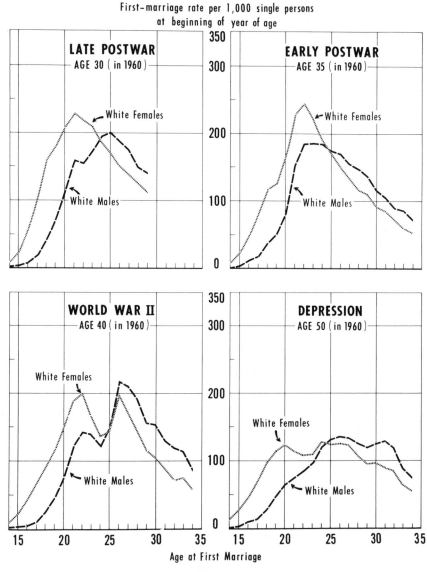

First-marriage rate per 1,000 single persons
at beginning of year of age

LATE POSTWAR
AGE 30 (in 1960)

White Females

White Males

EARLY POSTWAR
AGE 35 (in 1960)

White Females

White Males

WORLD WAR II
AGE 40 (in 1960)

White Females

White Males

DEPRESSION
AGE 50 (in 1960)

White Females

White Males

Age at First Marriage

Fig. 3.2. First-marriage rates by age at marriage, for persons 30, 35, 40, and 50 years old in 1960: United States

Source: Table 3.3.

Recent rates by age at first marriage and remarriage. Highly contrasting age-specific first-marriage rates for persons between 14 and 44 years old — the age bracket comprising nearly all first marriages — are shown in Table 3.4. Few boys married during their eighteenth

Table 3.4. First marriages in 1958 and 1959 per 1,000 single persons
14 to 44 years old: United States, 1960

Age at marriage	Men	Women	Age at marriage	Men	Women
14-44 years	85.6	115.8	22 years	237.6	305.0
			23 years	230.9	260.6
14-16 years	4.2	30.5	24 years	217.3	227.8
17 years	24.2	109.7	25 & 26 years	213.0	190.5
18 years	61.8	204.8	27-29 years	164.7	143.9
19 years	108.2	243.9	30-34 years	102.9	81.7
20 years	156.2	274.2	35-39 years	61.5	47.3
21 years	213.7	306.4	40-44 years	38.5	27.1

Source: U.S. Bureau of the Census, U.S. Census of Population:
1960, Subject Reports, Age at First Marriage, Final Report PC(2)-4D,
table 17.

year of age, the rate being only about 1 in every 16 single males.
Thereafter the rate for males rose steadily until age 22, when almost
one-fourth of the single men entered married life. The rate was fractionally lower at age 23 and thereafter declined steadily until for
persons 40 to 44 years of age less than 1 eligible in 26 married for
the first time.

The pattern is different for women, with a much higher rate in
the younger ages, a far higher peak rate, and a greatly reduced rate
among eligible older persons. Thus, during age 17 more than 1 girl
in 10 married; at age 18, 1 single girl in 5 married, and by ages 21
and 22 the rate reached a peak as it approached 1 in every 3 of the
never-married women. By the time a cohort of single women reached
age 23 years, the pool of eligibles had been greatly depleted through
marriages at younger ages, but of the remaining never-married group
more than 1 in 4 married during the year and at age 24 the rate was
reduced only moderately. Thereafter the rate declined rapidly with
advancing age, and for the group 40 to 44 years of age the corresponding rate was only 1 in every 36 eligibles entering first marriage
within a year's time.

Marriage rates for the Marriage Registration Area in 1963 (including over 1 million marriages among 69 percent of the entire population) are shown in Table 3.5 and Figure 3.3. For all marriages,
the rate per 1,000 persons 14 years of age and over was 72.5 for men
and 61.7 for women. There were substantially more women than men
in the population who were eligible to marry, largely because of dif-

Table 3.5. Marriage rates per 1,000 persons, by age, sex, and previous marital status: Marriage Registration Area, 1963

Age	All marriages		First marriages	
	Women	Men	Women	Men
Total	61.7	72.5	82.0	66.6
14-17 years	26.9	2.8	26.1	2.7
18 & 19 years	181.0	68.4	175.7	67.3
20-24 years	264.5	195.1	249.7	189.1
25-44 years	111.6	149.7	84.8	112.9
45-64 years	19.3	45.2	8.4	12.7
65 & over	2.2	15.1	1.1	3.7

Age	All remarriages		Previously widowed		Previously divorced	
	Women	Men	Women	Men	Women	Men
Total	33.0	97.1	10.2	38.4	133.5	177.0
14-44 years	170.8	306.8	66.6	163.8	221.9	312.2
14-24 years	467.0	337.5	a	a	565.9	353.1
25-44 years	139.6	302.6	61.0	191.4	179.0	306.6
45-64 years	22.9	81.4	16.2	70.1	45.2	89.5
65 & over	2.3	18.7	2.0	17.4	9.7	26.5

Source: National Center for Health Statistics, Monthly Vital Statistics Report, Vol. 15, No. 3, Supplement, "Advance Report, Final Marriage Statistics, 1963," May 31, 1966, table 3, and records. See text for limitations of the data.

[a]Rate not shown where base is less than 40,000.

ferential mortality. Thus, for the previously widowed, the rate was 10.2 for women and 38.4 for men, but the *number* of widows who remarried in 1963 was actually higher than the number of widowers who remarried by a ratio of 10 to 9.

The individuals most likely to marry were the younger divorcees, especially the women. Of all the divorced persons 14 to 24 years of age, more than one-half of the women and one-third of the men were remarried within one year. In general, the marriage rate for divorced persons remarrying was substantially higher than for never-married persons of comparable ages. Likewise, widowed persons 25 years old and over, except for widows 25 to 44 years old, married at substantially higher rates than single persons of the same age. The presence of dependent children may have reduced the remarriage rate for young widows more than for young divorced women. In the age group

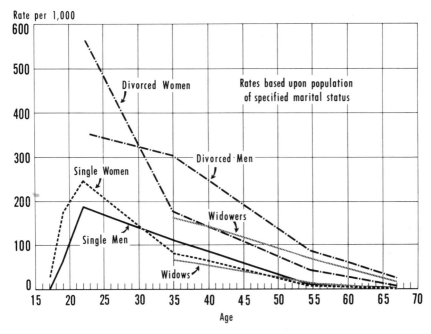

Fig. 3.3. First-marriage and remarriage rates by age at marriage: Marriage Registration Area, 1963

Source: Table 3.5.

25 to 44 years old, divorced women had a remarriage rate about three times as high as the widows, and divorced men had a remarriage rate half again as high as the corresponding widowers.

Of course, many persons obtain a divorce primarily so they can remarry. However, the marriage rate for the divorced was higher than for the widowed, at least in part for other reasons. One is the fact that widowed persons within a given age group were somewhat older than divorced persons; another is the typical attitudes of divorced and widowed persons toward their former spouse. The divorced person is more likely to have feelings of anger, rejection, guilt, frustration, and other negative attitudes. By contrast, the widowed person is more likely to have much less hostile feelings; with the passage of time, the familiar process of idealizing the departed spouse probably creates a serious barrier to remarriage among a substantial proportion of the widowed.

Among the other factors that influence the marriage rate is the mortality rate. Differential mortality was clearly an important element in the variation of remarriage rates by sex for persons 45 to 64 years old. For this age group the remarriage rate for widowers (70.1 per 1,000) was more than four times as high as the rate for widows (16.2); but in numbers of reported remarriages for persons in this age group, the approximately 27,000 widows who remarried exceeded the 22,000 widowers who remarried in 1963.

Differences in marriage patterns by color may be examined by considering the proportion of each group that had married before reach-

Table 3.6. Percent of persons first married in 1957 and 1958 by age at first marriage, by color and sex: United States, 1960

Age at first marriage	Men		Women	
	White	Nonwhite	White	Nonwhite
1958				
Percent less than:				
18 years	3.5	3.8	19.6	20.7
20 years	17.9	16.5	48.0	42.1
25 years	67.5	59.6	84.3	75.2
35 years	93.8	88.5	96.0	93.5
Median age	23.0	23.7	20.2	20.9
1957				
Percent less than:				
18 years	3.4	3.4	19.4	20.5
20 years	17.5	15.4	47.2	40.9
25 years	66.2	57.2	83.4	75.3
35 years	93.3	88.3	96.0	93.4
Median age	23.2	24.1	20.3	21.1

Source: U.S. Bureau of the Census, U.S. Census of Population: 1960, Subject Reports, Age at First Marriage, Final Report PC(2)-4D, table 3.

ing certain ages. Data in Table 3.6 show the cumulative percentages of persons who entered first marriages in 1958 and 1957 before reaching specified ages from 18 to 35 years. The table shows that nonwhite females had a larger proportion married under 18 years of age than did white females, but with advancing age a smaller proportion of nonwhite than of white women were married. The picture was essentially the same for men. One factor here is the lower average income of the nonwhite young adults, which could cause delay in establishing a household.

Recent rates by educational level and color. The first-marriage rate in 1958–1959 for persons who had completed 12 or more years of school (as a group) was significantly higher than that for persons with less than 12 years of education. The rates were highest for persons with four years of college and generally lowest for those who dropped out of high school as shown in Table 3.7. Those who stopped

Table 3.7. First marriages in 1958 and 1959 per 1,000 single persons 14 to 44 years old, by years of school completed and color: United States, 1960

Years of school completed		First-marriage rate			
		Men		Women	
		White	Nonwhite	White	Nonwhite
Total		86.8	77.0	117.3	106.2
Elementary:	0-7 years	62.5	63.9	94.9	96.2
	8 years	73.1	63.7	101.3	93.2
High school:	1-3 years	51.0	65.0	70.3	87.9
	4 years	125.0	114.5	178.6	146.0
College:	1-3 years	103.6	99.2	127.2	119.8
	4 years	176.8	134.1	189.7	159.9
	5 or more	154.6	134.0	89.6	117.3

Source: U.S. Bureau of the Census, U.S. Census of Population: 1960, Subject Reports, Age at First Marriage, Final Report PC(2)-4D, table 17.

their schooling after high-school graduation had higher marriage rates than those who went only part of the way through college. Men who completed graduate-school training were much more likely to marry than women with this level of schooling. For white women, in fact, the marriage rate for those with graduate-school training exceeded only that of high-school dropouts. Thus, the relationship between education and rate of first marriage is rather complex, but it is generally positive and is generally higher for those with the usual terminal levels of education than for those with a little more or a little less education than that.

Generally speaking, nonwhites had lower first-marriage rates than whites, especially at the upper educational levels. More of the marrying among nonwhites than whites was concentrated among those who had not completed high-school training. For the nonwhites who had graduated from high school, the marriage rates tended to be considerably lower than those for whites, except that the rate for nonwhite women with graduate-school training substantially exceeded that for white women with the same level of education.[1]

Seasonal variation in marriages. There are marked differences in the rate of marriage for various months of the year and different days of the week. Presumably because of typical work patterns a large proportion of marriages occur on weekends, but the month-to-month change in marriage rates is associated with many factors.[2]

Overall, in the United States the marriage rate is lowest during the first three months of the year, then rises during the second three months to a marked seasonal peak in June. After a sharp drop in July, the rates are somewhat higher for two months; the rates decline again for two months, but for December the rate again rises moderately. From this general pattern there are numerous variations. The four regions of the country differ, with the sharpest difference between the Northeast and the South. In the Northeast, there is a marked decline in marriages in March, an especially pronounced peak in June, and a noticeable decline in December. In the South, there was no decline in March, a less pronounced rise in June, and a marked rise in December.

In searching for an explanation of the regional differences, it may be noted that the percentage of the population reported as members of the Roman Catholic Church was highest in the Northeast and lowest in the South. Restrictions by the Catholic Church on marriage during Lent could account for the decline in marriages in the spring and the consequent marked rise in early summer. On the other hand, the rise in December marriages in the South is part of a long-standing regional pattern, perhaps associated with old harvest customs in an agricultural area and also associated with traditions of the Negro population. In the same way, the states with the highest proportion of the population residing in and near large cities (Standard Metropolitan Statistical Areas) showed a pronounced June peak and a decline in December, whereas states with the lowest proportion of population residing in SMSA's showed the opposite pattern.

The 1960 marriage records for the United States illustrate the marked difference between the seasonality of first marriages, with sharp monthly swings, and remarriages, with a smaller month-to-month change and a pronounced rise in fall weddings.[3] These records also show differences between white and nonwhite patterns. The nonwhite marriages are clustered in December to a greater degree than are white marriages.

The favorite day of the week for weddings in 1960 was Saturday, with 47 percent occurring on that day. Friday was next in popularity and then Sunday; 72 percent of the marriages took place during these three days. Persons in each of the four regions preferred Saturday weddings, but in the Northeast they placed Sunday in second place; in the South and West their second preference was Friday, and in the North Central region they showed no significant preference for Friday or Sunday.

Type of marriage ceremony. Marriage ceremonies are most frequently performed in church buildings, or in private residences with a church official performing the ritual and completing the legal documents before filing them with the appropriate local officials. Marriage ceremonies are also performed by a number of civil officials, including judges, mayors, and individuals authorized to issue marriage licenses. In some municipal buildings there is a room reserved for marriages; in New York City this room is reserved well in advance, and certain members of the City Clerk's staff perform numerous marriage ceremonies. In rural areas the ceremony may be performed in the residence of a Justice of the Peace or other local official. There are striking differences, regional and otherwise, in the proportion of weddings that are classified as "religious" or "civil."

Of all first marriages in 1960, about 16 percent were solemnized in civil ceremonies, and of all remarriages 37 percent were civil ceremonies.[4] In recent decades a substantial majority of remarriages have followed divorce rather than widowhood. Most churches frown upon divorce, some of them making it difficult for the divorced person to be married by a church official. Thus it is not surprising that more than twice as high a proportion of remarriages as of first marriages were performed by civil officials.

Until recently, 100 percent of Maryland marriages involved religious ceremonies; under an old law, recently modified, weddings could be solemnized only by church officials. In eight other states, more than 90 percent of the first marriages during recent years were classified as religious. On the other hand, there were civil ceremonies in more than half of the remarriages in eight states; in most of these states higher-than-average proportions of first marriages also were performed with civil ceremonies.

Doubtless there are many reasons for these state differences, such as the religious composition of the population and the proportion of a state's marriages that are remarriages. For instance, if a large proportion of a state's population is Roman Catholic, the proportion of church ceremonies will generally be high, since a sacrament — as a marriage is believed to be by members of this faith — can be performed only by a church official. In some states remarriages are relatively few — say, less than 20 percent of all marriages — as in Delaware, Maine, New Jersey, New York (excluding New York City), Pennsylvania, Rhode Island, Utah, Vermont, and Wisconsin. Seven of these nine states are northeastern states, mostly with large Catholic

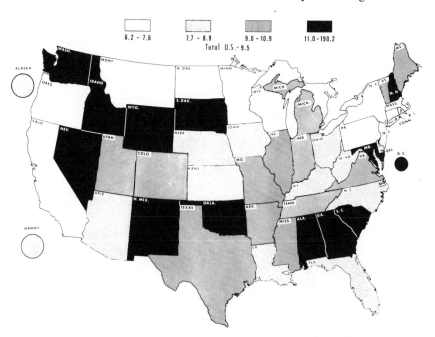

Fig. 3.4. Marriages per 1,000 population, by states: United States, 1966

Source: National Center for Health Statistics, Monthly Vital Statistics Report, Vol. 17, No. 11 Supplement, "Marriage Statistics, 1966," table 1.

populations; one is a far-western state (Utah) which is atypical since a large number of Mormons reside there. By contrast, four of the five states in which remarriages constituted over 30 percent of all marriages (Alaska, Idaho, Montana, and Wyoming) are far-western states, and the other (Florida) has an unusually high divorce rate.

As age at first marriage rises, there is an increasing tendency for the ceremony to be performed by a civil officiant.[5] For women under 45 years of age, remarriages by civil officials are common, but for older women (most of whom are widows) they are less frequent. For men, the proportion of civil ceremonies rises with age through age 44 and thereafter declines. This trend is also related to the fact that at ages over 50 years, and especially for men over 60, men who remarry are more likely to be widowers, but at younger ages they are usually divorced.

White women are more likely than nonwhite women to shift to a civil ceremony for their remarriage, as indicated by the following data for the District of Columbia:[6]

Type of marriage	Percent of women married in civil ceremonies
First marriages:	
White	6.4
Nonwhite	1.5
Remarriages:	
White	19.2
Nonwhite	3.3

Marriage rates by states. The number of marriages per 1,000 population of each state in 1966, shown in Figure 3.4, is affected by many factors. Among them are the age distribution of the population, especially the proportion of persons of marriageable age; the state marriage laws, including minimum age at marriage, waiting period to obtain a license, and physical-examination requirements; the racial- and national-origin composition of the population; and the occupational distribution, especially the proportion of men who are farmers or farm laborers.

The interplay of these factors results in a geographic distribution of marriage rates that does not show a clearly defined pattern. The Northeast region, in general, had low rates, although New Hampshire had one of the highest. The South had high rates, although lower-than-average rates were recorded for West Virginia, Louisiana, North Carolina, and Florida. The lowest rate recorded was for Delaware, a border state. In the North Central and Western regions the pattern was decidedly mixed. States with especially high rates included Nevada and Idaho, and those with especially low rates included Wisconsin, Rhode Island, and New Jersey.

Divorce Rates

The process of marriage disruption usually includes a period of separation before the divorce becomes final. This period of separation may last for a relatively short time, but usually continues for a year or longer. Many husbands and wives with serious marital problems are too impoverished to obtain a divorce; others obtain legal separations or simply live apart informally because their religious beliefs forbid divorce or strongly discourage it. Moreover, in the analysis presented here the statistics on divorces and annulments are generally combined, as in the reports published by the National Center for Health Statistics, without specific mention of this fact in the tables and text. (Annulments account for only about 3 percent of the combined total.)

Long-term trend of rates. The most meaningful analysis of the trend of divorce relates the number of divorces to the population at risk of becoming divorced, namely the married population. This rate per 1,000 married persons, by sex, for every tenth year from 1890 to

Table 3.8. Divorce rates per 1,000 married persons 15 years old and over, by sex: United States, 1890 to 1960

Sex	Year							
	1960	1950	1940	1930	1920	1910	1900	1890
Men	9.2	10.4	8.7	7.4	7.8	4.6	4.0	3.0
Women	9.2	10.3	8.8	7.5	8.0	4.7	4.0	3.0

Source: U.S. Bureau of the Census, U.S. Census of Population: 1950 and 1960, U.S. Summary, Detailed Characteristics; National Center for Health Statistics, Vital Statistics of the United States, 1950, Vol. I, and 1960, Vol. III.

1960 is shown in Table 3.8. During this 70-year period, there was a threefold increase in the rate of divorce, with most of the rise taking place during the first 30 years; between 1890 and 1920 the rate increased by two and one-half fold, but in the following 40 years it increased only moderately.

Many factors are involved in the rise of the divorce rate since 1890. During these years the United States has become increasingly an urban society, and divorce rates are substantially higher in city than in country. The position of women has changed drastically; the proportion who are farmers' wives and unpaid family workers has declined, while the proportion employed in business and industry has risen sharply. The education of women has advanced dramatically. Women who contemplated divorce in 1890 were unlikely to obtain a comfortable livelihood. If they sought employment, their limited education and training made the outlook, other than for unskilled or semiskilled work, anything but bright; if they returned with their children to the home of their parents, they might be placing a heavy responsibility on persons who were approaching retirement age. Remarriage following divorce was made difficult by the widespread disapproval of divorced persons. Thus the unhappy wives of 1890 were often constrained to tolerate conditions that wives of the 1960's would find intolerable. So, also, the unhappy husbands of 1890 were reluctant to seek divorce because of strong community disapproval of such action. And if the husband was a farmer, as so many were, the wife was an indispensable member of the production team; this fact was a strong economic motivation for avoiding a legal ending of the marriage.

A more intangible set of factors in the upward trend of the divorce rate, though difficult to document, is accepted by most students of the family. These factors include a rising expectation of happiness in marriage and an increasing unwillingness to tolerate an unhappy marriage. Much has been written about the "over-romantic attitude" of young people toward marriage, abetted by popular literature and songs with much to say about the blissful state that comes with the perfect marriage. These attitudes deserve at least some of the credit for the frequent development of disillusionment and increasing divorce.

Further refinement of the indicated change in the divorce rate by decades is given in the year-to-year change from 1920 to 1965 in Table 3.9 and Figure 3.5. Here, the number of married women 15

Table 3.9. Divorce rates per 1,000 married women 15 years old and over: United States, 1920 to 1965

Year	Rate	Year	Rate	Year	Rate	Year	Rate
1965	10.6	1953	9.9	1941	9.4	1929	8.0
1964	10.0	1952	10.1	1940	8.8	1928	7.8
1963	9.6	1951	9.9	1939	8.5	1927	7.8
1962	9.4	1950	10.3	1938	8.4	1926	7.5
1961	9.6	1949	10.6	1937	8.7	1925	7.2
1960	9.2	1948	11.2	1936	8.3	1924	7.2
1959	9.3	1947	13.6	1935	7.8	1923	7.1
1958	8.9	1946	17.9	1934	7.5	1922	6.6
1957	9.2	1945	14.4	1933	6.1	1921	7.2
1956	9.4	1944	12.0	1932	6.1	1920	8.0
1955	9.3	1943	11.0	1931	7.1		
1954	9.5	1942	10.1	1930	7.5		

Source: National Center for Health Statistics, Vital Statistics of the United States, 1962, Vol. 3, Marriage and Divorce, table 2-1 (for 1920-1962); Monthly Vital Statistics Report, Vol. 15, No. 5 (August 1966); and unpublished data from the National Center for Health Statistics and the U.S. Bureau of the Census.

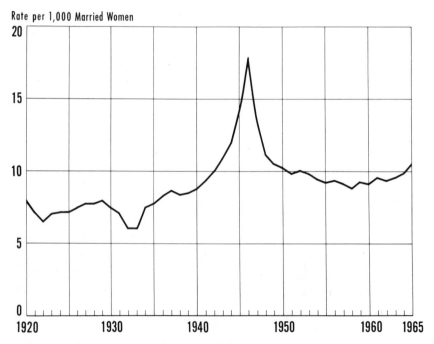

Fig. 3.5. Divorce rates per 1,000 married women 15 years old and over: United States, 1920 to 1965

Source: Table 3.9.

years old and over is taken as the base.[7] Within the framework of a generally upward trend in divorce over the 45-year period, significant deviations have occurred on a short-term basis. The divorce rate declined sharply from 1929 to 1932 as the country moved into the Great Depression. During this period, undoubtedly an increasing proportion of couples with marital troubles found divorce too costly and consequently resorted to permanent separation. During the war years, the divorce rate rose with unprecedented rapidity and reached an all-time high in 1946, the first postwar year. Beginning with 1947, however, the rate moved downward to 1955, by which time it had returned to about the same level as in 1941. It remained relatively stable for the seven years through 1962, then moved moderately upward through 1965, when the rate was at the same level as in 1949.

Preliminary figures for 1966 to 1968 indicate a continuing rise in the divorce rate, essentially in line with the long-term (45-year) trend.

Recent rates by age at divorce. Comprehensive data on divorce rates by age, color, and sex for the entire United States are not available because many states are not in the Divorce Registration Area and, of those which are in the DRA, many have incomplete reporting of age on divorce certificates. However, rates are available for four states — Hawaii, Iowa, Tennessee, and Wisconsin — and these are shown in Table 3.10. (The "total" column for this table

Table 3.10. Divorce rates per 1,000 married persons, by age, color, and sex: Four selected States, 1960-61

Age at divorce	Divorce rate for men			Divorce rate for women		
	Total	White	Nonwhite	Total	White	Nonwhite
Total	7.5	7.1	10.7	7.5	7.1	10.7
Under 20 years	24.8	26.6	7.7	29.0	30.7	13.4
20-24 years	22.0	22.3	15.5	18.9	18.8	18.1
25-29 years	15.5	15.2	17.6	11.1	10.7	14.6
30-34 years	10.2	9.5	16.0	9.0	8.3	13.1
35-39 years	7.5	6.8	13.3	7.1	6.8	9.9
40-44 years	6.9	6.5	11.4	5.9	5.6	8.5
45-49 years	5.6	5.4	7.2	4.2	3.9	7.0
50 & over	2.5	2.3	5.4	1.8	1.6	4.2

Source: National Center for Health Statistics, Series 21, No. 7, Divorce Statistics Analysis: United States, 1962, table 4.

appears as a row for men and a row for women in Table 2.6 of Chapter 2.) An examination of Table 3.10 makes it clear that rates show somewhat greater variability by age for women than for men. For persons under 20, rates are higher for women than for men; for those over 25, however, they are generally lower for women than for men.

For adults of all ages taken together, rates for nonwhites are half again as high as those for whites, and the distribution of rates by age is markedly different for the two color groups. The divorce rates for whites are clearly highest for those under 20 years of age and decline with advancing age; for nonwhites, however, the highest rates occur among those one or two age groups older. Thus for nonwhite men the highest rates are at ages 25 to 29 years of age and for women at ages 20 to 24 years old. Caution is appropriate in interpreting the relatively low divorce rates for nonwhite persons under 20 years of age. It seems reasonable to doubt that teenage marriages are more stable for nonwhite couples than for white couples, because the desertion rate is much higher for young nonwhite persons.

The reasons for the overall differences between white and nonwhite persons in the levels of divorce must be in part speculative. The factors involved, as discussed elsewhere in this monograph, include the long-term effects on Negroes of the experience of slavery, the historically low average income of nonwhite persons, the enormous volume in recent decades of Negro migration both from region to region and from country to city, and the practices of racial discrimination prevailing in many areas.

Divorce rates by states. The number of divorces per 1,000 population in each state in 1966, shown in Figure 3.6, is affected by such factors as the percent of the population that is Catholic, the strictness of the divorce laws, and the proportion of the divorces that are granted to temporary residents of the state. In general, divorce rates were found to be lower in the East than in the West, and lower in the North than in the South, although there are numerous exceptions. Along the Atlantic Coast, rates were low except for Georgia (slightly above the national rate) and especially Florida, where many decrees are granted to temporary residents. Along the southern border of the country, rates were high except for Louisiana, where there is a substantial Catholic population. Along most of the northern border east of Montana, divorce rates were fairly low. In the Rocky Mountain

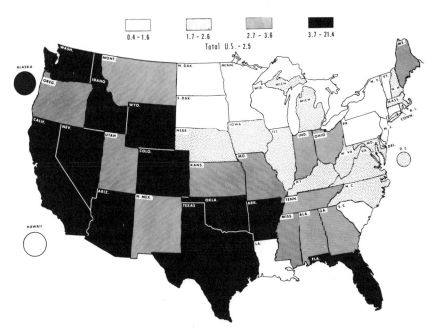

| 0.4 - 1.6 | 1.7 - 2.6 | 2.7 - 3.6 | 3.7 - 21.4 |

Total U.S. - 2.5

Fig. 3.6. Divorces per 1,000 population, by states: United States, 1966 (Louisiana, rate for 1963; New Mexico, rate for 1965)

Source: National Center for Health Statistics, *Monthly Vital Statistics Report,* Vol. 17, No. 10 Supplement, "Divorce Statistics, 1966," table 1.

and Pacific Coast states, the rates were high. In the middle of the country, divorce rates were higher in the South than in the North.

Marital Status

Long-term trend. During the 75 years between 1890 and 1965, the marked changes which occurred in the age and sex distribution of the population of the United States had an important bearing on the changing marital-status distribution. The adult population of the nation formerly had a relatively high proportion of young adults (20 to 29 years old), but by 1965 had a far larger proportion than ever before of persons in the middle and upper range of age (45 years old and over). Also, the ratio of men per 100 women among adults declined from the high level of nearly 110 in 1910, to 103 in 1930, and 95 in 1965. The earlier excess of men had turned into a deficit, but the deficit of men in 1965 was concentrated largely at the upper ages where marriages occur rather rarely. These changes in age and sex distribution were largely the result of declining birth and death

Table 3.11. Percent by marital status, for persons 14 years old and over, by sex, standardized for age and unstandardized: United States, 1960 and 1965, and conterminous United States, 1890 to 1955.

Year	Men					Women				
	Total	Single	Married	Widowed	Divorced	Total	Single	Married	Widowed	Divorced
STANDARDIZED FOR AGE[a]										
1965	100.0	24.3	70.3	3.1	2.3	100.0	18.8	65.2	11.9	3.1
1960	100.0	25.3	69.3	3.5	1.8	100.0	19.0	65.9	12.5	2.6
1955	100.0	25.5	68.5	4.2	1.7	100.0	19.1	65.4	13.2	2.2
1950	100.0	26.5	67.3	4.5	1.7	100.0	20.0	64.2	13.8	2.1
1947	100.0	27.4	66.4	4.7	1.6	100.0	21.4	62.7	13.8	2.0
1940	100.0	30.9	62.4	5.3	1.3	100.0	24.3	59.5	14.5	1.6
1890	100.0	32.1	61.5	5.9	0.3	100.0	23.8	58.3	17.4	0.4
UNSTANDARDIZED										
1965	100.0	26.6	67.9	3.3	2.2	100.0	20.7	63.9	12.5	2.9
1960	100.0	25.3	69.3	3.5	1.8	100.0	19.0	65.9	12.5	2.6
1955	100.0	24.1	69.9	4.2	1.8	100.0	18.2	66.9	12.6	2.3
1950	100.0	26.2	68.0	4.2	1.7	100.0	19.6	66.1	12.2	2.2
1947	100.0	28.2	66.2	4.1	1.6	100.0	22.0	64.2	11.6	2.1
1940	100.0	34.8	59.7	4.2	1.2	100.0	27.6	59.5	11.3	1.6
1890	100.0	43.6	52.2	3.8	0.2	100.0	34.1	54.9	10.6	0.4

Source: U.S. Bureau of the Census, U.S. Census of Population: 1960, Detailed Characteristics, U.S. Summary, Final Report PC(1)-1D, table 177; Current Population Reports, Series P-20, Nos. 10, 62, 105, 122, and 144.

[a]Standardized on the basis of the age distribution in 1960.

60

rates during the half-century from 1890 to 1940 and the sharp drop in the net immigration rate during the 1920's and 1930's, followed by only a moderate rise.

That the structure of the population by age and sex was more conducive to a higher percentage married in 1965 than in 1890 can be seen from a comparison of standardized and unstandardized figures in Table 3.11. For example, unstandardized census data show that only 52.2 percent of men 14 years old and over were married in 1890 as compared with 67.9 percent in 1965, an increase of 15.7 percentage points. Yet if the population in both 1890 and 1965 had had the same distribution by age and sex as in 1960, the percent married for men in 1890 standardized for age would have been 61.5, and the increase to 1965 would have been only 8.8 percentage points, or about one-half the unstandardized change. In other words, about half of the 1890–1965 rise in the unstandardized percent married for men is attributable to the aging of the population. The corresponding proportion for married women, however, is much smaller.

During the same period, about two-thirds of the decline in percent single for both males and females can be traced to the declining proportion of adults who were in the younger age groups. Among women, the observed increase from 10.6 percent widowed in 1890 to 12.5 percent widowed in 1965 actually becomes a decrease from 17.4 percent to 11.9 percent when the data are adjusted for changes in the age distribution. In short, the underlying trends in marital behavior appear in clearer perspective when shifts in the age distribution of the population are taken into account.

Events of the 1940's produced a greater decline in the percent single and a greater rise in the percent married than those of the half-century prior to 1940 or the 15 years after 1950, as is evident in Figure 3.7. Many new factors must have encouraged persons to marry during the 1940's. One important element was the much greater opportunity for women to combine paid employment and marriage. The labor shortage generated by World War II led to the large-scale hiring of married women to perform work in numerous fields — professional, clerical, and factory — where employment practices previously had tended to bar them. Once jobs in these fields were opened to married women, and once men grew accustomed to having their wives thus employed, more and more women followed the pattern of working for a few years before and after marriage. In addition,

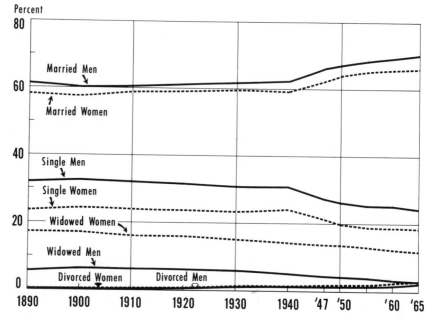

Fig. 3.7. Percent by marital status, for persons 14 years old and over standardized for age: United States, 1890 to 1965

Source: Table 3.11.

women with work experience before they bore children were more employable and evidently more interested in working after their children reached school age than women without such experience.

Events of the 1940's probably also caused young men to develop a more optimistic economic outlook and hence to be more willing to assume the responsibilities of marriage at an earlier age than before. The prospect of marrying a woman who would help share expenses through her employment was probably another contributing factor. At the same time, improving health conditions permitted an increasing proportion of couples to live into their fifties, sixties, and seventies and remain in the married state.

Changing attitudes toward the sanctity of marriage may have been developing during this period and generating more of an experimental approach, so that marriage became more readily entered, more readily terminated by legal procedures, and more readily re-entered with a different mate.

Although the foregoing rationale behind the upsurge in marriage during the 1940's must remain largely speculative, the basic fact in

ages at marriage, other factors besides years of schooling in preparation for their work are undoubtedly involved, because their schooling is generally completed long before the age of 24 or 25 years — the average age at which they marry. The amount of income men receive from their work and the extent to which their daily work depends on having a wife (as in the case of farm workers, especially farm operators) undoubtedly are additional factors which have much to do with the age at which men marry.

Among employed women of middle age who had married, those in professional occupations were about 25 years old when they married, on the average, and four to six years older at marriage than those employed in most of the other occupations. About half these women were in the teaching profession. Women in clerical positions also tended to be a year or so above the overall average age of 22 at first marriage, for those who had reached their forties or fifties by 1960.

Employed nonwhite men of middle age in 1960 were about one-half year younger than corresponding white men at first marriage. But nonwhite men in white-collar positions tended to have delayed marriage more than other nonwhite men; consequently, white and nonwhite men in white-collar positions differed less in regard to average age at marriage than white and nonwhite men in other occupational lines, notably farm work. In fact, nonwhite men in managerial and sales positions were actually older than white men at first marriage. Evidently nonwhite men took more time than white men to become established in these lines of work before they were ready to marry.

Employed nonwhite women of middle age had an average age at first marriage that was more than one-half year younger than that of corresponding white women. Yet for nonwhite women in several occupation groups — professional and clerical workers, craftsmen, operatives, laborers, and service workers (except private household) — it was older than for white women. In fact, the only occupation groups for which the average age at marriage was distinctly lower for nonwhite women were the farm-occupation groups, but only a small minority of women of either color group are farm workers.

The differences between white and nonwhite women in regard to age at first marriage by occupation group can be better understood by studying their occupational distributions by color and sex. Among women 45 to 54 years old, nearly one-half the nonwhite workers were employed in service occupations, whereas only one-sixth of the white workers were in these occupations. At the same time, only one-tenth of the nonwhite women were employed in professional or clerical occupations, as compared with more than one-third of the white women.

Another view of the relationship between occupation and age at first marriage is shown for white and nonwhite men in Table 4.11. The same occupation groups now are classified by four broad age-at-marriage categories: very young (14 to 20 years), oldest (34 years and over), most frequent (21 to 26 years), and relatively old (27 to 33 years). One is struck first by the marked difference in 1960 between the distribution of jobs for the two color groups; for example, professional, managerial, and sales workers included 30 percent of the white but only 7 percent of the nonwhite men, and craftsmen included 24 percent of the white but only 12 percent of the nonwhite men.

When attention is directed to the variation in job distribution by age at marriage, it becomes evident that professional workers among both color groups were most concentrated among the men who married at a relatively old age (27 to 33 years); laborers on the other hand tended to concentrate among those who had married at the very young or the oldest age. The explanatory principles mentioned above (amount of training for the job, amount of income from the work done, and dependence on a wife's help on the job) undoubtedly apply differentially to the occupation groups which are characterized by the several patterns of age at marriage.

To carry the analysis a step farther, men in some occupations show a distinct progression in age at marriage. Farmers and farm managers represent almost 7 percent of the white men marrying when very young but decline to 5 percent of those marrying when in the oldest age group. Corresponding figures for nonwhite men are roughly 6 and 3 percent. Clerical workers, in general, show an opposite progression with greatest concentration among those who were rather old at marriage.

For certain occupations the pattern differs by color. For instance, the largest proportion of white craftsmen married when very young, but the largest proportion of nonwhite craftsmen married at intermediate ages. White service workers were most frequently found among those who married very young or old, but among nonwhites they were especially overrepresented among those who were in the oldest age at marriage.

Table 4.11. Percent by major occupation group, for men ever married 45 to 54 years old with earnings in 1959, by age at first marriage and color: United States, 1960

Major occupation group	White men 45-54 years old					Nonwhite men 45-54 years old				
	Total ever married	Age at first marriage (years)				Total ever married	Age at first marriage (years)			
		14-20	21-26	27-33	34 & over		14-20	21-26	27-33	34 & over
Total with earnings	100.0	100.0	100.0	100.0	100.0	100.0	100.0	100.0	100.0	100.0
Professional, technical, & kindred workers	8.8	4.0	8.4	12.2	9.6	2.9	1.7	2.9	4.5	2.6
Farmers and farm managers	6.0	6.9	6.4	5.3	5.0	4.9	5.9	5.8	4.1	2.6
Managers, officials, & proprietors, except farm	14.8	13.4	15.7	15.0	11.9	2.9	2.8	3.2	3.1	2.5
Clerical & kindred workers	5.9	4.2	5.6	6.8	7.3	3.9	2.9	3.8	4.7	4.2
Sales workers	6.5	5.4	6.6	7.1	5.9	1.1	1.0	1.1	1.4	1.1
Craftsmen, foremen, and kindred workers	24.3	27.5	24.9	22.3	21.4	12.1	11.3	12.5	12.8	11.6
Operatives & kindred workers	19.3	22.0	19.4	17.6	19.5	23.5	23.4	24.7	22.2	23.2
Service workers, incl. private household	4.9	5.2	4.5	4.7	6.4	14.5	14.6	13.5	14.9	16.2
Farm laborers and foremen	1.4	2.0	1.3	1.1	1.6	6.2	8.1	5.8	5.0	5.6
Laborers, except farm and mine	4.8	5.5	4.4	4.5	6.5	21.1	22.3	20.5	20.3	21.8
Occupation not reported	3.3	3.9	2.8	3.4	4.8	6.8	6.1	6.2	7.0	8.6

Source: U.S. Bureau of the Census, U.S. Census of Population: 1960, Subject Reports, Age at First Marriage, Final Report PC(2)-4D, table 14.

Income level. The 1959 incomes of middle-aged persons are related, in the following five tables, to an event that had occurred up to three decades before — their original date of marriage. These tables show several variables cross-classified with income (or earnings), including place of residence, educational achievement, and occupation. The complex interplay of these factors is evident. But for both men and women, regardless of color, the underlying pattern is one of younger-than-average age at marriage for those in the lowest income levels and higher-than-average age for those in the higher income levels.

Some of the tables in this section show mean values of age at first marriage and earnings, whereas others show medians. Although median values tend to be preferred for analytical purposes, the means were computed instead wherever doing so would save substantial processing. A comparison of means in the first column of Table 4.12 with corresponding medians in the last column of Table 4.13 demonstrates that the patterns of high and low values are quite consistent, even though the mean values are higher than the medians by about one-half to two years.

Mean age at first marriage is shown in Table 4.12 for middle-aged persons in the United States as a whole, and for four contrasting areas: central cities of large urban agglomerations versus rural farm, and the Northeast versus the South. The greatest contrast was the very substantial difference between the high average ages at marriage for persons in the Northeast and the low average ages for persons on rural farms, amounting to about two years for the white population and three years for the nonwhite. Since the Northeast has the largest proportion of the population in central cities of urbanized areas, it is not surprising that the mean age at marriage of persons in central cities tended to be almost as high as that in the Northeast. Likewise, since the South is much more highly rural than any other region, it is not surprising that the mean age at marriage approximated the low level shown for the farm population.

For the United States as a whole, men in the highest income level ($10,000 or more) had married at the most advanced age and those in the lowest level (less than $1,000) at the youngest age. Within this general pattern, however, some noteworthy deviations occurred, in particular a primary or secondary peak in age at marriage among men in the middle of the income range in the Northeast and in the central cities of urbanized areas.

Mean age at first marriage, for persons ever married 45 to 54 years old, by income in 1959, color, sex, and type of residence: United States, 1960

Income, color, and sex	Mean age at first marriage				
	United States	Central cities of urbanized areas	Rural farm	North-east	South
Men 45-54					
White	26.3	26.9	25.5	27.2	25.5
ithout income	26.0	26.8	25.3	27.0	25.2
1-$999 or loss	26.0	26.8	25.6	27.2	25.2
1,000-$2,999	26.1	27.1	25.6	27.2	25.3
3,000-$4,999	26.4	27.3	25.5	27.3	25.4
5,000-$6,999	26.4	26.9	25.4	27.1	25.5
7,000-$9,999	26.3	26.6	25.3	27.1	25.8
10,000 & over	26.6	26.9	25.7	27.3	26.2
Nonwhite	26.6	27.2	24.7	27.8	25.9
ithout income	26.2	27.3	24.3	27.4	25.5
1-$999 or loss	25.8	26.6	24.7	27.0	25.5
1,000-$2,999	26.3	27.0	24.6	27.7	25.9
3,000-$4,999	27.0	27.3	25.3	28.0	26.3
5,000-$6,999	27.1	27.2	24.6	27.8	26.3
7,000-$9,999	26.9	27.1	a	26.9	26.3
10,000 & over	27.4	27.7	a	27.5	27.0
Women 45-54					
White	23.2	23.8	22.2	24.2	22.3
ithout income	22.9	23.6	22.0	23.9	22.0
1-$999 or loss	23.0	23.7	22.3	24.3	22.1
1,000-$2,999	23.0	23.6	22.2	23.9	22.2
3,000-$4,999	24.0	24.2	23.8	24.8	23.8
5,000-$6,999	25.3	25.4	25.2	26.2	24.9
7,000-$9,999	26.0	26.0	25.5	26.7	25.0
10,000 & over	24.7	25.3	24.5	25.6	24.1
Nonwhite	23.2	23.8	21.8	24.4	22.8
ithout income	23.1	23.8	21.6	24.5	22.7
1-$999 or loss	22.8	23.4	21.9	24.0	22.6
1,000-$2,999	23.4	23.7	22.2	24.3	22.9
3,000-$4,999	24.6	24.5	a	25.0	25.4
5,000-$6,999	25.7	25.8	a	25.2	26.0
7,000-$9,999	24.8	25.4	a	a	25.1
10,000 & over	a	a	a	a	a

Source: U.S. Bureau of the Census, U.S. Census of Population: 960, Subject Reports, Age at First Marriage, Final Report PC(2)-4D, able 13a.

aMean not shown where base is less than 1,000.

Among women, the pattern differs from that for men mainly in that the oldest age at marriage did not occur among those in the highest income bracket (with enough sample cases to show a value) but in the second-highest bracket. Although census data are not available to demonstrate it, the fact may be that women in the highest income category include an especially large proportion who have inherited a substantial amount of wealth from which they receive much of their income.

The difference between the incomes of middle-aged men and women in relation to their ages at marriage some 20 to 30 years earlier serves to underline the fundamental distinctions between their sources of income. A man may have married late because he used his income at a young age to amass enough capital to start a business, or he may have used his available resources to obtain professional training. If widowed or divorced before middle age, he probably continued in the same occupation. The woman's occupation before marriage is likely to be interrupted, at least temporarily, by marriage and the care of young children. If she becomes widowed or divorced, she may have to move to a new locality and change her work, perhaps rather suddenly. For these and other reasons, the woman's age at first marriage is less likely than that of her husband to have been closely associated with either early job training or current income.

Further insight into the relationship between income and age at marriage is given in Table 4.13 for men and women 45 to 54 years old in 1960. A glance down the column reveals that the highest figure for white men 14 to 17 years old at marriage, 5 percent, is for those "without income," and the next highest figure, 4.9 percent, is for those with the lowest reported income. Thus there was a strong concentration in very low income classes for those who married very young. At the base of this column the median income — $4,453 — is the lowest for any of the age groups among white men. This is the income distribution one would expect for marriages in early youth, where education and job training prior to marriage must have been extremely limited.

Continuing analysis of white men shows that the highest median income — $5,855 — is for those who had married in the broad age group 25 to 29 years old. In this group were found 38 percent of the white men with incomes of $10,000 and over by the age of 45 to 54 years. There was also overrepresentation in the next highest income class. These and other figures in the table make it clear that for white

Table 4.13. Percent by income in 1959, for persons ever married 45 to 54 years old, by age at first marriage, color, and sex: United States, 1960

Income, color, and sex	Total ever married	Age at first marriage (years)							Median age
		14-17	18 & 19	20 & 21	22-24	25-29	30-34	35 & over	
Men, 45-54									
White	100.0	2.6	7.0	13.8	24.9	30.0	12.9	8.8	25.3
Without income	100.0	5.0	9.6	15.7	23.4	24.9	11.4	10.0	24.5
$1-$999 or loss	100.0	4.9	10.5	15.9	22.9	23.7	11.6	10.5	24.4
$1,000-$2,999	100.0	4.1	9.5	15.5	23.7	25.0	11.9	10.2	24.6
$3,000-$4,999	100.0	2.8	7.6	14.7	24.3	27.6	12.8	10.3	25.1
$5,000-$6,999	100.0	2.2	6.5	13.8	25.2	30.5	13.3	8.5	25.4
$7,000-$9,999	100.0	1.9	5.7	12.8	26.3	33.4	12.9	7.0	25.5
$10,000 & over	100.0	1.4	4.3	10.2	25.7	38.2	13.6	6.6	26.1
Median income	$5,483	4,453	4,800	5,189	5,593	5,855	5,582	4,967	...
Nonwhite	100.0	7.1	10.7	14.5	18.9	21.6	12.7	14.4	24.8
Without income	100.0	7.6	10.9	16.4	19.5	20.6	11.5	13.6	24.3
$1-$999 or loss	100.0	8.6	12.8	16.2	18.5	20.1	11.5	12.3	24.0
$1,000-$2,999	100.0	8.2	11.9	14.7	18.5	20.3	12.0	14.4	24.5
$3,000-$4,999	100.0	6.4	9.6	14.1	18.6	21.8	13.7	15.8	25.3
$5,000-$6,999	100.0	4.7	8.7	12.6	20.5	24.7	14.3	14.5	25.7
$7,000-$9,999	100.0	4.2	6.8	13.2	21.6	28.3	13.4	12.5	25.7
$10,000 & over	100.0	3.5	5.2	9.6	17.8	36.2	17.8	9.9	26.9
Median income	$2,879	2,438	2,514	2,713	2,940	3,091	3,119	3,024	...
Women, 45-54									
White	100.0	15.6	17.7	17.5	20.1	17.4	6.8	5.0	21.9
Without income	100.0	16.6	18.3	17.8	19.9	16.8	6.4	4.3	21.7
$1-$999 or loss	100.0	17.3	17.9	16.8	19.3	17.4	6.7	4.7	21.8
$1,000-$2,999	100.0	16.8	18.7	17.7	19.5	16.3	6.4	4.7	21.6
$3,000-$4,999	100.0	12.0	16.0	17.5	21.2	19.2	7.7	6.5	22.6
$5,000-$6,999	100.0	8.0	12.3	15.0	22.0	23.0	10.5	9.2	24.0
$7,000-$9,999	100.0	7.2	10.3	13.7	22.8	24.4	10.5	11.0	24.5
$10,000 & over	100.0	8.4	11.4	17.0	25.8	21.1	9.0	7.2	23.5
Median income	$2,236	1,881	2,073	2,222	2,343	2,419	2,507	2,748	...
Nonwhite	100.0	24.7	16.4	13.6	14.4	15.0	7.9	8.0	21.3
Without income	100.0	25.4	16.8	13.8	14.1	14.2	7.6	8.0	21.1
$1-$999 or loss	100.0	27.6	17.1	13.4	13.1	13.9	7.5	7.5	20.8
$1,000-$2,999	100.0	23.3	16.3	13.5	15.3	15.8	8.1	7.8	21.6
$3,000-$4,999	100.0	16.5	13.2	14.1	17.9	18.1	9.6	10.5	23.0
$5,000-$6,999	100.0	10.2	10.7	10.6	18.0	28.7	13.2	8.6	25.1
$7,000-$9,999	100.0	12.2	10.6	15.2	19.0	22.6	12.2	8.3	23.9
$10,000 & over	a	a	a	a	a	a	a	a	a
Median income	$996	880	945	999	1,252	1,254	1,192	1,151	...

Source: U.S. Bureau of the Census, U.S. Census of Population: 1960, Subject Reports, Age at First Marriage, Final Report PC(2)-4D, table 13.

[a]Percent not shown where base is less than 1,000.

men interested in high income the best age to marry was 25 to 29 years old. For those who had married below 25 or over 29 years the median income in middle age was lower. Those who married after their thirtieth birthday evidently included a considerable number of the less competent, but these "late bloomers" did considerably better, as measured by the income they eventually received, than did the group who married as teenagers.

The picture is quite different for white women; they received less than half as much income as did white men and had their highest income among those who were 35 and older at first marriage. Lowest median incomes were received by those who married as early teenagers, followed by the late teenagers, and with each advance in age at marriage there was a slight advance in average income. Moreover, it was only among those marrying at 35 or older that the women's median incomes were more than one-half that of men marrying at the same age. It must be emphasized that these are incomes of persons, not family incomes; also that in most families it is the husband's income, not the wife's, that is the major source of family support. The higher average income for the atypical women who married after reaching 35 years of age may reflect the fact that many of these women were established in professional or business careers at the time of marriage.

The relationship between income and age at marriage for the nonwhite population is quite different from that for the white population. Not only are incomes of nonwhites drastically lower, but the distribution by age at marriage of nonwhites shows less concentration for both men and women. Among nonwhite men, highest incomes were received by those who married at 30 to 34 years of age, but the incomes of those in the two adjacent age categories were only slightly lower. Thus nonwhite men who received the highest incomes were those who married somewhat older than the corresponding white men. Perhaps the economic competition faced by nonwhite men was such that they tended to delay marriage longer than white men in order to maximize their earnings before marriage.

Nonwhite wives (or ex-wives) had incomes less than one-half those of nonwhite men, and those with the highest incomes were those who had married when they were between 22 and 29 years old. Doubtless most of the nonwhite women held jobs that required less education and training than those held by white women. Also, a larger proportion of the nonwhite women were divorced, separated, and widowed than the white women, and this may have required more of them to make an emergency entry into the labor market. Another possible factor is the slightly higher remarriage rate among nonwhite than among white women; women who remarry are more likely to have little or no income than women who remain widowed or divorced. It is also possible that a larger proportion of the nonwhite women who married at age 35 or older had ceased to be employed after they married.

The final three tables in this chapter relate exclusively to men and show data on mean earnings for men ever married, 45 to 54 years old at the census date, classified by age at the time of first marriage. Table 4.14 presents such data by educational level of the man; Table 4.15, by major occupation group; and Table 4.16, by selected occupation groups within each educational level.

As shown in Table 4.14, white men in every educational level had the highest mean earnings by middle age if they married for the first time when they were 21 to 26 years old; this was their best age to

Table 4.14. Mean earnings in 1959 and percent distribution, for men ever married 45 to 54 years old with earnings, by age at first marriage, years of school completed, and color: United States, 1960

Years of school completed and color	Age at first marriage (years)				
	Total	14-20	21-26	27-33	34 & over
Mean earnings					
White men	$6,563	$5,542	$6,766	$7,052	$5,914
Elementary: 0-8 years	4,602	4,442	4,729	4,671	4,214
High school: 1-3 years	5,913	5,766	6,056	5,954	5,338
High school: 4 years	6,924	6,945	7,132	6,872	6,100
College: 1-3 years	8,890	8,543	9,384	8,679	7,538
College: 4 or more	13,340	11,551	14,020	13,347	11,453
Nonwhite men	$3,195	$2,832	$3,269	$3,458	$3,218
Elementary: 0-8 years	2,778	2,568	2,812	2,892	2,908
High school: 1-3 years	3,669	3,499	3,827	3,699	3,509
High school: 4 years	4,182	4,000	4,307	4,396	3,777
College: 1-3 years	4,545	4,092	4,652	4,691	4,460
College: 4 or more	6,598	5,819	6,747	6,926	5,869
Percent by age at first marriage					
White men	100.0	15.4	47.4	26.6	10.5
Elementary: 0-8 years	100.0	20.5	46.4	22.5	10.6
High school: 1-3 years	100.0	17.6	48.7	24.3	9.4
High school: 4 years	100.0	11.6	48.8	28.7	10.9
College: 1-3 years	100.0	8.9	48.8	31.8	10.6
College: 4 or more	100.0	3.9	43.8	40.0	12.2
Nonwhite men	100.0	24.8	36.1	22.5	16.6
Elementary: 0-8 years	100.0	27.4	35.6	20.7	16.2
High school: 1-3 years	100.0	22.7	36.9	23.5	16.8
High school: 4 years	100.0	16.1	38.7	26.5	18.8
College: 1-3 years	100.0	15.3	37.6	29.8	17.3
College: 4 or more	100.0	8.5	33.9	41.2	16.3

Source: U.S. Bureau of the Census, U.S. Census of Population: 1960, Subject Reports, Age at First Marriage, Final Report PC(2)-4D, table 14.

marry in terms of later income. But the highest mean-earnings level for all education groups combined was that for men who had married at ages 27 to 33. The superficial contradiction between these two observations is a consequence of the greater concentration of men with low education among those who married at ages 21 to 26 than at ages 27 to 33, as the lower section of the table demonstrates.

In like manner, the lowest earnings for white men were those where marriage occurred before age 21; yet at each educational level these men had higher mean earnings than those who had first married at ages 34 and over. Again, men with low education were more highly concentrated among those who married when quite young than among those who first married when relatively old.

Education emerges from an analysis of Table 4.14 as a much more significant discriminator between those with high and low earnings by middle age than does age at first marriage. The range of mean earnings among the educational levels of white men overall is considerable — from $4,602 for the least educated to $13,340 for the most educated — whereas among the groups by age at first marriage the range is far more moderate — from $5,542 for the youngest to $7,052 for the next-to-oldest age at marriage.

Even so, white men with no college education who managed to enter first marriage during the optimal age range for first marriage — in terms of eventual earnings level — were shown to be likely to fare up to one-eighth better in their earnings than those who first married while still minors or after they had reached bachelor age (defined here as 35 years old or over). White men with college education appeared likely to fare about 10 to 20 percent better in eventual earnings if they married during the optimal range of age at first marriage.

For white men who married before 21 and did not graduate from college, the earnings differential by age at marriage diminished sharply as the amount of education increased. But for white men who postponed marriage until they were 34 or older, the earnings differential by age at marriage increased sharply as the amount of education increased. These men probably include a substantial proportion who lack one or more significant qualifications of a successful marriage partner.

The findings show, furthermore, that white men who continued their education until they had graduated from high school and then went no farther in school had very little difference in their eventual earnings according to their age at marriage, provided they married before they reached far into their thirties. Those who had gone to college, however, tended to reach the highest earnings level if they had, in addition, delayed marriage until age 21.

Nonwhite men exhibited the same tendency as did white men to vary much more widely in mean earnings by middle age according to how much education they had received than according to when they had first married. Differences between the white and nonwhite patterns in Table 4.14 reflect the smaller increment to earnings from a given increment to education for the nonwhite men and the markedly flatter distribution of ages at first marriage for the nonwhite men, as seen in the second part of the table.

More specifically, the nonwhite men in each education level had a much larger proportion who married early instead of waiting until they were better established in a job and more capable of providing a comfortable home for their wife. In addition, the nonwhite men in each education level were much more likely to have reported the postponement of first marriage until age 34 or older.

The relationship between age at first marriage and mean earnings by major occupation group is considered in Table 4.15. White men who were professional or managerial workers ranked clearly above those in other occupational groups with regard to mean earnings. The same conclusion is also appropriate for men in each group according to age at marriage. Sales workers ranked next in earnings, then clerical workers and craftsmen — again, for those in each group by age at marriage. Operatives, service workers, and laborers were consistently at or near the lowest earnings levels for men in nonfarm occupations. Farm workers had still lower earnings.

In each occupation group, white men who married when they were in either of the two intermediate age-at-marriage groups had higher mean earnings by middle age than those who married at a very young or quite old age. The earnings disadvantage recorded for those who were not of intermediate age at marriage varied from less than 10 percent (for farmers, operatives, and nonfarm laborers who married after age 34) to more than 30 percent (for professional and technical workers who married before age 21). As for the low earnings of professional and technical men who married before they were 21, a plausible factor may be a concentration of technicians and marginally successful professional men among those who married very young.

Occupation, like education, differentiates more between white men with high earnings and those with low earnings than does age at first

Table 4.15. Mean earnings in 1959, for men ever married 45 to 54 years
old with earnings by age at first marriage, by major
occupation group and color: United States, 1960

Major occupation group and color	Mean earnings by age at first marriage (years)				
	Total	14-20	21-26	27-33	34 & over
White men	$6,563	$5,542	$6,766	$7,052	$5,914
Professional & tech. wkrs.	11,139	8,805	11,225	11,793	10,119
Farmers & farm managers	3,641	3,234	3,747	3,751	3,565
Managers, off'ls., prop'rs.	10,374	8,961	10,772	10,719	9,244
Clerical & kindred wkrs.	5,775	5,430	5,911	5,882	5,347
Sales workers	7,760	6,643	7,933	8,205	7,051
Craftsmen & foremen	5,739	5,369	5,883	5,884	5,304
Operatives & kindred wkrs.	4,918	4,686	5,034	4,993	4,614
Service workers	4,366	4,006	4,518	4,538	4,003
Farm laborers & foremen	2,294	2,063	2,435	2,396	2,027
Laborers, exc. farm & mine	3,908	3,602	4,031	3,997	3,759
Nonwhite men	$3,195	$2,832	$3,269	$3,458	$3,218
Professional & tech. wkrs.	6,052	4,583	6,219	6,749	5,430
Farmers & farm managers	1,394	1,088	1,374	1,871	1,518
Managers, off'ls., prop'rs.	4,843	3,498	5,398	5,949	3,713
Clerical & kindred wkrs.	4,470	4,292	4,667	4,514	4,203
Sales workers	4,339	3,749	4,606	4,713	3,862
Craftsmen & foremen	3,706	3,352	3,814	3,868	3,722
Operatives & kindred wkrs.	3,447	3,311	3,481	3,505	3,498
Service workers	2,923	2,733	2,983	2,998	2,976
Farm laborers & foremen	1,243	1,173	1,210	1,299	1,403
Laborers, exc. farm & mine	2,777	2,611	2,846	2,821	2,835

Source: U.S. Bureau of the Census, U.S. Census of Population:
1960, Subject Reports, Age at First Marriage, Final Report PC(2)-4D,
table 14.

marriage. Yet regardless of occupation group, those who succeeded in
waiting to marry until they were legally of age but did not wait until
they were bachelors came out ahead, on the average, with respect to
eventual earnings.

Among nonwhite men, marriage while in the intermediate range
of ages shown in Table 4.15 was likewise associated with relatively
high earnings by middle age.[11] Earnings by this age for nonwhite men
who married very young and were in a white-collar job (except clerical) or who were farm operators fell far below the earnings of those
who married at an intermediate age. The "penalty" for youthful marriage was especially great for farm operators and sales workers, among
whom the earnings gap amounted to three-fourths of their income,
as compared with the earnings of those in the same occupation who

married when they were 21 to 33 years old. How much the factor of youthful marriage was the root cause of the difference is not known; many other factors having varying degrees of correlation with marriage at an early age may also have been significant.

Nonwhite men at the lower end of the occupational listing had consistently low earnings regardless of how old they were at marriage. In this respect they showed less difference than white men in comparable occupational levels.

Table 4.16. Mean earnings in 1959, for men ever married 45 to 54 years old, by years of school completed, selected major nonfarm occupation groups, age at first marriage, and color: United States, 1960

Selected major occupation groups and years of school completed	Mean earnings by age at first marriage (years)									
	Total		14-20		21-26		27-33		34 & over	
	White	Percent less for nonwhite	White	Percent less for nonwhite	White	Percent less for nonwhite	White	Percent less for nonwhite	White	Percent less for nonwhite
Elementary, 0-8 years										
Managers, off'ls., prop'rs.	$6,965	46.1	$6,886	53.1	$7,135	39.7	$6,950	39.4	$6,158	52.1
Craftsmen & foremen	5,073	33.8	4,906	38.5	5,185	33.0	5,152	32.8	4,693	25.3
Operatives & kindred wkrs.	4,556	28.4	4,384	27.7	4,658	30.3	4,600	28.1	4,339	22.2
Service workers	3,856	28.4	3,623	27.7	3,946	29.7	4,028	29.0	3,623	21.9
Laborers	3,669	27.0	3,410	25.5	3,773	27.3	3,753	28.1	3,562	23.2
High school, 1-3 years										
Managers, off'ls., prop'rs.	8,479	47.4	8,377	51.4	8,632	35.0	8,523	---	7,578	---
Clerical & kindred wkrs.	5,448	17.1	5,390	13.1	5,544	16.9	5,166	18.0	5,106	17.9
Sales workers	6,764	35.0	6,341	---	6,855	---	6,979	---	6,428	---
Craftsmen & foremen	5,841	27.8	5,657	28.3	5,955	27.1	5,897	27.7	5,385	25.6
Operatives & kindred wkrs.	5,221	25.1	5,131	26.2	5,302	23.4	5,283	26.4	4,814	22.3
Service workers	4,537	31.0	4,297	31.3	4,744	31.7	4,564	30.5	4,075	23.4
High school, 4 years										
Professional & tech. wkrs.	8,037	28.0	8,453	---	8,223	29.9	7,894	---	7,228	---
Managers, off'ls., prop'rs.	9,766	41.1	9,749	---	9,985	45.4	9,726	27.0	8,600	---
Clerical & kindred wkrs.	5,872	18.1	5,982	17.2	6,008	20.1	5,825	15.5	5,447	16.2
Sales workers	7,696	33.1	7,314	---	7,917	---	7,822	---	6,620	---
Craftsmen & foremen	6,293	28.3	6,219	25.1	6,449	29.0	6,232	26.4	5,806	27.8
Operatives & kindred wkrs.	5,535	26.0	5,407	27.3	5,686	24.9	5,513	25.9	5,072	23.5
College, 1-3 years										
Professional & tech. wkrs.	8,957	48.8	8,452	---	9,395	50.4	8,743	---	7,931	---
Managers, off'ls., prop'rs.	12,171	47.4	12,005	---	12,757	41.4	11,784	---	10,225	---
Clerical & kindred wkrs.	6,486	22.4	6,052	---	6,863	19.0	6,353	23.3	5,745	---
Sales workers	9,377	---	9,389	---	9,686	---	9,316	---	8,098	---
Craftsmen & foremen	6,912	37.5	6,510	---	7,166	40.5	6,929	37.3	6,096	---
Operatives & kindred wkrs.	5,850	27.2	5,394	---	6,151	31.9	5,733	22.2	5,340	---
College, 4 years & over										
Professional & tech. wkrs.	13,687	46.2	11,760	44.3	13,920	44.5	14,099	47.2	12,053	43.8
Managers, off'ls., prop'rs.	16,479	52.5	15,184	---	17,663	---	15,702	---	14,077	---
Sales workers	11,534	---	9,404	---	12,110	---	11,532	---	10,160	---
Craftsmen & foremen	9,624	47.2	8,177	---	10,162	---	9,585	---	8,168	---

Source: U.S. Bureau of the Census, U.S. Census of Population: 1960, Subject Reports, Age at First Marriage, Final Report PC(2)-4D, table 14.

Table 4.16 shows the combined effect of three factors — age at first marriage, educational attainment, and occupation group — on the amount of earnings white men received by middle age. It also shows, where a sufficient number of sample cases permitted, the percentage by which the mean earnings of nonwhite men fell below that of corresponding white men. The major nonfarm occupation groups chosen for presentation are those with at least 5 percent of the white male earners 45 to 54 years old in the specified education level. Comparable data for farmers and farm laborers are available in the source cited in the table.

Managers, officials, and proprietors (except farm) outranked all other major occupation groups with respect to mean earnings by middle age, within each educational level of white men overall. Moreover, this occupation group, referred to for brevity as managerial workers, had the highest mean earnings at every educational level of white men who married for the first time in each of the four age groups. The highest mean earnings shown in Table 4.16 is $17,663 for white men college graduates who married between the ages of 21 and 26 and were managerial workers by middle age. This is more than $3,500 above the highest mean earnings for white professional men (those who were college graduates with first marriage between the ages of 27 and 33 years). It is also nearly $2,000 above the earnings level of white managerial college graduates who married when they were 27 to 33 years old. In other words, white men who a generation ago were on their way to becoming managerial workers offered the best prospects of becoming husbands with a peak level of earnings.

Professional and technical workers who graduated from college ranked uniformly second in mean earnings by middle age among those in the several groups of white men by age at first marriage. No doubt a larger proportion of professional than managerial college graduates went on to graduate school and thus delayed their marriage. Perhaps this is one of the reasons why the mean earnings of college graduates was slightly higher for professional (but not managerial) workers who married at 27 to 33 than for those who married at 21 to 26.

Sales workers ranked third in earnings among white men who were college graduates and second among white men who attended college but did not complete the four years. To earn $10,000 or more by middle age, white sales workers had to have graduated from college and to have married at 21 or older, and white craftsmen had to be college graduates and to have married at 21 to 26 to reach that earnings level. Similarly, white professional workers averaged above $10,000 earnings only if they were college graduates, whereas white managerial workers attained this earnings level even if they had started but did not complete a four-year college education.

When account is taken of both educational level and occupation group (as in Table 4.16), the remaining variation in mean earnings by age at first marriage is only slightly smaller than when account is taken of education alone (as in Table 4.14) or occupation alone (as in Table 4.15). Within this framework, the relationship between age at first marriage and eventual earnings appears to reflect most the financial deprivation of white men *without* college education who married comparatively *late* rather than early, and by the even greater relative financial deprivation of white men *with* college education who married *either* comparatively early or late rather than at an intermediate age.[12]

Nonwhite men had consistently smaller mean earnings by middle age than white men, in all the detailed cross-classifications shown in Table 4.16 where the sample was large enough to make such a comparison. The average deficiency of nonwhite earnings (as a percent of white earnings) was smaller among the men who reported that they postponed first marriage until they were 27 or older than it was among those who reported a younger age at first marriage. The unweighted average of the nonwhite deficiencies in earnings shown in the table was about 28 percent for those reported as 27 years old or older at first marriage and 32 percent for those under this age.[13]

The greatest deficiencies of earnings for nonwhite men, by a considerable margin, were found among managerial and professional workers, amounting in most instances to approximately one-half the corresponding earnings for white men. These are occupations in which the cumulation of considerable capital, managerial skills, or advanced college training are generally required.

Clearly the smallest deficiencies of earnings for nonwhite men were found among clerical workers, amounting to about 16 percent among those who married relatively young or relatively old and about 19 percent for those who married at an intermediate age. As amount of education increased, however, the deficiency in mean earnings for the nonwhite clerical workers tended to increase. Apart from experience, clerical workers generally require only those qualifications which can be obtained from high-school training, perhaps supplemented by vocational training in a business or trade school.

Explanations of the differential earnings by color, and reasons why these differences were greater in some occupations than in others, must be partly speculative. The white professional may have graduated from a better medical or law school, for example, than did the nonwhite professional; he probably interned in a better hospital or had an opportunity to join a better-known law firm; if he established his own office, he was probably able to attract patients or clients who were financially able and accustomed to paying higher fees than could the nonwhite professional of comparable training. The white craftsman was more likely than his nonwhite counterpart to have belonged to a trade union and to have gone through an apprenticeship training program and thus to have benefited from the relatively high wage scale bargained by a union. On the other hand, the white clerical worker, whose earnings differential was lowest, may have worked for a large-scale employer who had standard wage rates that applied to everyone.[14]

Discussion

In the foregoing presentation, the long-term downward trend of age at marriage in the United States, especially among men, has been interpreted as a consequence of the declining proportion of the population of foreign birth or parentage, the increasing ease with which married women can find employment outside the home, and numerous other factors. Moreover, the proportion of persons who eventually marry has been increasing to the point where all but 3 or 4 percent of today's young adults may expect to marry. The amount by which the age of men at marriage exceeds that of women has been diminishing, and from this standpoint the average husband and wife should live jointly for a correspondingly longer period of their lives.

In recent years, the proportion of women who marry as teenagers has been decreasing, and the proportion of first marriages postponed until bachelorhood or spinsterhood has likewise decreased. In short, marriage is occurring increasingly during the "preferred age range," not too young and not too old. Of course, there will always be a range of a few years in which people of somewhat different preferences and varying lengths of preparation for adult activities decide to leave the single state.

The "best" age for men to marry, from the standpoint of earnings level at middle age, has been shown to be the intermediate range — after the man has become legally of age but before he becomes a bachelor. This finding remained relatively constant regardless of amount of education or type of occupation. Men whose life work depended on a long period of college training or the cumulation of considerable capital or managerial skill tended to have higher eventual earnings if they married toward the upper part of the generally preferred range of age at first marriage, whereas most of the other occupation groups fared better financially if they married during the younger part of the preferred range. Within the range of "best" ages to marry, those men who are the most promising marriage partners, from the viewpoint of attractiveness and competence to earn a good living, probably marry at a younger age than the less promising.

The findings are interpreted as showing that nonwhite men were at a competitive disadvantage, because they evidently had to postpone marriage longer than white men of similar education and occupation in order to have earnings by middle age that were relatively near those of their white counterparts. Although the findings provide no direct evidence, the interpretation here implies that this postponement of marriage by nonwhite men probably was not by choice.[15]

5 / INTERMARRIAGE AMONG EDUCATIONAL, ETHNIC, AND RELIGIOUS GROUPS

The analysis in the preceding chapter showed the extent to which husbands and wives tend to have the same age, in relation to their previous marital status and their place of residence. In the present chapter, the education, race, national origin, and religion of husbands and wives are compared. The underlying hypotheses being tested are that "like tends to marry like" and that husbands and wives with similar demographic characteristics are more likely to have stable marriages than those with dissimilar demographic characteristics. The results presented here, as well as earlier studies of mate selection,[1] tend strongly to support these hypotheses.[2]

A marital partner's date of birth, education, ethnic origin, and religious preference tend to be relatively "permanent" or "irreversible" social characteristics. A person cannot reduce his chronologic age, though he may do something about how old he looks; he cannot diminish the highest grade of school he has completed, though he may add an extra level of schooling after marriage; he cannot change his racial or ethnic ancestry, though people may alter their attitudes about the social rankings of ethnic groups; and he cannot change his religious background, though an increasing proportion of persons change their religious affiliation at or near the time of marriage. The less permanent economic characteristics of husbands and wives, such as their employment, occupation, and income,[3] are compared in Chapter 7.

Education of Husband and Wife

Among the social characteristics of husband and wife, one of the most appropriate for analyzing the process of mate selection is education. Because of the high degree of correlation between education of children and that of their parents,[4] data on education tend to reflect not only the cultural values of the spouses themselves but also the parental backgrounds of the partners in a marital union. Moreover, educational attainment applies to both husband and wife,

112

Table 5.1. Percent distribution of married couples with husband and wife married once, by years of school completed by husband and wife: United States, couples married between 1950 and 1960

Years of school completed by husband	Total couples, husband and wife married once	Years of school completed by wife										
		Elementary			High school		College			First quartile	Median	Third quartile
		0-4	5-7	8	1-3	4	1-3	4	5+			
Total, married 1950 to 1960	100.0	1.5	4.6	6.6	22.4	45.4	11.8	6.2	1.5	10.8	12.3	12.9
Elementary: 0-4	2.7	0.7	0.7	0.4	0.6	0.3	0.0	0.0	0.0	4.9	7.7	10.2
5-7	6.9	0.4	1.7	1.1	2.2	1.5	0.1	0.0	0.0	7.5	9.5	11.9
8	9.2	0.2	0.8	1.9	3.0	3.1	0.3	0.1	0.0	8.7	10.8	12.4
High school: 1-3	20.9	0.2	0.8	1.7	8.1	8.9	1.0	0.2	0.0	9.9	11.9	12.5
4	33.0	0.1	0.5	1.3	6.7	20.8	2.8	0.7	0.1	11.9	12.4	12.8
College: 1-3	12.3	0.0	0.1	0.2	1.4	6.3	3.2	1.0	0.2	12.2	12.7	14.2
4	8.7	0.0	0.0	0.1	0.4	3.1	2.6	2.3	0.3	12.6	13.9	16.2
5+	6.3	0.0	0.0	0.0	0.2	1.5	1.8	2.0	0.8	12.9	15.3	16.6
First quartile	9.9	2.7	5.2	8.1	9.0	11.2	12.5	14.7	16.0	...	...	...
Median	12.3	5.6	7.8	9.0	11.0	12.4	14.6	16.5	17+	...	...	...
Third quartile	13.6	8.6	10.0	11.8	12.4	13.0	16.6	17.4	18.1	...	...	...

Source: U.S. Bureau of the Census, U.S. Census of Population: 1960, Subject Reports, Marital Status, Final Report PC(2)-4E, table 11.

113

Table 5.2. Ratio of actual number of couples with specified years of school completed by husband and wife to expected number if couples married at random, for married couples with husband and wife married once: United States, couples married between 1950 and 1960

Years of school completed by husband		Years of school completed by wife							
		Elementary			High school		College		
		0-4	5-7	8	1-3	4	1-3	4	5+
Elementary:	0-4	17.5	6.2	2.2	0.9	0.2	0.1	0.1	0.0
	5-7	3.6	5.2	2.4	1.4	0.5	0.2	0.1	0.1
	8	1.1	1.8	3.1	1.4	0.7	0.3	0.1	0.1
High school:	1-3	0.6	0.9	1.2	1.7	0.9	0.4	0.2	0.1
	4	0.2	0.3	0.6	0.9	1.4	0.7	0.3	0.3
College:	1-3	0.2	0.1	0.3	0.5	1.1	2.2	1.3	0.9
	4	0.1	0.1	0.1	0.2	0.8	2.5	4.2	2.2
	5+	0.1	0.0	0.1	0.1	0.5	2.5	5.0	9.1

Source: U.S. Bureau of the Census, U.S. Census of Population: 1960, Subject Reports, Marital Status, Final Report PC(2)-4E, table 11.

whereas occupation and income are valuable demographic character-istics primarily when applied to the husband.[5]

Tables 5.1 and 5.2 show the extent to which marital partners tend to have a similar level of educational attainment. The data in these tables relate to recently married couples with relatively stable mar-riages, inasmuch as the average duration of marriage had been about five years.

Although the median educational attainment of both husbands and wives was the same (12.3 years), the lower quartile was one year higher for wives than husbands, with the upper quartile one grade higher for husbands than wives. Figure 5.1 shows this observation graphically. To carry the analysis further, one-third of the husbands but almost one-half of the wives had terminated their education with high-school graduation, with the men graduates from high school more likely than the women graduates to enter and complete college. As a consequence of these educational patterns, many persons at the prime marriageable ages must choose between marrying someone outside their own educational (or age) level and remaining unmarried.

Table 5.2 shows how far recently married couples deviate from marrying at random with respect to their partner's educational level. All entries in the table would be 1.0 if there were no deviations from the "expected value."[6] Entries above 1.0 show a greater concentra-tion of marital partners with specified combinations of education than a random distribution would produce.

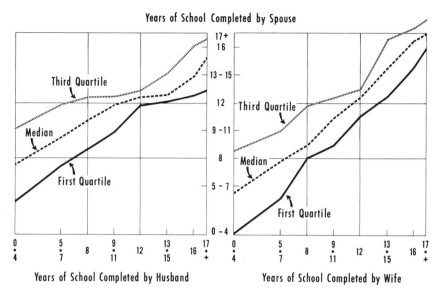

Fig. 5.1. Quartile of years of school completed by husband and wife: United States, 1960

Source: Table 5.1.

The most frequently occurring combination of marital partners, as shown by Table 5.1, is 12 years of school for both husband and wife; 21 percent of all couples were in this category. According to Table 5.2, this combination occurred 1.4 times as often as expected in random marriage. This means that high-school graduates with no college education were about 40 percent more likely to marry someone with the same amount of education as themselves than someone with either more or less education.

Of special interest are the exceptions to the general rule that the highest values in the rows and columns are those where the spouses were in the same educational level, and the next highest are those where they were in an adjacent level.[7] One of these exceptions is the value 5.0 for husbands with graduate training and wives with only four years of college, which exceeds the value 4.2 for both husband and wife with exactly four years of college.

This specific finding suggests the interesting hypothesis that such a combination of educational levels is mutually preferable: the women "terminal college graduates" prefer husbands with the skill and initiative to obtain graduate training that will increase their earning potential and the cultural side of their lives; and the men with graduate training prefer a wife with a bachelor's degree only, because such women may be more ready and willing to perform the roles of wife and mother, whereas women with more advanced university training may be more likely to possess drives for personal achievement which detract from their potential home-making roles. Another hypothesis deserving mention is that college-educated men in general may prefer not to marry women who have a greater amount of education than themselves. Nevertheless, women with graduate-school training are very rapidly disappearing from the ranks of spinsters, as pointed out in Chapters 3 and 10.

Another exception occurred at the lower end of the educational range: the value on the diagonal for spouses with five to seven years of schooling is smaller than when the wife had this amount but the husband had less education. This particular combination has a greater probability of occurring among nonwhite than white couples, as indicated by the following summary of data on the educational levels of married couples classified by color of the husband (not shown in Table 5.1):

Among every 100 white couples:
   40 husbands and wives were in the same educational level;
   21 husbands were one level higher;
   12 husbands were two or more levels higher;
   17 wives were one level higher; and
   10 wives were two or more levels higher.
Among every 100 nonwhite couples:
   37 husbands and wives were in the same level;
   15 husbands were one level higher;
    8 husbands were two or more levels higher;
   21 wives were one level higher; and
   19 wives were two or more levels higher.

The above tabulation shows that white men are more likely than nonwhite men to have outdistanced their wives in educational attainment. However, to an even greater extent, the education of nonwhite wives tends to exceed that of nonwhite husbands. This fact may be better understood in the context that the educational attainment of nonwhite adults of marriageable age falls largely below the level of high-school graduation; among white adults in this educational stratum, wives tend likewise to have more education than their husbands.

Race of Husband and Wife

In the 1960 census, for the first time, national data on race of husband were classified by race of wife for all married couples in the United States.[8] These data are shown in Tables 5.3 and 5.4. Despite the potential weaknesses in the data, different races (in terms of the seven-category classification shown in Table 5.4) were reported for the husband and wife in a substantial number of cases — 163,800 married couples, or 0.4 percent of the 40,491,000 married couples in the United States in 1960. There was a total of 141,500 white-non-white couples; about 81,200 white husbands were married to non-white wives, and 60,300 white wives were married to nonwhite husbands. Thus about 20,900 more white men than white women had a nonwhite spouse; this difference might have been near zero if there had not been 21,700 white husbands married to Japanese wives. Nearly all of these white-Japanese marriages occurred between 1940 and 1960, when approximately 20,000 Japanese war brides were brought to the United States by American men in military service.

Table 5.3. Married couples by race of husband and wife: United States, 1960

Race of husband	All married couples	Race of wife		
		White	Negro	Other
Total	40,490,998	37,132,013	3,061,342	297,643
White	37,152,907	37,071,672	25,913	55,322
Negro	3,063,673	25,496	3,033,122	5,055
Other	274,418	34,845	2,307	237,266

Source: U.S. Bureau of the Census, U.S. Census of Population: 1960, Subject Reports, Marital Status, Final Report PC(2)-4E, table 10.

Table 5.3 gives a broad classification of all married couples in order to place in context the really small number of couples involving unlike races. Within this framework, Table 5.4 highlights only those married couples in 1960 who comprised husbands and wives of different races.

White-Negro combinations were clearly the most numerous in terms of the seven detailed categories of race, comprising 51,400 couples or 31 percent of all 163,800 couples with racially mixed marriages.

Table 5.4. Married couples with husband and wife of different races, by race of husband and wife: United States, 1960

(Numbers in thousands)

Race of husband	All couples involving mixed races	Race of wife							
		White	Negro	Other, total	Am. Indian	Japanese	Chinese	Filipino	All other
Total	163.8	60.3	28.2	75.3	20.1	27.2	4.7	6.2	17.0
White	81.2	...	25.9	55.3	17.3	21.7	2.9	4.5	9.0
Negro	30.6	25.5	...	5.1	2.2	1.7	0.1	0.5	0.6
Other, total	52.1	34.8	2.3	14.9	0.6	3.7	1.7	1.3	7.5
Am. Indian	13.4	12.0	1.1	0.3	...	0.1	0.0	0.1	0.1
Japanese	5.6	3.5	0.1	2.1	0.0	...	0.0	0.3	1.1
Chinese	6.4	3.5	0.3	2.6	0.0	1.1	0.6	0.3	1.2
Filipino	15.5	11.2	0.5	3.8	0.4	1.1	0.2	...	2.1
All other	11.1	4.7	0.3	6.1	0.2	1.4	0.9	0.6	3.0

Source: U.S. Bureau of the Census, U.S. Census of Population: 1960, Subject Reports, Marital Status, Final Report PC(2)-4E, table 10.

These combinations involved only slightly more white husbands than white wives. White-"other" (nonwhite except Negro) combinations considered as a totality, however, involved 90,200 couples or 55 percent of the couples with mixed marriages; 3 out of 5 of these mixtures were white-Japanese or white-American Indian. The preponderance of white-Japanese couples involved a white husband, as did a majority of the white-American Indian couples. Among the less numerous combinations involving a white spouse, two-thirds of the white-"all other" (Hawaiian, Eskimo, Asian Indian, etc.) combinations likewise involved a white husband, but white-Chinese pairs included a majority with a white wife and about three-fourths of the white-Filipino pairs included a white wife.

In summary, white-nonwhite combinations of spouses more often involved a white husband in all of the racial pairings except white-Filipino and white-Chinese; and the number of white-Negro combinations was more nearly equally divided as to which spouse was Negro than any of the other racial mixtures.

Of the 58,800 mixed couples at the time of the 1960 census involving a Negro spouse, 7 out of 8 were Negro-white couples; the similarity in numbers of white husbands with Negro wives and white wives with Negro husbands has already been noted. The most frequently occurring combinations among the 7,400 couples involving a Negro and a spouse of "other (nonwhite) races" were:

> 2,200 Negro husbands with American Indian wives;
> 1,700 Negro husbands with Japanese wives; and
> 1,100 Negro wives with American Indian husbands.

Although quite small, these figures are of interest in showing that nearly one-half the 7,400 were Negro-Indian couples, divided in a 2-to-1 ratio in favor of Negro husbands married to Indian wives. Moreover, the 1,700 Negro husbands with Japanese wives constitute approximately 0.1 percent of all Negro husbands, just as the 21,700 white husbands with Japanese wives constitute 0.1 percent of all white husbands. Most of the Negro-Japanese couples probably resulted from marriages of servicemen in Japan or of Negro migrants from the South to the western coastal cities.

Of the 14,900 couples with husband and wife of unlike "other races" (column 4, line 4 of Table 5.4) about two-thirds involved a spouse in the category "all other" races (Hawaiian, Eskimo, Asian

Indian, etc.). Filipino men and Japanese women were the most numerous of the six specified groups who married spouses of "all other" races. Imbalances in the sex ratios of adults in localities where these groups generally live undoubtedly contributed to this outmarrying. In order to complete the presentation of detailed races, an arbitrary but conservative estimate of 3,000 was made for interracial marriages among couples with both husband and wife in the "all other" races category.

Proportion of spouses of same race. The volume of interracial mixtures is made still more meaningful when analyzed in terms of the *proportion* of all husbands (or wives) of a given race who have married a spouse of the same race as their own. A summary of such proportions is presented in Table 5.5.

By contrast with white spouses, who had nearly complete racial endogamy (99.8 percent), and Negro spouses, who had nearly as high a value (99.0 percent), "other races" as a whole had a rate of only 79 percent.[9] Wide variations existed in the figures for specific minor races, notably the quite high proportion of Japanese husbands married to Japanese wives (94 percent) and relatively high endogamy figures for both Chinese husbands and Chinese wives (86 and 89 percent, respectively); the intermediate values (around 75 percent) for wives who were American Indians, Japanese, and Filipinos; and the quite low values for Filipino husbands (53 percent) and wives of "all other" races (57 percent).

Wives had slightly higher racial-endogamy rates than husbands among the white, Negro, and Chinese groups, and Filipino wives had a much higher endogamous rate than Filipino husbands. Husbands had substantially higher racial-endogamy rates than wives among the remaining groups — American Indian, Japanese, and "all other."

The historical antecedents of the data in the first two columns of Table 5.5 are shown in the other columns, which classify married couples into broad first-marriage cohorts, corresponding roughly to the postwar, World War II, and prewar periods. The totals for all married couples show a small decline during the 1940's in the percentage with husband and wife of the same race, and a larger (yet still quite small) decline during the 1950's. The same generalization applies also to husbands of each race except Filipinos. For wives, the same generalization applies to whites, Japanese, Chinese, and Filipinos. Among Negroes, the trend for husbands (downward) was op-

Table 5.5. Percent of married couples with husband and wife of same race, by period of husband's first marriage: United States, 1960

| Race | All married couples | | Period of husband's first marriage | | | | | |
| | | | 1950-60 | | 1940-49 | | Before 1940 | |
	Husband	Wife	Husband	Wife	Husband	Wife	Husband	Wife
Total	99.60	99.60	99.24	99.24	99.64	99.64	99.73	99.73
White	99.78	99.84	99.62	99.76	99.82	99.84	99.85	99.88
Negro	99.00	99.08	98.73	99.13	99.10	99.09	99.14	99.03
Other races	82.13	75.72	80.08	67.94	82.38	80.09	84.15	81.60
Am. Indian	82.45	75.80	81.40	75.94	82.50	79.51	83.30	73.28
Japanese	93.92	76.31	90.62	61.66	95.14	84.12	96.72	92.44
Chinese	85.85	89.21	82.39	85.69	86.93	90.84	88.61	91.57
Filipino	53.06	73.76	57.78	67.20	50.97	75.33	49.27	84.40
All other	69.43	56.64	66.14	55.98	70.42	55.56	73.22	58.51

Source: U.S. Bureau of the Census, U.S. Census of Population: 1960, Subject Reports, Marital Status, Final Report PC(2)-4E, table 10.

121

posite that for wives; this was also true among Filipinos, except that the downward trend was among the wives.

Observed versus random racial mixture. Table 5.6 shows the extent to which husbands and wives are of like or unlike racial category. The table was derived by the same method as Table 5.2 (see reference 6). Here the diagonal values compare the actual frequencies of husbands and wives of the same race with those expected if they had married at random with respect to race. The value 1.09 for white-white couples means, for example, that married couples in that racial combination were found 1.09 times as often as would have happened if the persons involved had married at random with respect to race. A value below 1.00 means that the racial combination occurred less often than expected, and suggests a tendency for persons of the races involved to avoid one another in the process of selecting a marital partner.

The table shows only a very small proportion of white and Negro persons married to persons of any other race. For all the other (mostly Asian) racial groups involving at least 100 couples, however, there is more than a chance rate of intermarriage among couples in every combination of these groups except Japanese wives married to American Indian husbands. These two generalizations apply also to corresponding values, not shown in the table, for married couples with the husband's first marriage occurring between 1950 and 1960.

The measures of endogamy on the diagonal of the table tend to increase sharply as the size of the racial group decreases. This tendency may be interpreted mainly as the joint consequence of two inseparable factors; namely, the degree of access to persons of any race except one's own for consideration as a marital partner, and the premium placed on marrying a person of the same race (or of avoiding marriage to a person of a particular different race). The first factor includes the situations in some states where certain types of racial intermarriage were prohibited by law before the United States Supreme Court overruled the legal barriers against such marriages in 16 states in 1967. It also includes the tendency for racial groups to cluster in certain localities and hence to be available only rarely for marriage to persons living far away.

The values on the diagonal have changed in opposite directions for whites and Negroes during recent decades, as the following figures show. The "total" column contains the same figures as those on the

Table 5.6. Ratio of actual number of couples with specified race of husband and wife to expected number if couples married at random, for married couples by race of husband and wife: United States, 1960

Race of husband	White	Negro	Other, total	Am. Indian	Japanese	Chinese	Filipino	All other
				Race of wife				
White	1.09	0.01	0.20	0.23	0.21	0.07	0.20	0.30
Negro	0.01	13.09	0.22	0.35	0.20	a	0.27	0.23
Other, total	0.14	0.11	114.90	112.57	112.70	125.25	116.25	93.67
Am. Indian	0.17	0.19	112.00	390.00	0.40	a	a	1.50
Japanese	0.04	a	130.24	a	308.86	7.50	9.00	13.50
Chinese	0.09	0.10	113.56	a	9.33	959.00	7.00	29.00
Filipino	0.37	0.19	88.00	4.50	14.00	6.00	866.00	52.00
All other	0.19	0.16	105.60	6.00	17.00	21.00	37.50	452.00

Source: U.S. Bureau of the Census, U.S. Census of Population: 1960, Subject Reports, Marital Status, Final Report PC(2)-4E, table 10.

aRatio not shown where fewer than 100 married couples.

diagonal of Table 5.6 above and were derived from the same source. The values indicate the ratio of the actual number of couples with white-white or Negro-Negro marriages to the expected number if couples married at random:

Race of husband and wife	Period of husband's first marriage			
	Total	1950–60	1940–49	Before 1940
White	1.09	1.11	1.09	1.05
Negro	13.09	11.28	13.41	19.91

The underlying reasons for the opposing trends of the measures of endogamy for whites and Negroes are complex and not readily susceptible to the desired type of further analysis from available 1960 census tabulations. In any case, the change for white couples shown in the table is extremely small and probably not very significant. The substantial decline in the index of endogamy for Negroes is consistent with the downward trend in the percentage of Negro husbands married to Negro wives, as shown in Table 5.5, but the values in that table move in the opposite direction for Negro wives. Conceivably, the results for Negro wives in the two situations would have been consistent if the classification by period of first marriage had related to the wife. The discrepancies in the findings presented here tend to weaken — but not necessarily neutralize — the argument that the sharp decline in the index of endogamy for Negroes provides evidence that the marriages which have lasted the longest are those in which the husband and wife were of the same (Negro) race.

Comment on racial intermarriage. Many of the proportions of race mixture are small — but by no means all of them; and many of the changes in race mixture have been so slight that they may be regarded as inconsequential — yet several are substantial. The directions and sources of the differences merit careful scrutiny, with due regard for their magnitudes.

The classification of racial-endogamy rates by period of husband's first marriage was designed to throw light on the joint effects of two factors, which unfortunately could not be identified separately — or isolated from still other factors — on the basis of data available from the 1960 population census. The two factors may be stated in terms of the following hypotheses: (1) the relative stability of racially mixed marriages over a period of two or more decades is less than that of unmixed marriages; and (2) there has been a trend during the last generation toward an increasing tolerance of racially mixed marriages. The overall findings are consistent with both hypotheses. With a few exceptions, married couples with the husband's first marriage dating back before 1940 have the highest rate of racial endogamy and those dating back only to the 1950's have the lowest.

Some of the spouses among the married couples in 1960 were in remarriages; but by making comparisons within the period of first marriage of the husband, the several racial groups were at least standardized with respect to the period of possible exposure to remarriage.[10] Additional factors certainly must have contributed to differences in the relative frequency of racial intermarriage from one period of husband's first marriage to the next. Perhaps the most obvious factor is the substantial influx of Japanese war brides after World War II. Incidentally, there was evidently also a significant (but much smaller) number of Filipino war brides who entered the United States during the same postwar period.

With the passage of decades since most of the Asian groups migrated to the United States, the original generation (particularly among Filipinos), with its high proportion of men, has given way gradually to younger generations with much more nearly equal sex ratios. This development has very likely increased the feasibility of intraracial marriage among such groups during recent decades. Admonitions of the elders of these groups for their youths to "marry their own kind" must accordingly be easier to follow at the present time. Where the pattern of intermarriage among the older generation had been previously established, however, the examples of successful mixed marriages probably tend to counteract the usual parental admonition to practice endogamy.

Still another factor affecting the trend of racial intermarriage may have been a heightened racial consciousness arising out of World War II. Japan at that time was an enemy, and Japanese in the western part of the United States mainland were isolated in camps. This condition most probably minimized Japanese-white intermarriage here in the 1940's. During the 1950's, however, there may have been a sympathetic reversal of this antipathy. As a matter of record, there were four times as many white-Japanese couples with the first marriage of the husband in the 1950's as in the 1940's which remained intact in 1960 — 18,500 versus 4,600.

One-fourth again as many white-Negro couples with the first marriage of the husband in the 1950's as in the 1940's — 17,300 versus 13,500 — were still intact in 1960. Most of the increase of white-Negro couples in the 1950's consisted of Negro husbands with white wives. The increase in number of white-Negro couples may be one of the social consequences of steps taken in various sectors of American society during the 1950's to reduce racial barriers. Selectivity among these white-Negro marriages during the 1950's with respect to place of residence and education of husband and wife is discussed in the next section.

White-Negro Married Couples

A special table from the 1960 census (see source note on Table 5.7) shows the number of married couples who survived from primary marriages occurring between 1950 and the census date which involved at least one white or Negro spouse but no spouse of "other races." The data are cross-classified in considerable detail, according to the race of husband and wife, whether residing in the South or in an urbanized area in 1960, and by education of husband and wife. Of the 9,224,834 married couples in the universe covered, the racial combinations were as follows:

8,430,979	or	91.41	percent — white husband, white wife
780,239		8.46	percent — Negro husband, Negro wife
6,082		0.07	percent — white husband, Negro wife
7,534		0.08	percent — Negro husband, white wife
9,224,834		100.00	percent

Place of residence. For the country as a whole, as the above figures show, a little over half the recently married white-Negro couples involved a Negro husband and a white wife. Whereas a majority of the white-Negro couples in the North and West (62 percent) involved a Negro husband and a white wife, a majority of the white-Negro couples in the South (58 percent) involved a white husband and a Negro wife. For the North and West as a whole, 0.14 percent of the couples involved white-Negro combinations; for the South, the corresponding figure was very slightly higher, 0.16 percent. For the country as a whole, 0.16 percent of the couples in urbanized areas, and 0.14 percent in other areas, involved white-Negro combinations.

Further analysis of the regional figures by type of residence shows that the number of white-Negro couples (especially those involving a Negro husband and white wife) tended to be considerably above the national average in the urbanized areas of the North and West. By contrast, the number of white-Negro couples (especially those involving a white husband and Negro wife) tended to be above average in "other areas" of the South. In terms of proportions rather than numbers, the few couples with white-Negro combinations in "other areas" of the North and West also comprised Negro husbands and white wives in 2 cases out of 3, whereas the few mixed couples in urbanized areas of the South comprised white husbands and Negro wives in nearly the same ratio.

These findings on differential interracial marriage by region call attention once again to the subject of common-law marriage, which was discussed in Chapter 1 (see particularly note 21). Evidently most of the Negro-white married couples in the South in 1960 were living in consensual unions, because at that time Negro-white marriage was outlawed throughout the South. However, some Negro-white couples may have married in the North or West before they moved to the South, and some persons may have migrated out of the South before they married a person of a different race.

Education of husband and wife. Table 5.7 throws light on the extent to which white-white and Negro-Negro marriages differ from white-Negro marriages with regard to social status, as measured by educational level. The central hypothesis being tested here is that a Negro who marries a white person tends to have superior qualities (specifically, a higher educational level) as compared with a Negro who marries another Negro; and that a white person who marries a Negro tends to have inferior qualities (educational level) as compared with a white person who marries another white person. The data in Table 5.7 are generally consistent with the hypothesis, but they include some secondary relationships worthy of special note.

At the lower end of the educational range, white husbands married to white wives included only one-half as large a percentage with no high-school training (17) as those married to Negro wives (34). Yet white husbands married to Negro wives included a smaller per-

Table 5.7. Percent distribution by years of school completed by
husband and wife, by race of husband and wife:
United States, 1960

Years of school completed by husband and wife	White husband		Negro husband	
	White wife	Negro wife	White wife	Negro wife
All married couples[a]	100.0	100.0	100.0	100.0
Husband:				
No high school (0-8)	16.9	34.4	30.2	40.0
High school (9-12)	54.2	48.1	49.7	49.9
College (13 or more)	28.9	17.5	20.1	10.1
Wife:				
No high school	11.3	24.8	25.4	27.0
High school	68.4	60.6	59.1	62.3
College	20.3	14.6	15.4	10.7

Source: U.S. Bureau of the Census, U.S. Census of Population:
1960, Subject Reports, Marital Status, Final Report PC(2)-4E, table 12.

[a]Married couples with husband and wife in first marriage, married
between 1950 and 1960, and excluding couples with either spouse other
than white or Negro.

centage with no high school (34) than Negro husbands married to
Negro wives (40).

At the upper end of the educational range, contrary relationships
are found. Negro husbands married to white wives included twice as
large a percentage with college training (20) as those married to
Negro wives (10). But Negro husbands married to white wives included a smaller percentage with college education (20) than white
husbands married to white wives (29).

The same kinds of differences can be cited from the standpoint
of the wife's education, but the differences are generally smaller
because of the uniformly greater concentration of wives in the middle
education group. Hence the conclusions to be drawn from the data
for wives are similar but less emphatic than those drawn from the
data for husbands.

Another way of generalizing the data in Table 5.7 is to observe
that the parties in recently contracted primary marriages involving
a white spouse and a Negro spouse tend to have educational levels
intermediate between those involving white spouses only and those

involving Negro spouses only. This does not contradict the hypothesis originally stated, but offers less intuitive insight into the underlying social processes which culminate in white-Negro marriages.

Perhaps the most plausible explanation of observed differences in the relative status of partners in white-Negro marriages is that, with the existing social relationships between Negroes and white persons in the United States, the Negro who sets out to marry a white person probably will have to offer a premium in order to attract the white person into marriage; here this premium is measured in terms of more education than would be required to attract another Negro into marriage. Contrariwise, a white person would probably be able to marry a Negro with higher qualifications than would be required to attract another white person into marriage. Sociologists refer to this process as the "compensation principle," or the "exchange theory" of intermarriage.[11]

The data suggest that the initiative in white-Negro marriages tends to be taken by the Negro. Also, from the fact that somewhat more of the recently married Negro men were married to white wives (7,534) than Negro women were married to white husbands (6,082), it seems to follow that Negro men tend to take more initiative than Negro women in seeking a white mate. This narrow margin may actually be the result of far more effort on the part of Negro men than Negro women, inasmuch as white persons probably tend to be more tolerant toward Negro women who marry white men than toward Negro men who marry white women. Available data do not indicate the motives Negro men have in seeking to marry white women. Some may believe that a white wife would be less domineering than a Negro wife; some may hope to enhance their social status by taking a white wife; and some — possibly the majority — may be motivated primarily by elementary attraction quite independent of other considerations.

Although the present number of white-Negro marriages is extremely small, coming decades may show substantial increases; the foregoing insights may point the directions this growth is likely to take.

National Origin of Husband and Wife

National origin of the prospective mate is another demographic characteristic to which some persons attach more value than others when looking for marital partners. Attention is focused here on the origin of mates where one or both, or their parents, were born outside the United States. Although there is some interest in more distant origins, the available census data permit analysis of husbands and wives of foreign origin only in terms of the last two generations (first generation, or foreign born; and second generation, or native of foreign or mixed parentage).

Most of the relevant results of the 1960 census on this subject have been further simplified in tabulation by grouping all spouses of foreign stock; that is, by the combination of the foreign born and the native of foreign or mixed parentage. All natives of third or higher generation are grouped under the heading "native of native parentage." Almost all of the husbands and wives of foreign stock in the United States in 1960 were white. Similarly, about 2.9 million (95 percent) of the 3.1 million Negro married couples were native of native parentage and are so considered in the discussion below.

Nativity and parentage of husband and wife. As shown in Table 5.8, nearly 3 out of every 4 married *persons* living with their spouse in 1960 were natives of native parentage, with 1 out of 4 of foreign stock. There were about 650,000 more native persons of native par-

Table 5.8. Married couples by national origin of husband and wife: United States, 1960

(Numbers in thousands)

National origin	Number of husbands	Number of wives	Percent of husbands	Percent of wives
All married couples	40,491	40,491	100.0	100.0
Native of native parentage	29,519	30,171	72.9	74.5
Foreign stock	10,973	10,320	27.1	25.5
United Kingdom	871	847	2.2	2.1
Ireland	501	466	1.2	1.2
Canada	892	913	2.2	2.3
Germany	1,408	1,275	3.5	3.1
Poland	986	950	2.4	2.3
U.S.S.R.	861	797	2.1	2.0
Italy	1,665	1,483	4.1	3.7
Other	3,788	3,589	9.4	8.9

Source: U.S. Bureau of the Census, U.S. Census of Population: 1960, Subject Reports, Families, Final Report PC(2)-4A, table 62.

entage among wives than husbands, doubtless in large part as a consequence of the excess of men among past migrants to the United States. Groups which contributed most to the 650,000 excess of husbands of foreign stock were the Germans, Italians, and "others."

To the extent that people have a strong preference for marriage within their own origin group, wherever there is an excess of spouses within the group (German husbands, for example) one might expect to find an excess of single persons in that group, because some of the persons involved may prefer bachelorhood or spinsterhood to out-marriage. Pertinent information on this matter will be found in Chapter 10, "Group Variations Among Bachelors and Spinsters."

About 2 out of 3 married *couples* in 1960 comprised a husband and wife who were "native of native parentage"; that is, both were citizens of third or higher generations of residence in the United States. (In some places in this section and the next, these persons are referred to as "native-native.") About 1 out of 10 couples comprised a husband and wife of the same foreign country of origin, in terms of the seven specific countries listed in Table 5.8 and an estimate for the "other" group. The percentage distribution, including couples of different national origins, is summarized as follows:

All married couples		100.0
Husband and wife of same national origin		74.3
Both native of native parentage	64.3	
Both of same foreign country of origin	10.1	
Husband and wife of different national origin		25.7
Husband native-native, wife foreign stock	8.6	
Husband foreign stock, wife native-native	10.3	
Husband and wife of different foreign country of origin	6.8	

Of the 64.3 percent with both spouses native of native parentage, about 7.2 percent were Negro couples and the remaining 57.1 percent were preponderantly white couples.

A substantial minority of married couples — 35.7 percent — included one or both spouses of foreign stock, here defined as first or second generation in the United States. Of the 35.7 percent, roughly one-half comprised couples with both spouses of foreign stock — 16.9 percent; 10.1 percent, or a clear majority of the 16.9 percent, were of the same detailed national origin and the other 6.8 percent were of mixed foreign origins. Thus, there is close to a 50–50 chance that a spouse of foreign origin is married to a person who is likewise of foreign stock; but the odds are even greater that, if both spouses are of foreign stock, they will be of the same national origin. About 18.9 percent of the married couples included one native spouse of native parentage and one spouse of foreign stock; of these, over half (10.3 percent) involved a husband of foreign stock and a native wife of native parentage, a fact related to the greater number of married men than married women of foreign stock.

Inmarriage and outmarriage by national origin. The extent to which spouses of a given national origin are married to spouses of the same national origin varies widely. As Table 5.9 shows, only 1

Table 5.9. Percent of husbands and wives of same or different national origin: United States, 1960

National origin	Percent of husbands with wives of--				Percent of wives with husbands of--			
			Different origin				Different origin	
	All origins	Same origin	Native-native	Foreign stock	All origins	Same origin	Native-native	Foreign stock
All married couples[a]	100.0	74.3	10.3	15.4[b]	100.0	74.3	8.6	17.1[b]
Native of native par.	100.0	88.2	...	11.8	100.0	86.2	...	13.8
Foreign stock (any)	100.0	62.2	37.8	...	100.0	66.1	33.9	...
Detailed foreign stock	100.0	37.1	37.8	25.0	100.0	39.5	33.9	26.6
United Kingdom	100.0	18.0	55.5	26.5	100.0	18.5	52.8	28.7
Ireland	100.0	25.9	47.3	26.8	100.0	27.9	43.3	28.8
Canada	100.0	27.6	50.8	21.6	100.0	26.9	48.7	24.4
Germany	100.0	27.2	50.6	22.2	100.0	30.0	45.6	24.4
Poland	100.0	44.7	25.1	30.2	100.0	46.4	20.7	32.9
U.S.S.R.	100.0	48.2	20.9	30.9	100.0	52.1	15.6	32.3
Italy	100.0	57.4	27.1	15.5	100.0	64.4	21.7	13.9
Other	100.0	35.6[c]	36.6	27.8	100.0	37.6[c]	32.9	29.5

Source: U.S. Bureau of the Census, U.S. Census of Population: 1960, Subject Reports, Families, Final Report PC(2)-4A, table 62.

[a]Calculated with the use of figures on detailed foreign stock.

[b]Includes 6.8 percent with husband and wife of different foreign stock.

[c]Estimated as average of percentages for the specific foreign stocks of husbands.

of 8 native husbands (or wives) of native parentage had a spouse of foreign stock, but 1 of 3 husbands (or wives) of foreign stock had a native spouse of native parentage. These differing proportions really are two ways of placing the mixed marriages in perspective; they differ in size because the base for native spouses of native parentage is about three times as large as the base for spouses of foreign stock.

The first three foreign countries listed in the table — United Kingdom, Ireland, and Canada — are English-speaking countries. These three countries and Germany are the national origins of spouses with the lowest proportions (only 18 to 30 percent) married to persons of the same origin. For spouses from the remaining three specific countries of origin — Poland, U.S.S.R., and Italy — the proportions married to persons of the same origin were much higher (45 to 64 percent). Most of the difference between these two sets lay in the proportion of spouses married to native persons of native parentage. In the second set, only about 15 percent of the spouses of Italian origin had married persons of foreign stock from countries other than Italy, whereas over 30 percent of the spouses of Polish and Russian origin had married persons of foreign stock with national origins other than their own. Interestingly enough, spouses with the United Kingdom and Ireland as their countries of origin actually had a larger percentage married to persons of other foreign countries of origin than their own.

These facts update and quantify well-known divergencies in the rate of assimilation of different nationality groups, as measured by the amount of intermarriage after residence in this country for less than one or two full generations. The comparatively rapid assimilation of English-speaking persons of foreign stock is less surprising than that of persons of German origin. Yet relatively more of the spouses of German than of Russian or Italian foreign stock had been in the United States for two generations and hence had a longer time to become adjusted to other nationality groups. Data available for four of the specific national-origin groups show that married family heads of Irish and German foreign stock included about 80 percent who were second-generation Americans, as compared with about 70 percent for married family heads of Russian and Italian extraction.

First-generation German husbands were even less likely than the Irish to have married a wife of their own foreign stock. Both Irish and German second-generation husbands were less than one-half as likely to have married a wife of their own foreign stock as were Russian and Italian husbands of the same cohort. Italian husbands of both first and second generation stood out as the most endogamous of the foreign-origin groups for whom such data are available; 82 percent of the first-generation and 46 percent of the second-generation Italian husbands married Italian wives.

In summary, the data confirm the hypothesis that first- and second-generation Irish and German men — of Northern and Central European origin — assimilated more rapidly than Russian and Italian men — of Eastern and Southern European origin — as measured by marriage to a wife of a different origin from their own; and

Italian husbands were the most persistent, among those analyzed, in marrying into their own nationality group.

Of even greater significance from some points of view may be the high rate of decline in the amount of endogamy from the first generation to the second. The preponderant inmarriage rate of 62 percent for first-generation husbands changed to a preponderant outmarriage rate of 61 percent for second-generation husbands. Even for the husbands of Italian stock, over one-half (54 percent) outmarried in the second generation.

Intermarriage of national-origin groups. Within the framework that each national-origin group indulges in considerable outmarriage, the fact remains that this outmarriage is far from random, as the figures in Table 5.10 demonstrate. Moreover, most of the deviations from

Table 5.10. Index of intermarriage of national-origin groups, for married couples with husband and wife of foreign stock: United States, 1960

National origin of husband	National origin of wife							
	Ireland	Canada	U.K.	U.S.S.R.	Germany	Poland	Italy	Other
Ireland	2,707	135	178	11	81	32	34	36
Canada	127	814	160	21	59	29	24	41
United Kingdom	184	168	689	36	100[a]	33	26	55
U.S.S.R.	10	25	44	618	31	99	9	53
Germany	88	60	101	29	542	46	16	59
Poland	22	32	36	103	41	540	22	48
Italy	43	30	34	12	23	27	463	26
Other	34	44	54	52	59	49	24	204

Source: U.S. Bureau of the Census, U.S. Census of Population: 1960, Subject Reports, Families, Final Report PC(2)-4A, table 62.

[a]A value of 100 for this cell of the table means that husbands of United Kingdom foreign stock married wives of German foreign stock at a rate equivalent to random intermarriage. Values over 100 mean greater than random tendency toward inmarriage.

randomness are sociologically meaningful; explanatory principles include the number of generations in the United States and the consequent degree of similarity or dissimilarity of the spouses' prevailing linguistic, religious, and other historical and cultural variables. In the table, a value of 100 indicates the equivalent of intermarriage at random with respect to national origin, a higher value meaning excess inmarriage and a lower value meaning excess outmarriage. The figures relate to all married couples in 1960 with both husband and wife of (first- or second-generation) foreign stock; data unfortunately are not available by generation.

The language factor appears to explain the high values (all over 100) for the nine combinations of the first three national-origin groups with one another — Ireland, Canada, and United Kingdom — inasmuch as all are English-speaking countries.

Of special interest is the fourth group, the U.S.S.R. Nearly all first- and second-generation persons in the United States whose origin is the U.S.S.R. are of Jewish cultural background. The relatively low rate of outmarriage for Jewish people (discussed in a later section of this chapter) is probably a decisive factor in causing the diagonal value to be high for persons of Russian origin. All four of the values in Table 5.10 which are 12 or smaller, denoting very low outmarriage, are for combinations of U.S.S.R. origin and Irish or Italian origin — the latter two being very largely of Roman Catholic heritage.

The only national-origin group other than the U.S.S.R. which combined with persons of U.S.S.R. origin to yield a value in the table near 100 was persons originating from the adjoining country of Poland. About 8 percent of the husbands or wives of Polish origin were married to persons of Russian origin, and about 9 percent of those of Russian origin were married to persons of Polish origin. A plausible hypothesis is that most of the couples with these combinations of spouses involved a Jewish husband and a Jewish wife. No other origin group in the table combined with persons of Polish origin to produce a value above 50.

Persons of German origin had a larger number of substantial intermarriage rates (values over 50 in the table) than any other group except the United Kingdom. In fact, the only values under 40 for persons of German origin were those for the U.S.S.R. and Italy. Only about 41,000 couples comprised a German person with a Russian spouse, whereas nearly 150,000 couples comprised a Polish person with a Russian spouse.

Persons of Italian origin were the only group having no intermarriage rates of substantial magnitude. Though small, the highest values for the Italians are for couples involving Italian and Irish partners, both largely of Catholic religious antecedents.[12]

Socioeconomic status and composition of mixed- and unmixed-origin groups. Table 5.11 shows that husband-wife families with both

Table 5.11. Selected characteristics of husband-wife families
with head of foreign stock, by whether wife was
of same foreign stock: United States, 1960

| Family characteristic | Husband-wife families with head of foreign stock | | |
	Total	Wife of same foreign stock	Other families
Percent with head who completed high school or more	38.8	28.5	45.1
Percent with head a professional or managerial worker	21.3	16.7	24.2
Percent with family income $10,000 or more	20.4	18.1	21.9
Percent with one or more own children under 6 years old	25.6	20.6	28.7
Average number of own children under 18 years old	1.2	1.0	1.3
Percent with one or more subfamilies "living in"	2.1	2.8	1.6

Source: U.S. Bureau of the Census, U.S. Census of Population:
1960, Subject Reports, Families, Final Report PC(2)-4A, table 59.

spouses of the same foreign stock in 1960 tended to have lower socioeconomic status than husband-wife families with the husband of foreign
stock but the wife of different origin (a different foreign stock or
native of native parentage). The "same-foreign-stock" families tended
to have fewer children, but were more likely to share their home with
a (related) subfamily than were the mixed-stock families. Parentheti-
cally, 38 percent of the husband-wife families with the head of foreign
stock had a wife who was of the same foreign stock.

These findings are probably affected by differences between the
age distribution of family heads with wife of same foreign stock and
that of other family heads. The smaller proportion of the former group
with young children and the smaller average number of children for
that group provide a basis for inferring that heads of families with
wife of same foreign stock are *older*, on the average, than heads of
other families. Additional evidence is the fact that the heads of "other"
families under question included some (perhaps as many as one-half)
who had married native women of native parentage; and those hus-

bands were undoubtedly younger, on the average, than the ones who were married to wives of foreign stock.[13]

Large socioeconomic differentials were found among mixed and unmixed Russian, Irish, German, and Italian heads (for whom the most detail was tabulated from the 1960 census). Differences were especially large with respect to education of the head, as Table 5.12

Table 5.12. Percent of husband-wife family heads of foreign stock who had at least completed high school, by national origin of husband and whether wife was of same foreign stock: United States, 1960

National origin of head	Percent of family heads who completed high school or more		
	Total	Wife of same foreign stock	Other families
Total[a]	38.8	28.5	45.1
Russian	52.0	45.8	57.9
Irish	43.5	33.5	47.0
German	32.8	24.8	35.8
Italian	30.9	22.2	42.5
Other	40.0	28.2	46.3

Source: U.S. Bureau of the Census, U.S. Census of Population: 1960, Subject Reports, Families, Final Report PC(2)-4A, table 59.

[a]Husband-wife families with head of foreign stock.

reveals. The outstanding percentages of heads of Russian foreign stock who had at least completed high school undoubtedly reflect the high value which persons of Jewish heritage tend to place on education, insofar as Russian stock in the United States is equated with Jewish cultural background. The particularly low percentage for heads of Italian foreign stock with wives of the same stock reflects, no doubt, the peasant backgrounds of a substantial proportion of the older couples of first-generation Italian origin in this country. However, family heads of Italian origin made the greatest "gain" in educational level in a generation; this so-called gain is an inference based on heavy weighting of "same-stock" couples with first-generation heads and of "other" couples with second-generation heads; the percentage of high-school graduates is nearly twice as large in the younger as in the older generation.

If occupation of family heads is used as a measure of socioeconomic level, those of Russian foreign stock again ranked highest, with 15 percent employed as professional or technical workers and 21 percent as managers, officials, or proprietors. Corresponding figures ranged downward to 7 percent for the professional category and 11 percent for the managerial category of Italian heads. Likewise, husband-wife families with heads of Russian foreign stock included more than half again as high a proportion with family income of $10,000 or more (31 percent) as those of Italian stock (18 percent); intermediate were the Irish (25 percent) and German (20 percent).

Families with heads of Russian stock had the smallest proportion (1 percent) with subfamilies,[14] and those with both spouses of Italian stock had by far the largest (4 percent). Despite the small amount of doubling among families of Russian stock and their low fertility rates,[15] the average size of family for this group, 3.4 related members of all ages and degrees of kinship, was intermediate between that of families with a head of German stock, only 3.1 members, and that for heads of Italian stock, 3.8 members.

These figures on composition of the family suggest that the families with heads of Italian stock tend most often to have married sons or daughters living in with them, and those of Russian stock tend more often to live by the commandment to "honor thy father and thy mother" by sharing their homes with their elderly widowed parents; those of German stock tend not to share their homes with relatives of either the younger or the older generation.

Religion of Husband and Wife

Nationwide data on religious preference of all persons 14 years old and over were collected by the Bureau of the Census in March 1957 in connection with its Current Population Survey. From this source a special tabulation was made of married couples to show the extent to which Protestant, Roman Catholic, and Jewish married persons had spouses of the same or different religious preference. Marriages across denominational lines within the Protestant or

Jewish groups were counted as unmixed. The tabulation covered the estimated 36,576,000 married couples with spouses reporting the three major groups only and excluded the remaining 2,364,000 couples with one or both spouses reporting other religions or no religion, or making no report on religious preference. The full detail published for the married couples in the study is presented in Table 5.13.

Table 5.13. Married couples and spouses living together, by religion: United States, 1957

(Numbers in thousands)

Religion	Married couples		Spouses living together	
	Number	Percent	Number	Percent
Total	36,576	100.0	73,152	100.0
Husband and wife of same religion	34,223	93.6	68,446	93.6
Protestant	24,604	67.3	49,208	67.3
Roman Catholic	8,361	22.9	16,722	22.9
Jewish	1,258	3.4	2,516	3.4
Husband and wife of different religion	2,353	6.4	4,706	6.4
Protestant-Roman Catholic	2,255	6.2	4,510	6.2
Protestant-Jewish	57	0.2	114	0.2
Roman Catholic-Jewish	41	0.1	82	0.1

Source: Adapted from Paul C. Glick, "Intermarriage and Fertility Patterns Among Persons in Major Religious Groups," Eugenics Quarterly, Vol. 7, No. 1, p. 35, 1960. Basic data originally published in U.S. Bureau of the Census, "Religion Reported by the Civilian Population of the United States: March 1957," Current Population Reports, Series P-20, No. 79, table 6; see also page 2 of text.

Whereas 93.6 percent of the married couples (and thus of husbands and wives) were members of unmixed unions with respect to religious preference, the remaining 6.4 percent were in mixed unions. The unmixed Protestant couples outnumbered the unmixed Catholic couples by a ratio of 3 to 1 and outnumbered the unmixed Jewish couples 20 to 1. Nearly all of the mixed couples consisted of a Protestant and a Catholic spouse. All Catholics and Jews could theoretically have married Protestants, but only about half of the Protestants could marry Catholics or Jews, because Protestants comprised about two-thirds and the others one-third of all persons 14 years old and over.

The problem faced in analyzing differences in intermarriage rates among the major religious groups, as revealed by these basic data, is how to eliminate the distorting effect of the overwhelming numbers of Protestants and the much smaller numbers of Catholic and Jewish persons. The method used here is to compare the actual intermarriage proportions with the expected intermarriage proportions if all persons involved were to choose a marital partner at random with respect to religion.

As a first step in developing actual and expected proportions of intermarried persons, the information in Table 5.13 was reorganized in Table 5.14 to show the total number of persons of a given religious preference classified by religion of the spouse. In the process, some differences develop between the percent distribution of *married couples*

Table 5.14. Protestant, Roman Catholic, and Jewish married couples and constituent spouses living together: United States, 1957

(Numbers in thousands)

Religion of husband and wife	Married couples			Spouses living together		
	Number	Percent of total	Percent of group	Number	Percent of total	Percent of group
Total	36,576	100.0	...	73,152	100.0	...
One or both Protestant	26,916	73.6	100.0	51,520[a]	70.4	100.0
Prot.-Prot.	24,604	...	91.4	49,208	...	95.5
Prot.-R.C. or Jewish	2,312	...	8.6	2,312	...	4.5
One or both Roman Cath.	10,657	29.1	100.0	19,018[b]	26.0	100.0
R.C.-R.C.	8,361	...	78.5	16,722	...	87.9
R.C.-Prot. or Jewish	2,296	...	21.5	2,296	...	12.1
One or both Jewish	1,356	3.7	100.0	2,614[c]	3.6	100.0
Jewish-Jewish	1,258	...	92.8	2,516	...	96.3
Jewish-Prot. or R.C.	98	...	7.2	98	...	3.7

Source: Table 5.13.

[a]Protestant spouses.
[b]Roman Catholic spouses.
[c]Jewish spouses.

with one or both spouses of a given religion and that of *persons* of the specified religion, because of unlike weighting of mixed and unmixed couples, on the one hand, and of persons in mixed and unmixed couples, on the other.

From Table 5.14 it can be inferred that 56 percent of the married couples would have comprised spouses of like religion and 44 percent would have comprised spouses of unlike religion if all persons involved had completely disregarded religion as a factor in mate selection (and no new disturbing element were introduced). This inference relates to all *persons* in the universe covered and is based on the assumption that 70.4 percent of the Protestants involved would have married Protestants, 26.0 percent of Catholics would have married Catholics, and 3.6 percent of Jews would have married Jews. The sum of the squares of these three values, carried to four decimal places, equals 56.4886 percent. Values for "actual" and "expected" percentages of both married couples and spouses in religiously unmixed and mixed marriages when the religion of one spouse is "fixed" (for example, is known to be Protestant) are given in Table 5.15.

The meaning of these actual and expected values can be illustrated in the following manner: Of all *married couples* with at least one

Table 5.15. Actual and expected (if random) proportions of mixed and unmixed Protestant, Roman Catholic, and Jewish married couples and constituent spouses living together: United States, 1957

Religion of husband and wife	Married couples			Spouses living together		
	Actual per-cent	Ex-pected per-cent	Inter-marriage ratio (A/E)	Actual per-cent	Ex-pected per-cent	Inter-marriage ratio (A/E)
One or both Protestant	100.0	100.0	...	100.0	100.0	...
Prot.-Prot.	91.4	54.4	1.68	95.5	70.4	1.36
Prot.-R.C. or Jewish	8.6	45.6	.19	4.5	29.6	.15
One or both Roman Cath.	100.0	100.0	...	100.0	100.0	...
R.C.-R.C.	78.5	14.9	5.27	87.9	26.0	3.38
R.C.-Prot. or Jewish	21.5	85.1	.25	12.1	74.0	.16
One or both Jewish	100.0	100.0	...	100.0	100.0	...
Jewish-Jewish	92.8	1.8	51.56	96.3	3.6	26.75
Jewish-Prot. or R.C.	7.2	98.2	.07	3.7	96.4	.04

Source: Table 5.13.

Protestant spouse, the proportion in which actually both spouses were Protestant (91.4 percent) amounted to fully 1.68 times as large a proportion as that expected (54.4 percent) if the spouses involved had married at random with respect to religious preference of their prospective marital partner. Equally true is the observation that the proportion in which actually one spouse was Protestant and one was not amounted to only about one-fifth (0.19) as large a proportion as that expected under random marriage. The value corresponding to the one just cited was slightly higher (0.25) for couples with a Catholic spouse who intermarried and far lower (0.07) for couples with a Jewish spouse who intermarried.

If the unit of analysis is the *person* (husband or wife) rather than the married couple, the actual percentage of intermarried Protestants was about one-seventh (0.15) as large as the percentage expected under conditions of random marriage. The corresponding intermarriage value for Catholics was of about the same magnitude (0.16) and that for Jews was again far lower (0.04).

The conclusion one can appropriately draw from these results on religious-group intermarriage is that the tendency to intermarry is similar and moderate for Protestants and Roman Catholics but that for Jewish persons it is very slight by comparison with the levels for the other groups. Such an inference could not be properly drawn from the "actual" proportions alone, because they reflect no adjustment for differences in the size of the groups.

Discussion

In the interpretation of the foregoing results on intermarriage, the reader is cautioned against attaching undue significance to *specific* levels of intermarriage values; more confidence can be placed appropriately in the *relative* levels of the values for the groups involved. The values are different depending upon whether one refers to unmixed or mixed marriage, and whether one concentrates on couples or persons. The interpretation of the absolute values depends on whether they refer to surviving married couples exclusive of couples of the same marriage cohorts whose marriages have been broken by divorce, disrupted by separation or residence apart from the spouse for other reasons, or dissolved by death; it also depends on whether the values relate to all current couples without regard to period of marriage or whether first-generation, second-generation, or higher-order generation stock. Furthermore, in view of the probable upward trend of intermarriage during recent decades, those groups which are heavily weighted with relatively old persons of foreign stock (such as Italian Catholics and Russian Jews) tend more than other groups to comprise marriages consummated abroad many years ago under the strong influence of Old World ideas, rather than to marriages contracted under the influence of several generations of living in the United States.[16]

Finally, although the reader should be fully aware of the limitations of the data shown here, he would not be justified in concluding that the intermarriage facts are subject to so many reservations that they are entirely inconclusive. In the absence of nationwide data on *marriages* rather than *married couples* by education, ethnic origin, and religious preference of the husband and wife, the results presented may be accepted as useful indications of general relationships but not definitive analyses.

In future nationwide studies of intermarriage among religious groups, in particular, it is suggested that the interpretation would be greatly improved if the data (1) showed more detail on religious denomination; (2) covered complete marriage cohorts; and (3) included not only current religious preference of each spouse but also religion of each at the time of (or shortly before) marriage, and religion of the father and mother of each spouse. Such data would throw light on the extent to which one spouse in the younger generation brings his or her religious identification into agreement with that of the other spouse, and the degree to which couples change their religious identification to a denomination in keeping with their current station in life (such as joining the "more respectable Episcopalians"). Moreover, the factor of locality in which the persons live should also be controlled if possible; many localities have relatively few persons of Roman Catholic or Jewish preference as potential marital partners, and some have few Protestants.

6 / FAMILY COMPOSITION AND LIVING ARRANGEMENTS OF MARRIED PERSONS

During the cycle of married life, the structure and residential arrangements of a family usually undergo a number of substantial changes. Some of these changes are uniform enough to fall into typical patterns, yet they may vary widely in detail from one stage of married life to another and from one social group to another. This chapter brings out some of the uniformities and some of the diversities of family composition and living arrangements throughout the span of married life.

The chapter begins with an analysis of the long-term changes in the usual ages of women when their children are born and when their children marry. It continues by showing how wide the differences are among age, racial, and income groups of married couples with respect to the decisions they reach about maintaining separate living quarters or sharing their home. Among the most interesting material is that on "who lives with whom" when couples share the living quarters of someone of their own generation or of a younger or older generation. Finally, a close relationship is demonstrated between the age of the couple and such characteristics as its residential movement and the likelihood of owning its home.

An attempt is made to throw light on the way in which lifetime changes in family structure and residential patterns are related to the social and economic circumstances in which married couples are situated, since these circumstances tend to modify the couples' goals with respect to privacy and marital stability. In later chapters, briefer discussions are presented on some comparable aspects of the living arrangements of divorced, widowed, and older single persons.

Children in the Home

Although nearly all women at the height of the reproductive age in the 1960's had children of their own, the situation only a generation or two earlier was quite different. Among women born in the first decade of the 1900's, fully 26 percent remained childless until they were too old to have children; of these, 8 percent remained single but the other 18 percent had married. By contrast, only about 10 percent of the women born in the 1930's and 1940's are expected to remain childless, including about 4 percent who will remain single and childless.[1] These very marked changes reflect a growing tendency for the childbearing and childrearing process to be shared by more nearly all women.

Table 6.1. Median age of women at selected stages of the family life cycle, for women born from 1880 to 1939, by year of birth: United States

Subject	Year of birth (birth cohort) of women					
	1880 to 1889	1890 to 1899	1900 to 1909	1910 to 1919	1920 to 1929	1930 to 1939
First marriage	21.6	21.4	21.1	21.7	20.8	19.9
Birth of first child	22.9	22.9	22.6	23.7	23.0	21.5
Birth of last child	32.9	31.1	30.4	31.5	30.0-31.0	---
First marriage of last child	56.2	53.5	51.9	53.0	51.5-52.5	---
Death of one spouse: For all couples	57.0	59.4	62.3	63.7	64.4	64.4
For couples surviving to first marriage of last child	69.2	68.1	67.8	68.2	67.2-68.2	---

Source: Paul C. Glick and Robert Parke, Jr., "New Approaches in Studying the Life Cycle of the Family," _Demography_, vol. II, 1965, pp. 187-202, table 1.

In Table 6.1 and Figure 6.1, it is seen that the interval between marriage and birth of the first child varies around a central value of about 1.5 years. For couples who entered marriage during the depression years of the 1930's the interval was somewhat longer, and for those who married in the much more prosperous 1950's it was somewhat shorter. Thus the spacing of children is affected by the level of economic conditions; it is affected also by the eventual size of the family, with closer intervals between marriage and the birth of successive children in large families and wider intervals in small families.

The age of the mother at birth of her last child was about 33 for

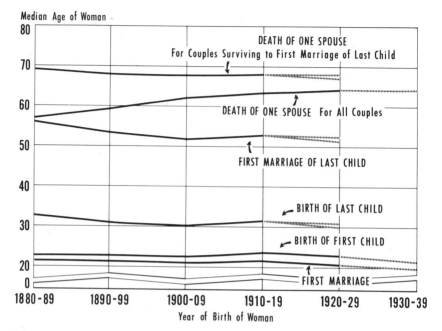

Fig. 6.1. Stages of the family life cycle, for women born in 1880 to 1939: United States

Source: Table 6.1.

women born in the 1880's, but fell to about 30 for women born two decades or nearly a generation later; the latter women were at the height of childbearing during the 1930's when birth rates were quite low. Among women still two or three decades younger, most of whose children were born in the high-fertility period of the 1950's, the factor of relatively young average ages at first marriage tended to offset the factor of larger family size; the net result was to minimize the effect of higher fertility on average age of mother at birth of last child. Hence, since the depression days of the 1930's, the average age of women at the birth of their last child has been one to three years younger than that of women a generation or two earlier. This change has given the typical mother a few additional years in her late thirties when she was free to engage in activities other than the rearing of young children.

When women are in their thirties and forties, their period of bearing children has generally ended, and the time for their children to marry arrives. For women of the oldest cohort shown in Table 6.1, their last child could be expected to marry about 35 years after the women themselves had married. For the youngest cohort, the interval was closer to 30 years. This shortening of the span of childbearing and childrearing results largely from the decline in number of children from an average of about four to about two and one-half per family, and the decline in age at marriage of the youngest as compared with the oldest generation.[2]

After the children marry, most of them leave home to establish a household of their own, as will be shown in the next section. In this period, therefore, the married couple typically maintains an "empty nest" until one spouse or the other dies. One of the major findings in the demography of marriage[3] is the very considerable increase in the proportion of couples who have many years of married life remaining after their children have married (see the last three lines of Table 6.1).

Approximately nine years have been added to the average length of married life of couples in the present century. For the oldest group of women, there was a difference of 35.4 years between the median age at first marriage and the median age at which one spouse (generally the husband) died, but for the youngest cohort the corresponding difference is expected to be about 44.5 years. This is an addition of about one-fourth to the length of marriage.

For the older cohort, the median age of mothers at the first marriage of their last child, 56.2 years, was less than a year before their age when one spouse died, 57.0 years; the corresponding figures for the youngest cohort shown are about 52 and 64 years, or a span of 12 years between the median age of the mother at first marriage of last child and the death of the mother or her husband. This lengthening of the post-children period from a 1-year to a 12-year span, it should be emphasized, is based on the probabilities of joint survival of one-half the married couples from first marriage to the death of one spouse, quite independent of the intervening marriage of the last child.

For those couples who survived to the first marriage of their last child, there has been hardly any change during this century in the gap between the median age at first marriage of last child and the time when one-half the married couples of the parental generation were dissolved by death of one spouse. On this basis of calculation, there was a span of 13 years of married life left in the post-children period for couples in which the wives were born in the 1880's (69.2 years minus 56.2 years) but only a little longer, about 16 years,[4] for couples of the 1920 vintage (67.7 minus 52.0).

Behind the contrasting results just reported is the fact that only a small majority of couples of the older generation (about 52 percent) used to survive to see all their children marry, but today a large majority of couples (about 79 percent) do so. This means that the post-children period of married life now constitutes a significant part for a much larger proportion of married couples than it did formerly. As will be pointed out in the next chapter, these latter years of married life tend to include the time when the economic well-being of the family is at or near its peak.

Maintaining versus Sharing a Home

When two young people marry, they generally face a series of adjustments in their residential arrangements before settling down to a relatively steady mode of living. In taking steps toward establishing a separate household, the couple makes adjustments which typically include moving from one set of living quarters to another and, very likely, the eventual purchase of a home. The remainder of this chapter deals with the extent to which couples are involved in these adjustments at successive durations of marriage or at successive ages of the husband.

Couples who share the homes of others. In 1940, 93.2 percent of married men in the United States who were living with their spouse maintained their own home (that is, the husband was head of the household). By 1965, this figure had risen to 98.1 percent.[5] In other words, as seen in Table 6.2, of all married couples in 1940 — near the end of the depression — 6.8 percent were without their own household; at the height of the housing shortage in 1947, the corresponding figure reached the peak level of 8.7 percent; but by 1960, it had fallen to 2.2 percent and was tending to level off during the first half of the 1960's.

There is, of course, a lower limit on the doubling rate, because some couples will live with relatives in order to care for elderly family members (or to be cared for) regardless of how much the wages earned by young couples go up, how much social security is provided for persons in old age, or how abundant the supply of housing space

Table 6.2. Percent of married couples without their own household, by age of wife and color of husband: United States, 1940 to 1965

Age of wife and color of husband	Percent of married couples without own household				
	1965	1960	1955	1947	1940
Total[a]	1.9	2.2	3.5	8.7	6.8
Under 25 years	6.1	7.7	11.5	29.7	19.0
25-34 years	1.6	1.9	3.6	10.3	8.2
35-44 years	1.1	1.0	2.2	3.8	3.8
45-54 years	1.0	0.9	1.1	2.9	2.7
55-64 years	1.0	1.3	2.0	3.0	3.6
65 years & over	2.3	2.8	4.1	7.7	7.0
White	1.6	1.9	3.2	7.9	6.4
Nonwhite	4.0	4.8	6.2	15.1	11.3

Source: U.S. Bureau of the Census, Current Population Reports, Series P-20, No. 144, tables 3, 6, and 7; No. 67, table 3; No. 62, tables 5 and 7; No. 16, table 4; and No. 10, table 2; and 1940 Census of Population, Vol. IV, Characteristics by Age, Part 1, U.S. Summary, tables 9 and 10.

[a]Statistics for 1940 and 1960 are from decennial censuses and those for 1947, 1955, and 1965 from the Current Population Survey. The 1960 figure for total married couples without own household based on the Current Population Survey was 2.4 percent, as opposed to 2.2 percent from the census.

becomes. Yet the continued downward trend in the percent doubled at both the young and old ages through 1965 leads one to expect at least some further decline in the doubling rate for couples of all ages.

The percent doubled was a little less than twice as high for non-whites as for whites during the 1940's, about twice as high in the 1950's, and more than twice as high in the 1960's. This set of facts supports the conclusion that nonwhite married couples in the 1960's were falling behind white couples in securing relief from the lack of privacy implicit in doubling. Presented otherwise, nonwhite couples, with a doubling rate of 4 percent in 1965, had advanced their progress toward lower doubling rates no farther than white couples had advanced by the early 1950's.

From the foregoing discussion, it is apparent that numerous factors contribute to determination of the doubling rate. These factors have led to a quite low overall rate of doubling — in the vicinity of 2 per-

Table 6.3. Percent doubled, for married couples by years
since first marriage, age, and color of
husband: United States, 1960

Years since first marriage and age of husband	Percent doubled, by color of husband		
	Total	White	Nonwhite
All couples	2.2	1.9	4.9
Years since first marriage:			
Less than 1 year	13.1	11.5	26.6
1 year	8.6	7.4	18.4
2 years	6.4	5.6	13.8
3 or 4 years	4.2	3.6	9.2
5 to 9 years	2.3	2.0	5.5
10 years or more	1.2	1.2	2.3
Husband 14-17 years old	43.6	41.0	60.3
Married less than 1 year	46.8	44.5	63.0
Married 1 year	32.6	33.2	62.8
Married 2 years	31.1	26.8	58.9
Husband 18-24 years old	9.9	8.6	22.8
Married less than 1 year	15.3	13.2	35.7
Married 1 year	10.5	9.1	24.7
Married 2 years	8.3	6.1	19.8
Husband 25-34 years old	2.8	2.4	7.0
Husband 35-64 years old	1.1	1.0	2.2
Husband 65-74 years old	1.9	1.8	2.6
Husband 75 & over	4.2	4.2	5.1

Source: U.S. Bureau of the Census, U.S. Census of
Population: 1960, Subject Reports, Persons by Family
Characteristics, Final Report PC(2)-4B, table 24.

cent — yet in 1960 many subclasses of married couples had rates
ranging up well over 50 percent. In Table 6.3, for instance, substantial variation can be seen in the doubling rate when examined in
terms of duration of marriage. The high rates for nonwhites during
the early years of marriage are particularly noteworthy.

Although many couples make their first home with others, there
is a tendency for them to move into separate quarters as soon as

feasible. Thus, 13.1 percent of the couples married less than one year, with an average duration of marriage of about six months, did not maintain their own household but "lived in" with someone else, usually a close relative. The corresponding figure for couples married less than three months, if available, might very well be twice as high.

The doubling rate is much higher among couples with a quite young husband than among couples with a relatively old one. In only 1 percent of the couples in 1960 was the husband under 18 years old; nearly one-half of these couples, however, shared the homes of others. About 27 percent of the doubled couples included husbands under 25 years of age, and the proportion doubled among couples in this range was about one-tenth for whites and one-fourth for nonwhites. The doubling rate was only 1 or 2 percent for white couples and only 2 or 3 percent for nonwhite couples with the husband between 35 and 74 years old. White couples with the husband 75 and over had a doubling rate of 4 percent, or only about one-half as high as that where the husband was under 25. For nonwhite couples, the doubling rate for this oldest age group was 5 percent, or hardly any higher than that for white couples and only about one-fifth as high as that for nonwhite couples with the husband under 25.

The low doubling rates for both whites and nonwhites in the age range from 35 to 74 suggest that nonwhite, as well as white, couples who manage to live together until middle age almost invariably, under current economic and housing conditions, also manage to maintain a separate household. In other words, regardless of the substantial marital differences among white and nonwhite adults of the middle-age range, these differences are not manifest in the form of doubling rates for married couples.

The income of the husband is a key variable associated with the doubling rate. Yet statistics on the relationship of income to doubling rate for husbands of all ages combined in Table 6.4 showed less variation than the doubling rates presented above by duration of marriage and by age. These figures also demonstrate that doubling rates are much higher for nonwhites at each income level than for whites. It is appropriate to conclude, therefore, that factors other than income level of the husband contribute to the difference between white and nonwhite doubling rates. These factors undoubtedly include greater lack of suitable housing for nonwhite couples.

Husbands with youthful marriages and low incomes had the highest doubling rates, according to the 1960 census. Thus, about 52

Table 6.4. Percent doubled for married couples
by income, selected ages, and color
of husband: United States, 1960

Income and age of husband	Percent doubled, by color of husband		
	Total	White	Nonwhite
All couples	2.2	1.9	4.9
Under $2,000	5.1	4.8	6.8
14-17 years	54.8	52.1	69.2
18-24 years	22.6	20.0	30.8
65-74 years	2.9	2.9	2.7
75 & over	5.7	5.7	5.4
$2,000-$3,999	3.2	2.9	5.1
14-17 years	31.4	29.5	44.6
18-24 years	10.6	9.5	19.0
65-74 years	1.8	1.7	2.6
75 & over	2.8	2.7	4.2
$4,000-$7,999	1.6	1.5	3.4
Under 35 years	2.8	2.6	6.6
65-74 years	1.2	1.2	1.9
75 & over	2.0	2.0	3.4
$8,000 & over	0.8	0.7	2.6
Under 35 years	1.7	1.6	5.6
65-74 years	0.6	0.6	1.7
75 & over	1.2	1.2	-

Source: U.S. Bureau of the Census, U.S.
Census of Population: 1960, Subject Reports,
Persons by Family Characteristics, Final Report
PC(2)-4B, table 24.

percent of the 14,000 white couples and 69 percent of the 2,600
nonwhite couples with husbands 14 to 17 years old and in the lowest
income level (under $2,000 in 1959) were sharing the homes of
others. But couples in this youthful age range with husband's income

of $4,000 or more were only one-third as likely to double (about 17 percent for whites and 23 percent for nonwhites). Even among the 2.4 million couples with the husband 18 to 24 years old, that 1.1 million with the husband's income below $4,000 had quite high doubling rates. These rates, however, were less than one-half as high as those for couples of similar income with still younger husbands.

Contrary to the general tendency for nonwhites to have higher doubling rates than whites, Table 6.4 shows a slightly lower doubling rate for impoverished nonwhite couples at the older portion of the age range (husband 65 years old and over with income below $2,000). This finding suggests that elderly nonwhite couples evidently do not let the pinch of poverty cause them to live in with others as readily as do elderly white couples. The very lowest doubling rates were those for couples in the highest income bracket, $8,000 and over, with the husband 65 to 74 years old. Here, the doubling rate was under 1 percent for white couples and under 2 percent for nonwhite couples.

Most of the 873,000 doubled couples in the United States in 1960 were living with relatives, generally with one or the other sets of

Table 6.5. Doubled married couples, by relationship of husband to head of household and color: United States, 1960

(Numbers in thousands)

Relationship of husband to head of household	Total number	Color of husband		
		Total	White	Nonwhite
All doubled couples	873	...	710	163
Percent	...	100.0	100.0	100.0
Son-in-law of head	306	35.1	36.5	29.1
Son of head	255	29.2	29.5	27.6
Father-in-law of head	75	8.6	9.7	3.5
Father of head	69	7.9	8.7	4.9
Brother-in-law of head	56	6.4	5.9	8.4
Lodger	35	4.0	2.6	9.9
"Other relative" of head	32	3.6	2.7	7.7
Brother of head	26	3.0	2.7	4.3
Grandson of head	15	1.7	1.3	3.6
Resident employee of head	4	0.5	0.4	1.0

Source: U.S. Bureau of the Census, U.S. Census of Population: 1960, Subject Reports, Persons by Family Characteristics, Final Report PC(2)-4B, table 2.

parents (see Table 6.5). About 35 percent of the doubled couples were sharing the home of the wife's parents and 29 percent the home of the husband's parents. This suggests that, inasmuch as the association between the womenfolk tends to be very close in the doubling situation, the adjustment process is somewhat easier when mother and daughter, rather than mother-in-law and daughter-in-law, are involved.

Doubled white couples were more likely to live in a parental home than were doubled nonwhite couples, and the preference of young doublers for the home of the wife's parents was distinct for white couples but not for nonwhite. Moreover, among doubled white couples of the older generation there was a slight preference for living with the couple's daughter and her husband; however, among doubled nonwhite couples, there was a preference for living with the couple's son and his wife. Again, doubled couples clearly preferred living with the brother-in-law of the husband rather than the brother; in light of the foregoing discussion, it seems probable that this generally means the wife is living in with her sister.

Only about 3 percent of white couples without their own household lived with nonrelatives; most of them lived as lodgers (2.6 percent) and the remainder as resident employees (0.4 percent) — such as servants or hired hands. By contrast, about 11 percent of nonwhite couples without households lived with nonrelatives — again, mostly as lodgers (9.9 percent) but some as resident employees (1.0 percent).

Not only do sons-in-law who double up with their wife's parents outnumber married sons who double up with their own parents, but the sons-in-law are likely to stay longer with their in-laws than married sons stay with their parents.[6] Thus 53 percent of the white doubled sons-in-law in 1960 had been (first) married five years or longer; the corresponding proportion of sons was only 39 percent. But the situation varied somewhat by duration of marriage.

For couples who share the homes of others, the relationship of the couple to the head of the household varies according to the couple's stage of married life at the time of the study. Insofar as this stage is revealed by the age of the husband, Table 6.6 shows how the relative concentrations of doubled couples shift from one relationship to another during the cycle of marriage.

Couples are more likely to live with the husband's parents than with the wife's parents if the husband is under 25 years old. In 1960,

Table 6.6. Doubled married couples, by relationship of husband to head of household and age of husband: United States, 1960

(Numbers in thousands)

Relationship of husband to head of household	All ages		Age of husband (years)						
	Number	Percent	14-17	18-24	25-34	35-44	45-64	65-74	75+
All doubled couples	873	...	12	233	245	119	141	69	52
Percent	...	100.0	100.0	100.0	100.0	100.0	100.0	100.0	100.0
Son-in-law of head	306	35.1	26.0	37.7	45.0	48.2	31.6	3.4	0.8
Son of head	255	29.2	48.7	43.3	38.0	30.0	13.1	0.7	0.0
Father-in-law of head	75	8.6	0.2	0.5	0.1	0.9	15.6	40.3	42.5
Father of head	69	7.9	0.4	0.2	0.1	0.3	12.1	38.2	47.1
Brother-in-law of head	56	6.4	6.5	4.1	4.9	7.5	12.1	8.0	3.4
Lodger of head	35	4.0	1.6	3.0	4.4	4.4	5.7	3.0	1.9
"Other relative" of head	32	3.6	3.5	4.3	3.5	3.9	3.1	2.6	3.4
Brother of head	26	3.0	3.1	2.4	2.5	3.8	4.9	3.1	0.8
Grandson of head	15	1.7	9.9	4.3	1.2	0.5	0.2	-	-
Resident employee of head	4	0.5	-	0.1	0.3	0.6	1.7	0.5	0.0

Source: U.S. Bureau of the Census, U.S. Census of Population: 1960, Subject Reports, Persons by Family Characteristics, Final Report PC(2)-4B, table 2.

nearly one-half of the doublers with the husband in this youngest age range made their homes with his parents. Most of the others doubling at this age likewise lived with a close relative — the wife's parents, the husband's grandparents, or the husband's or wife's sister and her husband.[7]

While the husband is 25 to 44 years old, doubling couples are most likely to live in with the wife's parents. This is the time of life when there are generally young children in the family, and one of the implications of the statistics seems to be that doubling couples are more successful in leaving their children in the care of the wife's mother than with the husband's mother while she (the wife) works outside the home. During this period the home of the husband's parents is clearly the second most frequent residence for couples to share. Far less frequent, but next in line, is the home of a brother-in-law of the husband, after which comes the home of a nonrelative.

In old age (defined as the time when the husband is 65 years old and over), as at the youngest ages, nearly all doubling couples live in with close relatives. About 80 to 90 percent of these older couples in 1960 who shared the home of others lived in with one of their sons or daughters, the number living with a son being about equal to the number living with a daughter. For husbands throughout middle age and up to age 74 years old, however, there was a consistent tendency for the doubling couples to stay with a daughter (generally still married), whereas at ages 75 and over somewhat more doubling couples stayed with a son (and his wife). When the husband exceeds 75 years of age, there may be a tendency for him to require special attention which a son is better suited than a son-in-law to render.

Couples doubling at their middle and older ages were much more likely than at younger ages to prefer sharing the home of a sister of the husband or wife or of a brother of the wife (that is, sharing the home of a brother-in-law of the husband) rather than sharing the home of the husband's brother. Although this comparison is complex, one of the things it seems to suggest is that living in with a feminine relative is more common at the older ages than living in with a masculine relative; this may be explained at least partially by the greater longevity of women than men and the consequent greater availability of feminine kin with whom to live.

Families who share their homes with others. The reverse side of doubling is amenable to study, too; for census data also show the extent to which heads of families and their wives, if any, have a "subfamily" (a related married couple or parent-child group) living with them. Although available statistics on doubling, viewed from this vantage point, are much more limited than those described above, it is instructive to point out the magnitude of the problem at successive age groups of the head and to see how the phenomenon varies by color and structure of the doubling group.

Table 6.7 shows that about 812,000 families, or 2 percent of all families in 1960, had a related married couple sharing their home as a subfamily. One out of every 15 families with doubled couples present had two or more such couples living in. Among husband-wife families (families with a "married, wife present" head), only 1.3 percent had a doubled couple living in, but among "other families" a much larger proportion, 5.8 percent, had such a couple among its members. At the same time, 5 out of every 8 families with a doubled couple among their members were husband-wife families. Although twice as large a proportion of nonwhite husband-wife families as white had a doubled couple living in (2.5 versus 1.2 percent), the same proportion of white as nonwhite "other families" (5.8 percent) had a doubled couple living in. As figures below will indicate, nonwhites have much more doubling than whites comprising parent-child groups living in.

Table 6.7. Families with a married couple living
doubled up, by type of family, age,
and color of head: United States, 1960

(Numbers in thousands)

Type of family and age of head	All families with a doubled couple	Percent with a doubled couple		
		Total	White	Nonwhite
All families	812	1.8	1.6	3.3
Husband-wife families	498	1.3	1.2	2.5
Under 35 years	55	0.5	0.5	1.3
35-44 years	88	0.9	0.8	1.8
45-64 years	264	1.8	1.7	3.5
65 & over	90	1.9	1.8	3.8
Other families	314	5.8	5.8	5.8

Source: U.S. Bureau of the Census, U.S. Census of
Population: 1960, Subject Reports, Families, Final Report
PC(2)-4A, table 23.

A substantial majority of husband-wife families with a related doubling couple in 1960 had a head in middle age, here defined as 45 to 64 years of age. The *rate* at which husband-wife families shared their home with a doubling couple was equally high, however, for those with the head 65 years old and over. Moreover, the rate of sharing the home with another couple was far lower for families with the head under 45 years of age. These observations represent the complements of the observations made above about the characteristics of doubled couples; since most of the doubled couples include sons or sons-in-law of family heads, the host couples must generally involve natural or in-law parents of the doublers.[8]

Subfamilies which involve a parent-child group living in with relatives were found in 586,000 families in 1960, or about three-fourths the number with husband-wife subfamilies (see Table 6.8). The proportion of families with parent-child subfamilies is especially noteworthy for nonwhites. This type of doubling commonly reflects parental sheltering of a young mother and her child where the young mother is unwed or has a disrupted marriage. Such doubling occurred

Table 6.8. Families with a parent-child group living
doubled up, by type of family and color
of head: United States, 1960

(Numbers in thousands)

Type of family	All families with a doubled parent-child group	Percent with a doubled parent-child group		
		Total	White	Nonwhite
All families	586	1.3	1.0	2.9
Husband-wife families	353	0.9	0.7	2.6
Other families	234	4.3	3.6	7.4

Source: U.S. Bureau of the Census, U.S. Census of
Population: 1960, Subject Reports, Families, Final Report
PC(2)-4A, table 23.

at a rate nearly four times as large for nonwhite as white husband-wife families; doubling of couples, by contrast, occurred at a rate only twice as high for nonwhite as white husband-wife families.

Very few families contain among their members both husband-wife and parent-child subfamilies. Only 1.8 percent of the families in 1960 had one or more doubled couples, 1.3 percent had one or more parent-child groups, and (as a separately determined statistic) 3.1 percent had one or more of either type of doubled group. Accordingly, no significant error would be made by adding together the rates for the two types of doubling to make overall comparisons of the presence of subfamilies for families by color and type.

Ethnic differences in the percentage of families having one or more subfamilies among their members are quite large. Statistics from the same source as Table 6.9 make possible the following comparison of families in the United States with subfamilies: white, 2.7 percent; Negro, 7.0 percent; American Indian, 7.7 percent; other nonwhite races, 6.2 percent; families with head of Puerto Rican origin, 3.8 percent; and families with head of Spanish surname, 5.2 percent.

Three-generation families among ethnic groups. As shown in Table 6.9, white families comprising three generations in sequence living together — with no intermediate generation missing — constituted

Table 6.9. White families with three generations present, by type of family and family composition: United States, 1960

(Numbers in thousands)

Family composition	Total		Husband-wife families	Other families
	Number	Percent		
All white families	40,887	...	36,465	4,422
Percent	...	100.0	100.0	100.0
3-Generation families[a]	1,994	4.9	4.4	8.9
Parent-HEAD-child	1,245	3.0	3.0	3.1
HEAD-child-grandchild	775	1.9	1.4	5.9
Other families	38,892	95.1	95.6	91.1

Source: U.S. Bureau of the Census, U.S. Census of Population: 1960, Subject Reports, Families, Final Report PC(2)-4A, table 60.

[a]Includes 25,000 families with four generations consisting of parent-HEAD-child-grandchild.

about 5 percent[9] of the 41 million white families in 1960. Among white husband-wife families, about two-thirds of the three-generation type included the head in the middle generation and the other one-third included the head in the oldest generation. The typical family composition where the head and wife are in the middle generation is a married couple maintaining a home in which they provide joint living quarters for not only some or all of their own children, but also for one or both of the husband's or wife's parents. Where the head and wife are in the oldest generation, the typical situation is that the couple maintains a home which is shared by a subfamily containing children.

Among white "other families," the distribution of three-generation families is weighted in the reverse direction. In two-thirds of the three-generation "other families" the head was in the oldest generation, and in the other third in the middle generation. Here the typical family composition in the former situation is one where the head is a woman with no husband present who maintains a home which she shares with a subfamily containing children. In 1960 this type of three-generation family composition was found in 5.9 percent of the "other families" with a white head; although the corresponding proportion for similar families with a nonwhite head is unknown, it probably exceeds 10 percent.[10]

Table 6.10. Incidence of three-generation families among families of
selected race and ethnic groups as compared with white
families, by family composition: United States, 1960

Race or ethnic group of head	Index of parent-HEAD-child families	Race or ethnic group of head	Index of HEAD-child-grandchild families
White	100	White	100
Japanese	281	American Indian	475
Chinese	162	Negro	400
Puerto Rican origin	142	Mexican foreign stock	295
Italian foreign stock	139	Spanish surname	251
		Filipino	240
American Indian	127		
Mexican foreign stock	126	Chinese	199
		Japanese	141
Polish foreign stock	120		
Russian foreign stock	119	Puerto Rican origin	134
		Italian foreign stock	129
Spanish surname	117		
Filipino	114	German foreign stock	107
Negro	104	Irish foreign stock	101
Irish foreign stock	88	Polish foreign stock	80
German foreign stock	72	Russian foreign stock	52

Source: U.S. Bureau of the Census, U.S. Census of Population:
1960, Subject Reports, Families, Final Report PC(2)-4A, table 60.

Some illuminating differences among ethnic groups in the two
prevalent types of three-generation families in the United States in
1960 are shown in Table 6.10. The highest indexes[11] of parent-
HEAD-child families were those for the Japanese, 281, and the Chinese, 162. This finding coupled with relatively high indexes of HEAD-
child-grandchild families for these two groups (141 and 199, respectively) may be accepted as evidence of the persistence, to a limited
degree at least, of the extended family system which has been relatively frequent in the Asian countries from which these groups had
moved or descended. The fact that the index for Japanese families with
the head in the middle generation is about twice as large as the corresponding figure for families with the head in the oldest generation,
whereas the difference is smaller and reversed for Chinese families,
suggests that elderly impoverished Japanese parents do not insist on
retaining the role of head of the family but that there is a slight
tendency for Chinese parents to do so.

Families with heads of Polish or Russian foreign stock had three-generation composition of the parent-HEAD-child type at a somewhat higher rate than white families in general (indexes of 120 and 119, respectively) but at a lower rate for the HEAD-child-grandchild type (indexes of 80 and 52). These contrasting facts are consistent with the hypothesis that middle-aged family heads of these origin groups — heavily weighted with persons of Jewish culture — tend to "honor their (elderly) parents" by caring for them in their homes. These are groups which have shown quite rapid upward economic mobility from the first to the second generation in the United States.[12] The tendency seems to be for the more affluent second generation to provide shelter, care, and companionship for the less affluent first generation. Moreover, these are groups with a reputation for low rates of family disorganization and illegitimacy; therefore, there probably tend to be relatively few young mothers among them with no husband for a breadwinner and consequently few occasions for such mothers to become a part of a HEAD-child-grandchild family.

The reverse situation was found in extreme form among families with an American Indian or Negro head and also to a substantial degree among Mexican; Spanish-surname, and Filipino families — all with indexes of HEAD-child-grandchild three-generation families of 240 and over. These groups tend to have high proportions of young adults who are handicapped by poverty as well as marital disruption, and some are known to have high rates of parenthood outside wedlock. The frequent presence of subfamilies which include children serves as a clue to the existence of serious family troubles that lead young parents to seek refuge in the home of a relative.

Noteworthy in this connection are the relatively low indexes of three-generation families of both types where the head is of Irish or German foreign stock. Evidently there is little cultural precedent or need for doubling to be practiced among these groups. They tend to be readily assimilated and capable of self-reliance.

This discussion of doubling probably should not be concluded without noting once again that the great majority of even the young married couples in the United States establish separate households soon after marriage. Those who gain their share of the economic abundance which characterizes modern society in this country tend to choose private living in a house or apartment away from relatives as one of their ways to enjoy their economic well-being. To the extent that young people postpone marriage and establish themselves in good jobs so as to achieve economic independence from their parents, they are in a position at marriage to move directly into the company of adults who maintain their own household. Moreover, with the current social-security arrangements, couples in old age usually can afford to enjoy separate living in areas not far from relatives who can serve as companions and check in on them occasionally.[13]

Residential Movement

Typically, the cycle of married life either starts with movement of the bride and groom from their respective parental homes into a home of their own, or with temporary residence in a parental home followed soon afterward by movement into separate living quarters. For a substantial minority of couples, however, the groom or bride or both establish bachelor quarters or other living arrangements "away from home" prior to marriage. About three-fourths of the single persons 18 to 34 years of age in 1964 reported no residential movement during the year before the survey, but the other one-fourth moved during that 12-month period for one reason or another. Far more mobile are married persons of the same age, as the following discussion and accompanying tables will show.

Although about 1 couple in every 5 in the United States — regardless of length of marriage — changes its place of residence within a year's time, this type of movement (or "mobility," as census reports

Table 6.11. One-year residential mobility rates for husbands, by age: United States, 1963 to 1964

Age of husband	Percent by type of mobility, 1963-64					
			Different house in U.S.A.			Abroad in 1963
	Total	Same house	Total	Same county	Different county	
All husbands	100.0	80.9	18.6	12.6	6.0	0.4
14-17 years	a	a	a	a	a	a
18-24 years	100.0	34.5	64.0	45.2	18.8	1.4
25-34 years	100.0	66.6	32.4	20.8	11.6	1.0
35-44 years	100.0	83.4	16.3	11.1	5.2	0.3
45-64 years	100.0	90.6	9.2	6.7	2.5	0.2
65 & over	100.0	94.1	5.9	3.8	2.1	0.1

Source: U.S. Bureau of the Census, Current Population Reports, Series P-20, No. 141, table 6.

[a]Rate (percent) not shown where base is less than 150,000.

use the term) reaches its highest level before the husband is 25 years of age (see Table 6.11). About 2 out of 3 husbands under 25 make at least one residential move during a 12-month period, many of these comprising residence changes at marriage. The one-year mobility rate goes down to 1 out of 3 couples as the husbands advance to the age group 25 to 34 years, and continues to decline until it becomes only about 1 out of 17 by age 65 and over.

The mobility rate for married couples with the husband 35 to 44 years old is near the average for husbands of all ages combined. The rate for couples with the husband under 35 is above this average, and for couples with the husband 45 and over is below it. This generalization applies to both short- and long-distance movement, as Table 6.11 demonstrates for one-year movement between 1963 and 1964. It likewise applies to movement during the five years before the 1960 census, as Table 6.12 shows for movement between 1955 and 1960.

Within the age span of husbands below 25 years, the "internal" mobility rate, or percent living in a different house in the United States in 1960 from that in 1955, actually increased with age. While 74 percent of husbands 14 to 17 were in a different house at the end of the period, 87 percent of those 18 to 24 were in a different house. This observation reflects the fact, discussed at length in the preceding

Table 6.12. Five-year residential mobility rates for husbands, by age: United States, 1955 to 1960

Age of husband	Total	Same house	Percent by type of mobility, 1955-60			Abroad in 1955	Not re-ported
			Different house in U.S.A.				
			Total	Same county	Different county		
All husbands	100.0	49.6	47.6	30.8	16.8	1.4	1.4
14-17 years	100.0	21.5	74.0	54.9	19.1	1.4	3.2
18-19 years	100.0	9.7	87.0	57.7	29.3	0.4	2.9
20-24 years	100.0	6.6	86.9	51.8	35.1	3.0	3.5
25-29 years	100.0	11.4	80.5	46.1	34.4	5.1	3.0
30-34 years	100.0	29.0	67.6	42.2	25.4	2.1	1.4
35-44 years	100.0	48.0	49.6	32.4	17.2	1.3	1.1
45-64 years	100.0	65.8	32.7	23.3	9.4	0.5	0.9
65 & over	100.0	75.8	23.4	16.0	7.4	0.1	0.7

Source: U.S. Bureau of the Census, U.S. Census of Population: 1960, Subject Reports, Mobility for States and State Economic Areas, Final Report PC(2)-2B, table 7.

section, that a much larger proportion of the very young than of the somewhat older husbands (and their wives) live in the home of the husband's (or wife's) parents for a while after marriage.

The volume of intracounty movement at every age of husband exceeds the volume of intercounty movement, regardless of whether a one-year or a five-year period is involved. However, the movement within a five-year period that takes place during the years when the husband is under 20 is, as would be expected, heavily weighted with local, intracounty movement. When the husband is 20 to 34, the ratio of far-ranging, intercounty movement to local movement is about 2 to 3 and is higher than for any other period. This interval, when men are in their twenties and early thirties, generally encompasses not only the time during which most men marry but also that part of the cycle of adult life when couples usually reach basic decisions about residential location, in the light of emerging expectations regarding the husband's career and the size of the couple's family. This is also the period when immigration and the return of men from military service in foreign lands are most likely to occur; accordingly, movement from abroad to the United States is highest in this age span. As husbands pass through middle age and on into old age, the ratio of long-distance to short-distance movement tends to subside, so that for those 45 and older this ratio dips below 1 to 2.

Mobility rates for husbands (and wives) drop sharply during the mature adult years, with close to 90 percent at age 25 but only around 25 percent at age 65 changing residential addresses in a five-year period. Obviously, at the younger ages there are many more reasons for movement, and greater ease of mobility. The accumulation of household possessions, generally including a paid-for home in a familiar environment, and other conservative influences (such as the husband's development of seniority in a job or of good will relative to a self-employment occupation, and the couple's cultivation of a circle of local friends over the years) tend to discourage movement in the later years. Attention is centered here on married couples; the situation is quite different for divorced or widowed persons, as will be seen in subsequent chapters.

Home Ownership

When young couples establish a separate household, their first home is very likely to be rented; then as they accumulate enough savings to make the down payment on a house, the majority purchase a home of their own. The fact of owning a home very likely has a stabilizing effect on the marriage, partly because the home serves as an "object apart" which the husband and wife can develop jointly.

Two-thirds of the married couples in 1960 owned their homes, as shown by a later table (6.14). This was a somewhat larger proportion than the 62 percent owned for all households, including those without a married head. Historical changes from 1940 to 1960 in home ownership by color of head cannot be traced for married couples in the United States as a whole, but are shown in Table 6.13 for all

Table 6.13. Home ownership by color of head of household and region, 1960, and by color of head of household, 1950 and 1940: United States

| Color of head | Percent with owned home | | | | | 1950 | 1940 |
	Total	North-east	North Central	South	West		
		1960					
All households	61.9	56.1	67.0	62.0	61.3	55.0	43.6
White	64.4	58.2	69.1	66.4	62.5	56.9	45.7
Nonwhite	38.4	27.0	35.8	41.6	44.6	34.9	23.7

Source: U.S. Bureau of the Census, U.S. Census of Housing: 1960, Volume 1, States and Small Areas, United States Summary, Final Report HC(1)-1, tables H, 1, and 22.

households on the basis of data from housing censuses. These data show an increase of virtually one-half in the home-ownership rate between 1940 (44 percent) and 1960 (62 percent). About two-thirds of the change took place in the 1940's.

The home-ownership rate among nonwhites was nearly one-half again as high in 1950 as in 1940, whereas among whites it rose only one-fourth. During the 1950's, however, when the increase in percent married among nonwhites lagged, the growth in the home-ownership rate likewise was less rapid for nonwhites (one-tenth) than for whites (one-eighth).

Home ownership has for decades been low in the Northeast, as compared with the rest of the country. This fact is perhaps related primarily to the large proportion of metropolitan apartment dwellers in the Northeast; it may also be affected by the tradition of relatively late marriage in New England. Among whites, the home-ownership rate was highest in the North Central region; among nonwhites it was highest in the West, where the majority of nonwhite persons are not Negroes. For nonwhites in the South, where nearly all nonwhites are Negroes, the home-ownership rate in 1960 (42 percent) had climbed to about the same level as for whites in 1940 (46 percent). The comparatively high proportions of owned homes in the North Central region and the South are related to the heavy concentrations of farm population; for the nation as a whole, the home-ownership rate is about one-tenth higher for farm than for nonfarm households.

The amount of the 20-year increase in home-ownership rate from 1940 to 1960 for nonwhite families (15 percentage points) was almost as large as for white families; but it meant that the home-ownership rate for nonwhites was more than half again as large in 1960 as in 1940, whereas that for whites was less than half again as large at the more recent date.

Typical home-ownership rates by stage of married life can be inferred from data in Table 6.14 on the percentage of homes owned by husband-wife families distributed according to (1) age of the family head and (2) length of time since marriage of the head. The two distributions can be interpreted as showing roughly equivalent

Table 6.14. Home ownership by age, color, and time of marriage of head of household: United States, 1960

Age of head	Percent of homes owned			Period of, and age at, first marriage of head	Percent of homes owned		
	Total	White	Non-white		Total	White	Non-white
All husband-wife families	67.0	69.0	43.9	All husband-wife families	67.0	69.0	43.9
Under 20 years	14.1	14.5	8.9	1955-60	33.4	35.1	18.0
20-24 years	25.0	26.3	10.5	1950-54	59.0	61.6	31.8
25-29 years	44.3	46.5	20.8	1945-49	69.8	72.2	42.2
30-34 years	61.7	64.4	32.6	Under 22 at			
35-39 years	69.7	72.3	41.8	marriage	65.0	68.0	34.1
40-44 years	73.0	75.2	46.7	22-27 at mar.	72.6	74.6	45.2
				28+ at mar.	70.4	72.8	47.4
45-49 years	73.8	75.9	50.2	1940-44	73.6	75.7	48.7
50-54 years	74.4	76.1	53.7	1930-39	74.5	76.3	52.4
55-59 years	74.1	75.8	55.9	1920-29	76.0	77.4	58.6
60-64 years	75.7	77.0	59.1	1910-19	78.4	79.6	63.3
65 & over	77.7	78.8	62.8	Before 1910	77.2	78.8	59.6

Source: U.S. Bureau of the Census, U.S. Census of Population: 1960, Subject Reports, Families, Final Report PC(2)-4A, tables 5 and 44.

information where the rates are approximately equal. For example, 69.7 percent of the heads 35 to 39 years old owned their homes and 69.8 percent of the heads who first married in 1945 to 1949 owned their homes by 1960; in this respect, these birth and marriage cohorts are rough equivalents. Likewise, heads in their fifties, with about 75 percent home owners, were similar in home ownership to heads who first married in the 1920's (76 percent). The comparison is not as easy to make for the younger ages and more recent marriages, partly because the class intervals in these parts of the distributions are quite far from equal in size.

Table 6.14 provides a basis for reaching conclusions about the very different ages and durations of marriage by which white and nonwhite family heads can expect to own their home. Based on these 1960 census data, the findings indicate the following ages and numbers of years after first marriage when one-fourth, one-half, and three-fourths were home owners:

One-fourth were home owners —
   White: By age 23, or 2 years after first marriage
   Nonwhite: By age 30, or 5 years after first marriage
One-half were home owners —
   White: By age 29, or 5 years after first marriage
   Nonwhite: By age 47, or 19 years after first marriage
Three-fourths were home owners —
   White: By age 41, or 16 years after first marriage
   (Nonwhites never exceeded 63 percent home owners)

The relationship between these figures and the fact that the average age at marriage for men is around 23 years is somewhat complex. In essence, however, the figures tend to reflect the fact that those who marry at a quite young age generally have to postpone the purchase of a home until an older age than do those who marry at an intermediate age. The home-ownership values presented in Table 6.14 for husbands who first married 10 to 15 years before the census at ages under 22, 22 to 27, and 28 years or older provide good reason for believing that youthful marriage is symptomatic of a lowered probability of future ownership of a home. The low home-ownership rates for white families with the head married at age 28 and over may be heavily weighted by late-marrying metropolitan New Englanders.

Family income was found to be one of the most discriminating characteristics by which home ownership was classified in the 1960

Table 6.15. Home ownership by family income and color of head, for primary families with the head first married 10 to 19 years before the census: United States, 1960

Family income	Percent of homes owned			Ratio of nonwhite to white
	Total	White	Nonwhite	
Total with 10-19 years since first marriage of head	69.0	72.0	40.2	.56
Under $2,000	42.3	50.2	24.2	.48
$2,000-$3,999	49.5	53.4	33.9	.63
$4,000-$7,999	70.5	71.9	49.9	.69
$8,000 & over	82.8	83.3	67.6	.81

Source: U.S. Bureau of the Census, U.S. Census of Population: 1960, Subject Reports, Families, Final Report PC(2)-4A, table 15.

census, within the framework of a given duration of marriage. The illustrative home-ownership rates in Table 6.15 show that, for every family-income level, white families were considerably more likely than nonwhite families to own their home. Therefore home ownership is determined in part by factors other than current income. Such factors probably include a shortage of savings for use as down payment on a home, the limited availability of suitable private homes for purchase by nonwhites, traditional habits of renting a home, and recency of migration of nonwhites away from the South. Perhaps the most important fact brought out is that the ratio of nonwhite to white home-ownership rates approaches unity as the amount of family income increases.

7 / WORK EXPERIENCE AND INCOME
OF MARRIED PERSONS

This chapter deals with variations in worker rates, occupational affinities, and income levels of married persons. Since nearly all married men below retirement age are in the labor force, worker rates vary relatively little from group to group. By contrast, married women in some life situations are far more likely than others to work outside the home and thereby to affect the potentiality for the family to purchase consumer goods and services. In view of these considerations, attention is devoted especially to the circumstances under which married women join the labor force and to the demographic characteristics of nonworking wives.

A special feature of the analysis of work experience is the identification of occupations which attract relatively large proportions of married persons. (Occupational concentrations of unmarried persons are discussed in Chapters 8, 9, and 10.) The present chapter also provides illustrative examples of the tendency for husbands in given professions to be married to wives in certain occupations, and vice versa.

The final major section of the chapter shows how much smaller the incomes of unmarried men tend to be as compared with those of married men. Group differences in the contributions of wives to family income are discussed, and the relationship between size of family and the economic position of the family is shown for families of given income levels. Changes in level of income during the cycle of married life are presented for several economic strata of the population.

The discussion culminates in an analysis of the amount of education usually associated with given levels of earnings for white and nonwhite husbands employed in each of the major occupation groups. This section brings into sharp focus the very substantial gap between the racial groups in the earnings which men can reasonably expect by middle age if they work at a given type of occupation after having attained a given educational level.

A comparison of this chapter with subsequent chapters will help to bring out the full force of the evidence in this monograph to the effect that men of mature adult age but not past middle age are

increasingly likely to be married and decreasingly likely to be unmarried as their socioeconomic level rises.

Labor-Force-Participation Rates of Married Men

Between 95 and 99 percent of all husbands between the ages of
20 and 55 years were in the labor force in 1960 (see source of Table
7.1). Of the small number of husbands under 20 years old, 93 percent were in the labor force, and of those in the older age groups
the labor-force-participation rates were: 55 to 64 years old, 87 percent; 65 to 74 years old, 41 percent; and 75 and over, 19 percent.
During the 1950's substantial declines had occurred in the rates for
those 65 to 74 years old (from 57 percent in 1950) and for those 75
and over (from 25 percent in 1950).

These declines in employment at the upper ages undoubtedly reflect the increasing role of social-security pensions in the income
maintenance of older married couples. To some extent they probably
also reflect the displacement of older workers — who found ample
employment opportunities during the labor shortage of the 1940's —
by the millions of younger workers whose services during the 1950's
were devoted to civilian rather than military duties. Moreover, with
the increasing automation of industrial operations, the services of
older men, particularly those of marginal literacy, evidently became
increasingly dispensable. The changes in employment rates suggest
that more and more of these relatively unemployable men failed in
their attempts to find work and eventually came to regard themselves
as retirees, no longer candidates for jobs.

Nonwhite husbands at most age levels have had consistently lower
levels of labor-force participation than white husbands. The differences in participation rates for the two groups of husbands have been
minimal, however, between the ages of 20 and 55. Among the few
under 20 years of age, as well as among those 55 to 64, the disparity
in 1960 was 6 percent. In both 1940 and 1950, nonwhite husbands
over 65 had higher labor-force rates than white, but in 1960 the
rates for both groups were essentially the same.

The inability of some husbands to find work or to keep a job has
a close bearing on marital stability. For example, among white married men 55 to 64 years of age — when many of the marginal workers drop out of the labor market — only 9 percent of those living
with their wife in 1960 had not worked in 1959. The corresponding

figure for nonwhites was 14 percent. At the same time, among married men of the same age who were living apart from their wives, 27 percent of the whites and 29 percent of the nonwhites had not worked in 1959. Thus a substantial proportion of the husbands who were not earning a livelihood for their wife had evidently drifted away from home, or else the wife had done so.[1]

Labor-Force-Participation Rates of Married Women

Recent trends for married and unmarried women. The upsurge during the 1940's and 1950's in the proportion of married women engaged in gainful employment away from their homes was partly a reflection of the long-term trend toward living and working in cities rather than on farms. In addition, the labor shortage at the peak of World War II provided the necessary impetus for employers to accept married women as employees in many new lines of work in industry and government, especially women with a high-school education. Their husbands may have been reluctant at first, but came to accept the idea of having their wives employed in outside work as a means of providing a better livelihood for the family.

During the 1940's married women replaced single women as the group with the largest number of females in the labor force. By 1950, married women in the labor force were twice as numerous as in 1940, and by 1960 they were more than three times as numerous, as Table 7.1 shows. In the 20-year span, the number of single workers outside

Table 7.1. Marital status of women 14 years old and over in the labor force: United States, 1960, 1950, and 1940

(Numbers in thousands)

Marital status	Women in the labor force			
	1960	1950	1940	Increase, 1940-60
Total	22,296	16,553	13,007	9,289
Single	5,263	5,274	6,377	-1,114
Married, husband present	12,292	7,697	3,918	8,374
Other marital status	4,742	3,581	2,712	2,030

Source: U.S. Bureau of the Census, U.S. Census of Population: 1960, Subject Reports, Employment and Work Experience, Final Report PC(2)-6A, table 6.

Table 7.2. Marital status of women 14 years old and over in the
labor force, by color: United States, 1960 and 1940

(Numbers in thousands)

Marital status	Women in the labor force				1960 as percent of 1940	
	White		Nonwhite			
	1960	1940	1960	1940	White	Nonwhite
Total	19,494	11,166	2,802	1,841	175	152
Single	4,741	5,841	522	536	81	97
Married, husband present	10,978	3,265	1,314	653	336	201
Other marital status	3,776	2,060	966	652	183	148

Source: U.S. Bureau of the Census, U.S. Census of Population:
1960, Subject Reports, Employment and Work Experience, Final Report
PC(2)-6A, table 6.

the home actually declined by a million, whereas working women of
"other marital status" increased by three-fourths.

The decline in the number of single workers between 1940 and
1960 was both absolutely and proportionately much greater for white
than nonwhite women, as shown in Table 7.2. One reason may be
that a larger proportion of the increase in marriage among white
women during this period occurred among women who were well-
educated; such women are generally the most employable.

Worker rates are generally lower for married women than for other
women, partly because of the obvious fact that most of the former are
preoccupied with the care of children during many of their best years
for gainful employment. In addition, despite the observation just made
about recent increases in marriage among the more employable
women, evidence brought out later in this chapter and in later chapters
suggests strongly that, other things being equal, relatively unemployable women are more inclined than their more employable sisters to
marry. On the other hand, spinsters, widows, and divorced women of
working age appear much more able and inclined to maintain economic independence through employment outside the home.

For married women, the labor-force-participation rate was much
closer to that for other women in 1960 than in 1940 (see Table 7.3).
During these two decades, however, the rate for nonwhite women in
each marital category lost ground as compared with that for white
women. The increase in the rate was much greater for white than
nonwhite *married* women, and the decrease in the rate was much

Table 7.3.   Labor-force-participation rate of women 14 years old and
over, by marital status and color: United States, 1960
and 1940

| Marital status | Labor-force-participation rate | | | | | | 1960 as percent of 1940 | | |
| | Total | | White | | Nonwhite | | Total | White | Nonwhite |
	1960	1940	1960	1940	1960	1940			
All women	34.5	25.8	33.6	24.5	41.7	37.6	134	137	111
Single	42.9	45.5	43.9	45.9	35.5	41.9	94	96	85
Married, husband present	30.6	13.8	29.8	12.5	40.5	27.3	222	238	148
Other marital status	38.7	33.7	36.9	30.2	48.2	53.2	115	122	91

Source: U.S. Bureau of the Census, U.S. Census of Population: 1960,
Subject Reports, Employment and Work Experience, Final Report PC(2)-6A, table 6.

greater for nonwhite than white *single* women. As a net effect of these changes, the worker rate for married nonwhite women became even higher than that for single nonwhite women — the reverse of the situation in 1940 for nonwhites and in both 1940 and 1960 for whites.

Much of the expansion in labor-force participation of married women during the two decades was at the expense of the other marital categories. Specifically, for white women, the overall gain in the labor-force-participation rate was 37 percent, and for nonwhite women it was 11 percent, whereas corresponding growth figures for married women exceeded these levels.

Among white women, the pattern of labor-force participation throughout the cycle of married life has undergone a noteworthy change since 1940. As Table 7.4 shows, a secondary crest of the worker rate has developed for white married women 20 to 24 years old; this development typically reflects the employment of young women for a while after marriage, before the first child is born.

Following the crest at ages 20 to 24, the worker rate for white married women in 1960 was moderately lower throughout the age span of 25 to 34 years, when the majority had children who were below school age. For nonwhite married women, however, the labor-force-participation rate continued to climb during this phase of life, partly because a larger proportion of nonwhite than white married women remain childless, as will be shown below. Also, 18 percent of nonwhite mothers, as compared with only 9 percent of white mothers, with the husband aged 25 to 34 had an adult in the home who was not employed and thus presumably in a position to care for the children while the mother worked.[2]

Table 7.4.   Labor-force-participation rate of married women with husband present, by age and color: United States, 1960 and 1940

| Age of woman | Labor-force-participation rate | | | | 1960 as percent of 1940 | |
| | White | | Nonwhite | | | |
	1960	1940	1960	1940	White	Nonwhite
All married women with husband present	29.8	12.5	40.5	27.3	238	148
14-17 years	16.2	4.1	18.1	13.5	395	134
18-19 years	29.6	8.7	25.7	18.6	340	138
20-24 years	30.8	16.2	34.0	25.7	190	132
25-29 years	25.7	17.1	38.2	31.1	150	123
30-34 years	27.6	16.3	43.0	31.8	169	135
35-44 years	35.4	13.8	48.7	30.5	257	160
45-54 years	38.6	10.1	47.2	25.5	382	185
55-64 years	24.6	6.4	33.6	19.3	384	174
65-74 years	7.4	2.7	12.7	10.7	274	119
75 & over	2.9	1.1	6.5	4.7	264	138

Source: U.S. Bureau of the Census, U.S. Census of Population: 1960, Subject Reports, Employment and Work Experience, Final Report PC(2)-6A, table 6.

The increases in worker rates between 1940 and 1960 for married women aged 25 to 29 — 50 percent for white women and 23 percent for nonwhite women — were among the smallest for each color group, and yet they were still remarkably high in view of the large simultaneous increase in childbearing by women of this age group. These substantial relative increases were possible partly because the 1940 worker rates were so small. Even in 1960, the rates amounted to only 26 per 100 white, and 38 per 100 nonwhite, married women. This still leaves much room for additional increase in the worker rates for married women in the age group 25 to 29, if adequate means of caring for their children are found. At any rate, an increasing proportion of mothers of even quite young children have already decided that caring for their own children is not a full-time job for them.

The most striking changes of all, however, were the increases in labor-force-participation rates for married women in the middle years of life. These changes shifted the peak years of employment for married women of both color groups from the age bracket 25 to 34 years in 1940 to 35 to 54 years in 1960. For married women around 50, the worker rate for white women nearly quadrupled in the two decades and that for their nonwhite counterparts nearly doubled. Moreover, the elongation of working life for married women shifted upward by ten years the point in the upper age span where the worker rate dips below the average for all ages; this point was being reached at about age 45 in 1940 but rose to about 55 in 1960.

These changes reflect a marked increase in the tendency for married white women to return to work during a number of years after their children are in or through school and for married nonwhite women increasingly to work well into middle age. They also reflect a sharply increasing degree of employability of women in their middle years, partly because more of them were trained to perform needed skills and partly because more of them had already had work experience and were therefore confident that they could re-enter the labor market. Furthermore, an increasing proportion of the less employable women in their middle and upper years have evidently contributed indirectly to the growing employment of younger married women by caring for their grandchildren while their (younger, better-educated, and otherwise more employable) daughters or daughters-in-law have gone to work. Women of upper middle age may experience increasing difficulty in finding and keeping acceptable work as young women, born during or after the postwar fertility crest, compete with them for the available positions.

Rates among mothers of young children. Women with husbands 35 to 44 years old are singled out in Table 7.5 for a fuller discussion of their employment in relation to the presence, age, and average num-

Table 7.5. Absence of own children and average number of own children of specified age in the home, for husband-wife families with head 35 to 44 years old, by color: United States, 1960

Husband-wife families with head 35-44 by age of own children	Percent with no own children of specified age			Average number of own children of specified age		
	Total	White	Nonwhite	Total	White	Nonwhite
Any age	12.2	11.2	22.9	2.75	2.69	3.56
Under 18 years	14.0	12.9	26.3	2.68	2.62	3.47
Under 6 years	56.8	57.1	54.1	1.50	1.47	1.86

Source: U.S. Bureau of the Census, U.S. Census of Population: 1960, Subject Reports, Families, Final Report PC(2)-4A, table 4.

ber of young children of their own in the home. While married women are in this age group, they usually make the critical decision as to whether they should start to work (or return to work) outside the home.

The left half of the table makes two important points. First, twice as large a proportion of nonwhite as white families are childless, in the sense that they had no children of their own under 18 in the home in 1960 (26 versus 13 percent). Fertility experts explain that this difference is caused to some degree by the higher incidence of certain types of venereal disease among Negroes than whites, but perhaps to greater degree by other factors — for example, higher Negro than white infant-mortality rates, and more of a tendency among young Negroes to "farm out" their children to grandparents or other near relatives or to have no children at all because their presence would interfere with the parents' upward social mobility. Second, despite the first point made here, as large a proportion of nonwhite as white families continue to have preschool-age children in the home while the husband is 35 to 44 years of age; this fact is the net effect of several factors, including, on the one hand, much higher fertility rates among nonwhites than whites during their thirties and, on the other hand, the greater tendency for the nonwhite children to be dispersed or to die.[3]

The right half of the table may seem contradictory to the first point made above, but it is not. This part of the table shows that nonwhite families have more children, on the average, than white families. Because of the more extensive childlessness of nonwhite families, this differential is even greater when it applies to families with children than when it applies to all families.

The next table shows how the presence of young children affects the extent of employment of married women 35 to 44 years old. From Table 7.6 it can be seen that white married women with husband present in 1960 were about twice as likely to be employed full time during the census week — or to be unemployed — if they had no children of their own in the home than if they had some. For nonwhite women, the corresponding proportion was one and one-half times. However, within each color group, the women were about as likely to work part time whether they did or did not have young children in the home. And, within each color group, the women were roughly half again as likely not to be in the labor force if they had young children than if they had none. The proportions of women with

Table 7.6. Full-time and part-time employment of married women 35 to 44 years old with husband present, by presence of own children under 18 years old and color: United States, 1960

Employment status	Percent distribution						Percent with own children under 18	
	Total		No own children under 18		With own children under 18			
	White	Nonwhite	White	Nonwhite	White	Nonwhite	White	Nonwhite
Married women 35-44 with husband present	100.0	100.0	100.0	100.0	100.0	100.0	82.7	68.5
During census week:								
Employed	33.8	45.7	51.3	55.5	30.0	40.7	73.8	59.3
Full time	24.0	30.2	42.1	37.9	20.6	26.3	71.0	57.9
Part time	9.9	15.4	9.2	17.9	9.6	14.4	80.6	62.0
Unemployed	1.6	3.2	2.5	4.0	1.4	2.8	73.3	58.1
Not in labor force	64.6	51.1	46.3	40.5	68.4	56.5	87.6	73.4
During 1959:								
Worked full year	17.6	22.4	33.2	29.2	14.4	19.0	67.5	56.3
Worked part year	24.0	33.6	27.8	35.7	23.2	32.6	80.0	64.4
Did not work	58.4	44.0	39.0	35.1	62.4	48.4	88.5	73.2

Source: U.S. Bureau of the Census, U.S. Census of Population: 1960, Subject Reports, Employment and Work Experience, Final Report PC(2)-6A, tables 4, 8, 12, and 18.

children, therefore, were significantly higher for those not in the labor force or working part time than for those employed full time or unemployed. The similarity of the pattern with respect to presence of children for unemployed married women and that for women with full-time work suggests that most of the unemployed women were looking for full-time work.

The proportions of married women who worked full year, part year, and not at all in 1959 show approximately the same relationships between those with and without young children as described above for married women who worked full time, part time, and not at all during the census week. Considerably more women worked full time during the census week, however, than worked all of the preceding year. Additional discussion of the presence of children as a factor in the employment of married women is presented in relation to Table 7.9.

Rates among ethnic groups. Variations in the employment of women 35 to 44 years old in the United States by color, race, and national origin are presented in Table 7.7. The data relate to women of all marital-status categories combined, because statistics for this age group were not available for women who were married and living with their husband; accordingly, they show somewhat higher percentages employed than corresponding figures in the preceding table. In this age group, however, the percent married is at or near the

Table 7.7. Percent employed, for women 35 to 44 years old, by color, race, and national origin: United States, 1960

Color or race	Percent employed	Employment index	National origin (second generation)	Percent employed	Employment index
Women 35-44 years old	40.5	100	Irish	40.6	100
			German	40.3	100
Nonwhite	51.7	128			
White	39.2	97	Polish	39.9	99
Japanese	54.3	134	Italian	38.1	94
Negro	52.5	130			
Chinese	49.1	121	Russian	36.2	89
Filipino	37.7	93			
American Indian	27.5	68	Mexican	31.3	77

Source: U.S. Bureau of the Census, U.S. Census of Population: 1960, Detailed Characteristics, United States Summary, Final Report PC(1)-1D, table 195; Subject Reports, Nativity and Parentage, Final Report PC(2)-1A, tables 7 and 13; and Nonwhite Population by Race, Final Report PC(2)-1C, tables 37-41.

maximum. Statistics for women of foreign stock whose origins were in certain countries are more heavily weighted by those of the first-generation stock and others by those of the second generation. To reduce this source of heterogeneity, the figures for women of foreign stock are limited to native women of foreign or mixed parentage (second generation).

An employment rate well above the general average was recorded for nonwhite women, largely because of the high percent employed for Negro women, although the percentages for Japanese and Chinese women were also quite high. All three groups have had a history of relatively high employment at work outside the home. The particularly low employment rates for Mexican and Indian women reflect their high fertility rates, coupled with such other factors as below-average employability because of low educational levels, extensive rural residence, and general inaccessibility to the labor market.

Recent changes in employment rates for the several ethnic groups are featured in Table 7.8. The relevant data are available from the 1950 census only for women 25 to 44 years old. For these women, the percent employed increased from 31.9 percent in 1950 to 37.0 percent in 1960. Dividing 37.0 by 31.9 gives the index of change, 116.

Employment rates for both white and Negro women increased about

Table 7.8. Percent employed, for women 25 to 44 years old, by color, race, and national origin: United States, 1960, and change 1950 to 1960

Color or race	Percent employed in 1960	Index of change, 1950-60	National origin (second generation)	Percent employed in 1960	Index of change, 1950-60
Women 25-44 years old	37.0	116	Mexican	30.2	132
			Russian	33.0	122
White	35.6	117			
Nonwhite	47.8	111	German	37.3	118
Filipino	37.5	160	Polish	37.4	105
Chinese	46.0	148			
American Indian	25.4	139	Italian	35.6	104
Negro	48.7	112			
Japanese	45.2	98	Irish	38.2	101

Source: U.S. Bureau of the Census, U.S. Census of Population: 1960, Detailed Characteristics, United States Summary, Final Report PC(1)-1D, table 195; Subject Reports, Nativity and Parentage, Final Report PC(2)-1A, tables 7 and 13; and Nonwhite Population by Race, Final Report PC(2)-1C, tables 37-41; also 1950 Census of Population, Vol. IV, Part 3, Chapter A, Nativity and Parentage, tables 10 and 20, and Chapter B, Nonwhite Population by Race, tables 9-13.

5 percentage points during the 1950's; the effect was to show a greater relative gain for white women but to leave Negro women at the top of the list of 1960 employment rates. This high employment rate for Negro women can be better understood in the perspective that unemployment rates are high for Negro men. Among nonwhite families in 1960 with the wife of the head an employed mother (with one or more children under 6 years of age) and with an adult in the family who was not employed (hence a potential baby-sitter), nearly one-half of the husbands were not employed.[4]

Some of the smallest relative changes in the employment rates were made by women of national origins which are predominantly Roman Catholic (Irish, Italian, and Polish). Women with these backgrounds tend to have higher fertility rates than other women in areas of comparable urbanization.

All ethnic groups with indexes of change in the employment rate during the 1950's which exceeded the national average, 116, had lower employment rates than the national average at the beginning of the period, 31.9 percent. On the other hand, all ethnic groups with indexes below 116 had higher employment rates than the national average in 1950. These observations demonstrate a tendency for employment rates among women of various ethnic groups to converge toward a common level.

The employment rates in 1960 for American Indian and second-generation Mexican women were still only one-half to two-thirds as high as those for groups with the highest rates (Negro, Chinese, and Japanese). Not only are birth rates among Indian and Mexican Americans very high, but the literacy rate is relatively low. The close relation between amount of education and worker rates will be apparent in the next section.

Rates by educational level. Among women 35 to 54 years of age (when most women are married but have no infants to care for), there was a strong positive correlation between amount of education and percentage of women who worked during 1959. The pattern is somewhat more complex, however, when those who worked all year and those who worked part of the year are considered separately. For both white and nonwhite women, the following patterns emerge:[5]

Full-year work rates were —
    Lowest for those with 0–7 years of school
    Highest for those with 12–15 years of school;
Part-year work rates were —
    Lowest for those with no years of school
    Highest for those with 16 or more years of school;
"No-work" rates for the year were —
    Lowest for those with 16 or more years of school
    Highest for those with no years of school.

Within this framework the fact remains that about one-half to three-fourths of the white women 35 to 54 years old with varying amounts of education below college graduation reported having worked gainfully in no week during the calendar year before the 1960 census. This observation reveals a vast reservoir of additional workers in the event of a national emergency. Moreover, to the extent that these non-working women change their life patterns and choose to work at least part of the year, and can find appropriate employment, they are in a position to raise the living standards of the population considerably.

Rates by income of the husband. Married women in 1963 were least likely to be in the labor force if their husbands were in a relatively

Table 7.9. Labor-force-participation rate of married women with husband present, by income of husband in 1962, age of woman, and presence and age of own children in the home: United States, 1963

Age of wife and presence and age of children	Percent of wives in the labor force, by income of husband in 1962				
	Total	Under $3,000	$3,000-$4,999	$5,000-$6,999	$7,000 & over
All wives	33.7	33.5	36.9	36.1	28.1
No children under 18 years	37.4	31.1	40.7	43.8	38.3
14-34 years	58.7	51.2	60.5	62.4	59.4
35-54 years	51.9	57.0	54.7	52.2	44.8
55 & over	20.7	17.7	21.3	25.0	25.4
Children 6 to 17 years only	41.5	49.2	45.8	45.0	31.9
Children under 6 years	22.5	28.7	26.5	22.6	14.9

Source: U.S. Bureau of Labor Statistics, Special Labor Force Report No. 40, table L.

high income bracket ($7,000 or more), as indicated in Table 7.9 and Figure 7.1 (see also Columns 1 and 2 of Table 7.20). Moreover, married women who had young children of their own at home were most likely to be in the labor force if their husbands were in a low income bracket (under $3,000). Within this general framework, however, there were some crosscurrents in the patterns, particularly for married women in the several age ranges who had no young children at home.

Wives with no children of their own at home tended, overall, to be more likely to work as the amount of their husband's income increased. This generalization held true most consistently for women 55 and over, whose worker rates were low throughout. For this age group, wives who had no children at home and whose husbands had low incomes probably included the maximum proportion with few if any marketable skills, whereas those whose husbands' incomes were above average were not only likely to have more talent for doing paid work but also to have prospects of performing more interesting tasks on the job and of continuing to do so until the usual retirement age.

Wives 35 to 54 years old with no children at home had the contrary pattern, wherein worker rates for the wife varied inversely with the income of the husband. In this group the maximum worker rate was recorded for women with husbands in the so-called poverty level. These women were still young enough to find employment readily,

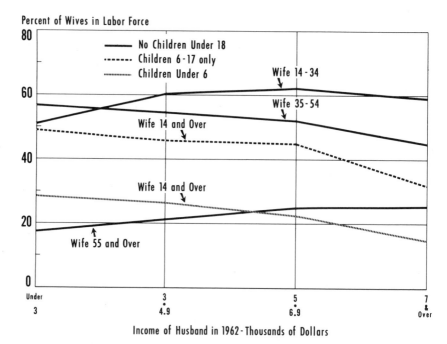

Percent of Wives in Labor Force

Fig. 7.1. Percent of wives working, by age of wife, presence of children, and income of husband: United States, 1963

Source: Table 7.9.

especially in view of the much higher educational level of women aged 35 to 54 than of those aged 55 and over.

Childless wives under 35 years of age had the highest labor-force-participation rates — around 60 percent — perhaps largely because they had more education and had no children to encumber them. In addition, however, it may be that the social contacts they made while working increased their enjoyment of outside work and provided a source for learning about how to prevent having children until the propitious time occurred, and how to space them after that.

Married mothers with children of school age but with no pre-schoolers had labor-force-participation rates nearly as high as those for women of roughly comparable age (35 to 54 years old) with no young children, at each level of the husband's income below $7,000. Moreover, childless wives 14 to 34 years old had far higher worker rates than the roughly comparable age group with children (those with children under 6); the rates for childless women ranged from about 22 percentage points higher where the husband's income was low to 44 percentage points higher where his income was high.

Married mothers with children of preschool age were only about one-half as likely to work as mothers with children of school age only, for the obvious reason that very young children require more care. Perhaps the most relevant consideration is that as many as 22.5 percent of the mothers of preschool-age children in 1963 managed to find nursery care or to make other arrangements for their children while they worked. For married couples with young children of either preschool or school level, there was a negative relationship between the employment of the mother and the amount of the husband's income. This relationship was moderate where the income was under $7,000, but a distinctly smaller proportion of mothers worked where their husband's income was above $7,000.

Rates by income of the wife and family. The typical effect of having the wife as an earner of money income is to elevate the family's total income toward the middle — but not the top — of the range. About 36.5 percent of all wives of family heads earned money from employment in 1959, although about 40 percent of all wives worked during that year. The difference represents those whose jobs consisted of unpaid work on the family farm or in the family business. The peak proportions of families with the wife as an earner occurred where the family income was between $6,000 and $15,000; within this range, 45 to 50 percent of the wives were earners (see source of Table 7.10). The proportion of family income contributed by earning wives varies widely from one income level to another but falls into a pattern which, in a number of respects, resembles the relationship between the education of women and their work experience in 1959.

Among the lower-income families, a relatively large proportion of the wives earned only a small part of the total family income. At the same time, a slightly larger than average proportion of the wives in these lower-income families earned more than half of the family income. Among families with incomes of $6,000 but less than $8,000, the proportion of wives in each of the three categories was close to the average for all families.

Among families with upper incomes but not the highest (that is, between $8,000 and $15,000), by far the largest proportion (65 percent) of the wives earned a substantial minority (one-fifth to one-half) of the family income, and relatively small proportions of wives

Table 7.10. Percent of wives earning given percent of family income, for husband-wife families with the wife an earner, by family income and work experience of head in 1959: United States, 1960

Family income and work experience of head in 1959	Number of families (000's)	Percent of wives earning given percent of family income			
		Total	Under 20 percent	20-49 percent	50 & over
Husband-wife families with the wife an earner	14,484	100.0	38.8	49.0	12.3
Head worked in 1959	13,778	100.0	39.8	50.0	10.2
Family income in 1959:					
Under $2,000	604	100.0	42.2	35.2	22.6
$2,000-$3,999	1,680	100.0	48.9	33.1	17.9
$4,000-$5,999	2,985	100.0	49.2	38.0	12.8
$6,000-$7,999	3,330	100.0	39.6	51.8	8.7
$8,000-$9,999	2,441	100.0	28.1	65.2	6.8
$10,000-$14,999	2,169	100.0	29.3	65.3	5.3
$15,000 & over	570	100.0	51.8	44.1	4.2
Head did not work in 1959	707	100.0	19.5	28.2	52.2

Source: U.S. Bureau of the Census, U.S. Census of Population: 1960, Subject Reports, Sources and Structure of Family Income, Final Report PC(2)-4C, table 14.

were in either of the other categories of earners. This family-income level, therefore, has an earner pattern for wives which resembles the work-experience pattern for wives who are high-school graduates or who have attended college but are not college graduates; wives in this group include an especially large proportion of full-year workers.

Among families with top incomes ($15,000 and over) and with the wife as an earner, the maximum proportion of wives earned only a small part of the family income and the minimum proportion earned a majority of the family income. Wives in this income level probably include many, if not most, of the women noted above as college graduates working part of the year.

Families at this top income level, however, had a below-average proportion of wives who were earners (only 29 percent; see source note of Table 7.10). Adding this fact to the knowledge that a little over one-half of the wives at this level earned less than one-fifth of the family income yields the broader perspective that actually 86 percent of all wives at this income level earned less than one-fifth of their family's total income. Curiously, it is equally true that, among families with less than $6,000, when wives earning less than one-fifth of the family's income are combined with wives who were not earners at all, fully 87 percent earned less than one-fifth of the total income for their families.

In contrast with these top and bottom family-income groups stand those in the $8,000 to $15,000 level; among these families, 78 percent of all wives earned less than one-fifth of the family income. The complements of these percentages make an even sharper contrast; about one-eighth of the wives in the top and bottom family income levels earned 20 percent or more of the family income in 1959, whereas nearly one-fourth of those in the upper-but-not-top level earned 20 percent or more.

Among families with the head 65 years old and over, a majority of the husbands do not work. And, as Table 7.10 shows, 52 percent of the earning wives earned one-half or more of the family income in those 707,000 families where the head (of any age) did not work during the preceding year.

During the decade before 1960, the rate of increase in the employment of wives had been largest among families in the middle range of family income. Thus, according to data from the Current Population Survey,[6] the trend line of the percent of husband-wife families with the wife in the paid labor force rose about one-fifth between 1949 and 1960 among families in the lowest quintile of family income. The corresponding proportion was nearly one-half among families in the second to fourth quintiles and about one-third among those in the highest quintile. These changes indicate a recent accentuation of the differentials discussed before in the work patterns of married women.

Occupational Selection Among Married Persons

Occupational concentrations of husbands. The distribution according to major occupational groupings for married men does not change substantially with advancement of age within the range of maximum family responsibility, 25 to 54 years. In fact, it is generally similar to the distribution for all men in the corresponding age groupings because married men constitute so large a proportion of the total within the age range (about seven out of eight for white men and three out of four for nonwhite).

Among white husbands aged 25 to 54 years, approximately one-fourth are craftsmen (skilled workers); one-fifth are operatives (semi-skilled workers — largely in factories); one-eighth are managers, officials, or proprietors; one-eighth are professional or technical workers; and the remaining three-tenths are scattered among the other categories, with the majority salesmen, clerks, or farm workers. Among nonwhites, the proportions are somewhat higher for the lower-status occupations and lower for the upper-status occupations.

To some extent, the selective factors that determine which men will marry and remain married evidently also help to determine which occupations married men have entered. Among married men 25 to 54 years old living with their wives, the following patterns emerged in 1960:

Men are *especially* likely to be married if they are employed as:
Farmers (if married only once)
Managers, officials, or proprietors (if married only once)
Craftsmen
Operatives (if nonwhite).
Men are *less* likely to be married if they are employed as:
Clerical workers (if white)
Private household workers (*much* less likely)
Other service workers (if married only once)
Laborers, except farm and mine (if white)
Farm laborers (if white, or if nonwhite and married only once).

In addition, at some ages men were especially likely to be married if they were employed as professional or technical workers (if married only once). The occupations in which married men are more likely to be employed are the kinds into which young men tend to shift as they become more mature. For instance, clerical workers may develop into managers or officials, and (now more rarely) farm laborers may eventually become farmers.

A tabulation of persons in the approximately 450 detailed occupations recognized in the 1960 census was made by marital status and sex but was not cross-classified further by age. Each occupation in this list was examined to determine whether it contained at least 50,000 "working men" (men in the experienced civilian labor force) and whether the proportion of men married with wife present was either 10 or more percentage points above or a like amount below that for the total 14 years old and over in all occupations combined (76.7 percent). For a selection of the occupations which met these criteria, and for the total in each major occupation group, the results are presented in Table 7.11. In the absence of a cross-classification by age, and in recognition of the fundamental importance of age for a fuller understanding of some of the occupations, the median age of all men in the occupational category is also shown. Aside from the major occupation groups, no occupation listed for men included as many as 5 percent of the entire 46 million men in the experienced civilian labor force.

Table 7.11. Percent married, wife present, and median age, for men in the experienced civilian labor force in selected occupations: United States, 1960

Occupation	Percent married, wife present	Median age	Occupation	Percent married, wife present	Median age
Working men, 14 & over	76.7	40.5	Craftsmen, foremen	85.3	41.9
Professional, tech. workers	81.3	38.2	Cranemen, derrickmen	88.4	41.9
Dentists	90.8	45.9	Foremen	92.6	44.7
Technical engineers	88.4	38.3	Inspectors	86.9	44.6
Lawyers, judges	86.9	45.3	Linemen, servicemen (tel.)	87.4	33.7
Musicians, music teachers	64.4	36.2	Locomotive engineers	90.8	54.2
Personnel, labor relations wkrs.	88.2	41.2	Millwrights	92.5	45.0
Physicians, surgeons	87.6	43.1	Plumbers, pipe fitters	87.4	42.6
			Stationary engineers	88.8	44.0
Farmers, farm managers	84.3	49.2	Toolmakers, die setters	88.3	42.3
Mgrs., officials, prop'rs.	90.2	45.4			
Banking & other finance	89.4	52.2	Operatives, kindred workers	77.5	38.2
Public-admin. officials	89.1	48.3	Apprentices	49.4	22.9
Purchasing agents, buyers	89.4	42.2	Attendants, auto service	52.4	25.3
Other--salaried	90.2	43.3	Brakemen, railroad	86.6	41.0
Other--self-employed	91.1	48.2	Oilers, greasers (exc. auto)	58.9	41.1
Clerical, kindred workers	70.9	37.9	Private hsld. workers	36.7	46.9
Cashiers	47.0	26.7	Service workers, other	66.7	43.3
Messengers, office boys	32.8	23.7	Attendants, hosp. & instit.	61.6	37.1
Office-machine operators	63.7	28.1	Cooks, exc. priv. hsld.	62.6	43.0
Stock clerks, storekeepers	63.3	34.6	Porters	60.7	43.4
Trade clerks	65.6	35.6	Firemen, fire protection	90.5	38.6
Finance, insur., real estate	61.5	34.7	Policemen, detectives	89.5	38.2
			Waiters	45.1	34.6
Sales workers	75.1	39.1			
Insurance agents, brokers	89.8	40.2	Farm laborers & foremen	44.4	31.2
Newsboys	5.5	15.7	Laborers, exc. farm & mine	63.6	37.2
Real-estate agents	86.9	50.4	Garage laborers	46.8	26.0
Salesmen: Manufacturing	88.0	40.2	Lumbermen, raftsmen	67.4	36.6
Salesmen: Wholesale trade	88.3	41.4	Construction, trade, railroad	60.2	37.2
Salesmen: Retail trade	69.7	38.3			

Source: U.S. Bureau of the Census, U.S. Census of Population: 1960, Subject Reports, Occupational Characteristics, Final Report PC(2)-7A, tables 6 and 12.

Some of the occupations within the category "managers, officials, and proprietors, including farm," had especially high percentages of married men with wife present. In addition, nearly all the detailed professional and technical titles were associated with high percentages of married men. The notable exception is musicians and music teachers, among whom the percent single was especially high, indicating a heavy weighting of young men in the profession. Musicians also had by far the highest percent divorced among the groups with 50,000 or more, suggesting that the way of life among musicians is hardly con-ducive to stability of marriage.

White-collar workers with the largest percentages of intact mar-riages tended to include men with positions which demand the great-est degree of public trust and confidence as well as the highest degree of training and skill. Some of the occupations conspicuously absent from the list by these criteria are those for which money income tends to be relatively low, whereas most of those listed as having a high proportion currently married are high-income positions. Among those absent are clergymen, who have one of the highest proportions single because of the inclusion of celibate priests; college teachers, who in-clude many single instructors and graduate assistants; and male ele-mentary-school teachers and technicians, for whom the percent single is also high.

White-collar workers outside the professional and managerial fields who had high percentages married with wife present were concen-trated among sales workers in high-income fields — insurance agents, real-estate agents, and salesmen in the manufacturing and wholesale trade industries. On the other hand, all the categories shown for clerical workers (who are also regarded as white-collar workers) were selected because of their low proportion married. Here the factor of age enters conspicuously, as it does in most extreme form in the "newsboy" category under sales workers. Other factors, in addition, such as educational background and certain more or less typical per-sonal characteristics, may also help to account for the low percent married among clerical workers.

"Craftsmen and foremen" tend to include the (occupationally) most talented and the (financially) most successful manual workers. It is perhaps not surprising, therefore, to find the percent of men married and living with a wife higher by far in this group than in any of the other manual-worker groups. The kinds of work performed by men in these occupations probably tend to yield more personal satis-factions and absorb the attention more fully than the jobs done by men in the other manual occupations. Not only would one expect these intrinsically satisfying positions to leave the workmen in a better frame of mind to enjoy his married life, but conversely the workman with a stable married life might be expected to have his mind in better condition to meet the more delicate demands of highly skilled work.

Among the other manual workers and the service workers, there are a few occupational types with a high proportion of married men in relatively stable positions — notably railroad brakemen, firemen, and policemen — and a very large number not shown in the list with marital-status distributions close to that for all men combined. Occupations at this level tend to be filled by persons of below-average amounts of education and by young or old men.

Members of the Armed Forces are classified as service workers, but Table 7.11 is limited to civilians. In 1960, 55 percent of the men on military duty in the United States were married, according to table 4 in the source of Table 7.1. Moreover, 49 percent of those stationed abroad were married (table 48, U.S. Summary, Volume 1 of the 1960 census). Between 1960 and 1968, the strength of the Armed Forces rose by about one million men, largely in their late teens and early twenties; meantime, the proportion of military men who were married fell by about 5 percentage points, according to information from the Defense Department. However, the typical period of military duty is only two or three years, and many men marry before or during their military service. Therefore, the effect of the expansion of the Armed Forces on the marital status distribution of the male population as a whole has been minimal.

Farm operators and farm managers had a relatively high percent married, wife present, despite their rather high average age and their quite low average income. Additional evidence of the quality of married life among farmers is the fact that, in 1960, they had consistently the lowest percentages at each age level who were separated or divorced or who had remarried — and a below-average percent widowed at nearly every age. The corresponding symptoms of family stability were not found among farm laborers and farm foremen. These men, unlike farmers, generally lack a joint economic enterprise with their wives. They probably also tend to measure up less favorably on those selective factors that determine which farm workers eventually acquire responsibility for running a farm — not the least of which may be the amount of accumulated or inherited wealth.

The statistics for farmers in particular, but to some extent also those for farm laborers, provide strong support for the hypothesis that the combined effect of social pressures against the disruption of marriage in farm communities and the economic needs of the farm (which, in the past at least, have held that the joint productive effort of husband and wife is virtually indispensable) tend to keep such workers from breaking their marriages. Moreover, if they do break (or are inclined to break) their marriages, they probably tend to move away

Table 7.12. Employed married women 25 to 54 years old, husband present, by major occupation group, age, and color: United States, 1960

Major occupation group	White, by age (years)			Nonwhite, by age (years)		
	25-34	35-44	45-54	25-34	35-44	45-54
Employed married women, husband present (percent)	100.0	100.0	100.0	100.0	100.0	100.0
Professional, tech. workers	14.3	11.6	13.9	11.2	8.6	7.7
Mgrs., off'ls., proprs.	2.5	4.2	5.6	1.0	1.5	2.0
Clerical, kindred workers	37.2	31.2	26.4	12.7	9.4	4.5
Sales workers	6.9	10.2	11.8	1.8	2.2	2.1
Craftsmen, foremen	1.1	1.5	1.6	0.7	0.8	0.7
Operatives, kindred workers	19.3	20.6	18.6	15.6	15.2	12.1
Private household workers	1.4	1.5	2.3	24.2	29.7	38.8
Service workers, other	11.3	13.2	13.2	21.8	22.3	21.3
Laborers, exc. farm & mine	0.5	0.5	0.4	0.8	0.7	0.9
Farmers, farm managers	0.3	0.4	0.6	0.3	0.5	0.8
Farm laborers & foremen	1.1	1.2	1.3	2.8	3.0	3.3
Occupation not reported	4.1	3.9	4.3	7.1	6.1	5.8

Source: U.S. Bureau of the Census, U.S. Census of Population: 1960, Subject Reports, Marital Status, Final Report PC(2)-4E, table 5.

from the farm and settle in a nonfarm area — and thereby exaggerate the greater amount of marital instability among nonfarm marriages.

Occupational concentrations of wives. The kind of work done by employed wives varies considerably with age and tends to be quite different for white and nonwhite women. Table 7.12 shows that among employed white women who were married and living with their husband in 1960, the largest proportion of those between 25 and 54 years old (about one-third) were doing clerical work. Of these clerical workers, however, the proportion who were young (hence better educated and more attractive, on the average) was high; it was low for women above age 45. Although the proportion of nonwhite women in the clerical occupations was uniformly far lower than that for white women, the relative concentration of nonwhite clerical workers in the youngest age group shown was especially marked. Among white women, those in the older groups were more likely than those 25 to 34 to do sales or managerial work; of the nonwhites, the older women were considerably more likely than their younger counterparts to do private household work. On balance, the occupational distribution by age in 1960 can be interpreted as evidence that young

wives, both nonwhite and white, have shared in an increasing opportunity to do more demanding yet more interesting types of work
with better pay and more comfortable working conditions.

At each age, the sharpest difference in the occupational patterns by
color was the far heavier concentration of nonwhite wives in private
household work and of white wives in clerical work. The second most
frequent type of work for the nonwhite wives was service work other
than private household work, whereas the second most frequent for
white wives was work as an operative (generally in a factory). At
each age, moreover, the proportion of nonwhite wives engaged in
sales work was only one-third to one-fifth as large as that for white
wives.

Noteworthy is the fact that at the younger ages the percentage of
professional and technical workers among employed nonwhite wives
was nearly as large as that among white wives. Insofar as differences
by age reflect changes over time, the advancement in percent employed as professional or technical workers has been much more
rapid in recent decades for nonwhite than white wives. This fact
stems in part from the increase in demand for school teachers to
match the increase in school enrollment among nonwhite children.
Nonwhite wives also made more progress than white wives in obtaining jobs as operatives. It remains a fact, however, that by 1960 the
proportion of nonwhite wives in the professional, operative, and especially clerical and sales categories had not come up to that of white
wives; even among employed nonwhite wives 25 to 34 years old,
whose educational level compared very well with that of white wives
of the same age, fully 46 percent were still engaged in service work,
as compared with only 13 percent for white wives.

Specific occupations which attract married women or which they
avoid to an exceptional degree are illustrated in Table 7.13. In the
list are all major occupation groups, as well as a selection of occupations reported by at least 5,000 women 14 years old and over in the
experienced civilian labor force in 1960, where the percent married,
husband present, was 10 or more percentage points above or below
the overall average (55.3 percent). As in the corresponding list for
men, the data are available only for white and nonwhite women combined; the median age of all women reporting the occupation is
shown.

The highest percent married and living with husband for any major
occupation group was found among women in the semi-skilled oc-

Table 7.13. Percent married, husband present, and median age, for women in the experienced civilian labor force in selected occupations: United States, 1960

Occupation	Percent married, husband present	Median age	Occupation	Percent married, husband present	Median age
Working women, 14 & over	55.3	40.2	Operatives, kindred workers	65.3	40.9
Professional, tech. workers	53.4	41.1	Assemblers	67.9	39.1
College professors--total	35.3	43.4	Bus drivers	84.5	40.6
College prof.--social science	34.3	45.6	Checkers, inspectors--mfg.	67.4	41.4
Librarians	43.2	45.8	Sewers, stitchers--mfg.	68.4	42.3
Recreation, group workers	40.2	33.8	Spinners--textile	76.4	42.3
Religious workers	25.8	45.5	Welders, flame cutters	66.6	36.5
Teachers, priv. elem. school	37.5	41.8	Pottery mfg.	72.8	42.1
Teachers, priv. sec. school	27.3	46.1	Canning, preserving	69.4	42.3
			Yarn, thread, fabric mfg.	73.6	41.7
Farmers, farm managers	54.7	51.7			
Mgrs., off'ls., proprs.	58.8	47.8	Private household workers	37.2	44.4
Clerical, kindred workers	54.9	35.9	Baby sitters	28.1	24.9
Attendants--library	39.6	31.1	Housekeepers	21.2	53.4
File clerks	44.1	29.8	Other	41.4	45.1
Postal clerks	68.4	45.2			
Ticket, station, express agts.	37.5	29.8	Service workers, other	54.7	41.4
			Bartenders	66.0	42.4
Sales workers	61.8	43.1	Elevator operators	42.2	38.3
Demonstrators	85.2	38.8	Housekeepers, stewards	40.8	51.3
Hucksters, peddlers	81.8	41.3	Watchmen--crossing	82.6	41.9
Real-estate agents	67.6	48.7			
Retail trade--food, dairy	67.9	43.2	Farm laborers & foremen	65.9	39.6
			Unpaid family workers	83.0	42.8
Craftsmen, foremen	59.6	43.2	Laborers, exc. farm & mine	52.5	38.1
Upholsterers	71.7	42.0	Nonmanufacturing	44.3	37.7

Source: U.S. Bureau of the Census, U.S. Census of Population: 1960, Subject Reports, Occupational Characteristics, Final Report PC(2)-7A, tables 6 and 12.

cupations identified as "operatives." Other occupational groupings qualifying for inclusion on the list which show higher-than-average percentages married are "managerial and sales workers," "craftsmen," and "farm laborers." Except for the farm laborers, these groups of women had in common, among other things, the fact that their median ages were above the general level (40.2) for working women in all occupations combined.

High percentages married, moreover, appear to be typical of women in occupations demanding special nonprofessional skills and the assumption of a high degree of responsibility, or involving the promotion of a family business. For example, special skills are demanded of women in such white-collar (usually high-salaried) positions as demonstrators and real-estate agents, in such (less high-salaried) jobs as retail food sales clerks, and in such blue-collar jobs as upholsterers, assemblers, bus drivers, factory inspectors, textile operatives, welders, and pottery makers. Some of these categories, notably demonstrators and bus drivers, are characterized by part-time work for women. Positions in the service trades requiring only a moderate degree of skill but calling for trust and reliability (to which stable married life might bear testimony) include bartenders and crossing watchmen. Women peddlers often sell goods produced by their husbands, and those who serve as unpaid workers on a family farm or in a family business are likewise usually engaged in a sort of occupational partnership with their husbands. All of these occupations are characterized by above-average median age of the women workers, except for demonstrators, assemblers, and welders — specialties in which the alertness of relatively young women would generally be a marked asset.

The lowest percent married and living with husband was that for women who were private household workers, all detailed categories of which likewise had low percentages married. These occupational groups included women of extreme ages — young baby sitters and relatively old housekeepers. The major occupation group with the lowest average age was the clerical group. Moreover, all detailed clerical occupations listed with low percentages married were associated with low average ages. Some of these detailed occupations tend to be preparatory for more responsible positions — for example, library attendants who may mature into librarians, and file clerks or ticket agents who may ultimately grow into a managerial or official position. Recreation and group workers, among the professional workers with a low percent married, tend also to be young, inasmuch as their work demands relatively vigorous physical activity.

All of the other professional workers listed with a low percent married were above the average age of working women in general, and all were women in career positions — college professors, librarians, teachers in private elementary and secondary schools, and religious workers. The low percent married among the private-school teachers and religious workers seems to be a consequence of the fact that women in these positions include many Catholic nuns.

A low percent married and a relatively young average age were also found among women in occupations involving manual labor in nonmanufacturing industries; among such women the percent "married, husband absent" (perhaps largely separated) and single was higher than the average for all women. This is a category with a larger proportion of nonwhite than white women. Likewise heavily weighted with nonwhite women are elevator operators, who tend to be relatively young and to have a low percent married; large numbers of these women are reported as separated, divorced, and widowed.

Occupations of spouses of professional workers. The relationship between the type of work performed by husbands and wives when both work outside the home tends to reflect the amount of education each has obtained, the types of occupations which draw men and women into close proximity during working hours, and the values which persons employed in a particular occupation tend to attach to persons of the opposite sex who are employed in a given occupation. Thus the pairing of marital partners who are in particular occupations may have arisen out of circumstances surrounding their original meeting or out of such other considerations as the type of work a man in an elevated position will "let" his wife do, or the type of work she considers appropriate for her to do. In the extreme case, the wives of men in some occupations appear to choose — or to be under pressure from their husbands — almost never to work; yet wives of men in other occupations seem attracted — or encouraged by their husbands — to be in the paid labor force.

Evidence related to these hypotheses can be found with respect to persons who were in one of the professional or technical occupations at the time of the 1960 census; corresponding data were not tabulated for persons in other occupational groups. The data relate to the experienced civilian labor force and are shown in Table 7.14.

The listings in the first column include most of the professional occupations in which 50,000 or more husbands were engaged in 1960. The listings in the second column show occupations of wives which

Table 7.14. Summary of types of work wives are more likely or less likely to do if their husbands are in specified types of professional work: United States, 1960

Having a husband in the following type of professional work	Increases the chances of the wife's being in the following type of work[a]	Decreases the chances of the wife's being in the following type of work[b]
In general	Professional, clerical	Sales, manual, service
Accountant, auditor	Clerical, sales	Professional
Clergyman	Service	Managerial, clerical, sales
College professor	Professional	Cler., sales, manual, service
Dentist		Prof., mgrl., cler., sales, man., serv.
Draftsman	Clerical, sales, manual, service	Professional
Elec., mech., sales engineer		Professional, mgrl., manual, service
Industrial engineer	Sales, manual	Professional, service
Lawyer, judge	Mgrl, not in labor force	Cler., sales, manual, service
Musician, music teacher	Prof., mgrl., sales, manual, service	
Personnel, labor relat. wkr.	Managerial, clerical, sales	Service
Pharmacist		Prof., cler., manual, service
Physician, surgeon	Managerial, sales	Mgrl., cler., sales, manual, service
Salaried	Professional	Mgrl., cler., sales, manual, service
Self-employed	Not in labor force	Prof., mgrl., cler., sales, man., serv.
Teacher, elementary school	Professional, service	Not in labor force
Teacher, secondary school	Professional	Manual, not in labor force
Technician, physical engin.	Clerical, sales, manual, service	Professional, managerial

Source: U.S. Bureau of the Census, U.S. Census of Population: 1960, Subject Reports, Characteristics of Professional Workers, Final Report PC(2)-7E, table 12.

[a]Underlined occupations were at least 50 percent above the expected.

[b]Underlined occupations were less than 50 percent of the expected.

were at least 20 percent more frequent than expected on the basis of the distribution of all working wives of professional men; underlined occupations were at least 50 percent above the expected. The third column lists corresponding occupations of wives at least 20 percent less frequent than expected; underlined occupations were less than 50 percent of the expected.

Married men in the professional and technical occupations, as anticipated, were much *more* likely to be married to a working wife who was also in one of the professional or technical occupations than they would be if the selection of occupation were by chance, and much *less* likely to be married to a working wife doing manual or service work. Moreover, these professional men were more likely to be married to a working wife in a clerical position and less likely to be married to one in a sales position. In 1960 the proportion of wives of professional men not in the labor force at all during the week before the census was about the same as that for wives in general (about 70 percent). In addition, extremely few professional men were married to farm workers; hence no listing was made of wives doing farm work.

Within this general framework, however, there is considerable variation in the relationship between the occupations of husbands and those of their wives. For instance, professional men with wives also in the professions were most likely to be in the teaching profession or salaried physicians. Also, as will be shown later, nearly one-half of the married men in the teaching profession with working wives in 1960 were, in fact, married to teachers. Salaried physicians were more likely than self-employed physicians and surgeons to be young and probably much more likely to be married to a wife who was working as a professional nurse.

At the same time, among professional men, those in teaching positions were most likely to have working wives. Most of these wives, as well as most of their husbands, were no doubt college graduates; the high correlation between college education and employment of women has been well documented above. Large proportions of men with working wives were found among elementary, secondary, and music teachers — groups known for their relatively low salaries.[7]

By contrast, among professional men, self-employed physicians and surgeons were unique for their high proportion with wives not in the labor force. Relatively high proportions, but below the standards for inclusion in Table 7.14, were also found for dentists and electrical, mechanical, and sales engineers. Many of the wives of men in these professions undoubtedly obtain their satisfaction in the performance of civic and philanthropic service, or in types of unpaid activity which do not involve a service motive, or in some combination of these activities. Pharmacists included an especially large proportion with wives engaged in sales work, presumably quite often in the family's own pharmaceutical business.

Close scrutiny of the table shows an affinity between occupations of the husband and wife in many, if not most, instances. Accountants tend to marry clerical and sales workers; clergymen tend to marry service workers. Likewise, draftsmen and technicians tend to marry clerical workers, industrial engineers tend to marry sales workers, and all these groups tend to marry manual workers — a fact which may reflect a lower prestige level of these occupations as compared with most of the other categories listed.

Table 7.15 Summary of types of work husbands are more likely or less likely to do if their wives are in specified types of professional work: United States, 1960

Having a wife in the following type of professional work	Increases the chances of the husband's being in the following type of work	Decreases the chances of the husband's being in the following type of work
In general	Prof., clerical, sales	Manual, farm
Accountant, auditor	Clerical, manual	Professional, farm
Librarian	Not in labor force	Farm
Musician, music teacher	Professional, managerial	Manual, service
Professional nurse	Manual, service	Professional, farm
Social & welfare work	Managerial, clerical	Manual, farm
Pub. elem.-school teacher	Farm	
Pub. sec.-school teacher	Professional, farm	Manual, service
Medical & dental tech.	Manual, service	Managerial, farm

Source: U.S. Bureau of the Census, U.S. Census of Population: 1960, Subject Reports, Characteristics of Professional Workers, Final Report PC(2)-7E, table 12.

A similar but briefer analysis is presented in Table 7.15, using the same criteria for inclusion and underlining, but with a reverse perspective — that is, the kinds of work husbands are performing while their wives are engaged in one of the professional occupations in which there were 25,000 or more working wives in 1960. Wives in the professions are, as expected, much more likely than other working wives to be married to a professional man. Professional women are somewhat more likely than other working wives to be married to a clerical or sales worker and somewhat less likely to be married to a manual worker.

Table 7.15 shows a great diversity in the patterns of positive and negative marital selection of wives in the several types of professions, a fact which suggests a substantial scattering of professional wives throughout the spectrum of occupations of husbands.

At the same time, the proportion of the occupations of husbands qualified for listing as an extreme (underlined) variation from the average distribution is larger than it would have been if this list, like the preceding one, had omitted farm husbands. About 4.6 percent of the professional wives were married to farm workers, and yet for about one-half of the professional men's occupations only 0.1 percent of wives were farm workers.

Perhaps surprising in this connection is the observation that wives who were public elementary-school teachers were *much* more likely — and public secondary-school teachers were *somewhat* more likely — to be married to a farm worker than the general distribution of occupations of professional women's husbands would lead one to expect. Evidently there remained in 1960 a conspicuous tendency for relatively well-educated farm wives to be teachers in local elementary schools in rural locations. Because of the trend toward locating secondary schools in the larger towns and cities within the largely rural counties, the proportion of farmers' wives who taught in such schools was not especially pronounced. Outside the teaching field, most of the listed professional occupations of wives were associated with a likelihood that the husbands were *not* farm workers.

It is equally surprising to find that wives who were accountants or auditors, professional nurses, or medical or dental technicians were much more likely to have married a manual worker than would have been expected from a chance distribution of the husbands of professional women. This finding, taken at face value, provides a basis for believing that many women are content to marry men in occupational levels below their own — and many men are content to marry women in occupations above their own. These women may include a disproportionately large number who miscalculated the eventual earning capacity of the men they married but remained with them all the same. The occupations involved are not among those with a large proportion of women who are nonwhite.

Only about one-half as large a proportion of professional husbands, as compared with husbands in general (8 versus 16 percent), were not in the civilian labor force in 1960. This may have been partially a result of the tendency for men in the professions to continue to work into old age. Women who were professional or technical workers in some of the occupational categories were nonetheless married in above-average proportions to men who were not in the labor force — notably wives who were librarians, whose average age was about 5 years above that of other professional women. Among wives who were nurses, welfare workers, or medical technicians, about 5 to 12 percent more than expected were married to men not in the labor force. Many of these wives may have been nonwhite, inasmuch as the proportion of women in health and welfare professions who are nonwhite greatly exceeds that of women in the other professions. Women may often be attracted to these professions because of health or employment problems which directly affect their own kinsmen.

Wives who were in certain positions which involved a great deal of record-keeping, such as accountants, auditors, and welfare workers, ranked high in the proportion of husbands in the more or less closely related lines of managerial or clerical work. Similarly, those who were accountants, auditors, welfare workers, and secondary-school teachers ranked moderately high in proportion married to salesmen, whereas librarians ranked moderately low. At the same time, women who were musicians or teachers at the secondary-school level were relatively unlikely to be married to a husband who was a manual worker or in the service trades.

Occupations of spouses of teachers. The teaching profession probably deserves the distinction of being the leading profession with respect to the proportion of married couples in which both husband and wife are engaged in the same general type of work. However, the teaching profession is the only detailed occupational field for which data in census publications show the detailed occupation of the husband and wife in cross-classification.

At the time of the 1960 census, 76.7 percent of all men in the experienced civilian labor force were married and living with their wife. For men who were professional and technical workers as a whole, the corresponding proportion was somewhat higher, 81.3 percent. Among women workers, the comparable figures were considerably lower, 55.3 and 53.4 percent, respectively; thus, among professional women the proportion "married, spouse present" (MSP) was slightly lower than that for all women. Within this general framework, the

Table 7.16. Percent of teaching married couples by level of school taught by husband and wife, for all couples and nonwhite couples: United States, 1960

Husbands teaching at--	Wives teaching at--			
	All levels	College level	Secondary school	Elementary school
White and nonwhite:				
All levels	100	5	?3	72
College level	15	4	3	8
Secondary school	54	1	17	36
Elementary school	31	0	3	28
Nonwhite:				
All levels	100	5	23	72
College level	10	4	2	4
Secondary school	49	1	15	33
Elementary school	41	0	6	35

Source: U.S. Bureau of the Census, U.S. Census of Population: 1960, Subject Reports, Characteristics of Teachers, Final Report PC(2)-7D, table 6.

well-known fact is worthy of documentation that women teachers at the college level deviate sharply in the direction of a low percentage married (see source of Table 7.16):

Percent of teachers "married, spouse present"

Sex	College level	Secondary school	Elementary school
Men	78.2	81.9	76.9
Women	35.3	53.3	59.4

In all, there were 1,860,000 persons in the teaching profession in 1960, of whom 64.6 percent were MSP. Although men constituted only 41 percent of the 1,201,000 MSP teachers in general, they held 89 percent of the teaching positions at the college level, as compared with only 35 percent of those below the college level which were filled by MSP persons. Compared with wives in general, of whom 31 percent were in the labor force, the wives of teachers included a larger proportion, 43 percent, who were in the labor force. About 92 percent of the husbands of women teachers were in the labor force.

The proportion of "teachers married to teachers," namely 16.3 percent, may not be so large as some would expect, perhaps partly because they overlook the point just made by implication, that 57 percent of the MSP men teachers in 1960 had wives who did not work, and partly because they may be thinking in terms of the proportion of teachers among spouses who are in professional work only. The following summary statement about teaching spouses should place the matter in clearer perspective than a single overall percentage:

16.3 percent of all MSP teachers were married to teachers

22.7 percent of all MSP teachers with working spouses were married to teachers

55.5 percent of all MSP teachers with spouses in *professional* work were married to teachers

47.2 percent of all MSP *men* teachers with working wives were married to teachers and six out of seven of the remainder were married to wives in other white-collar occupations

74.7 percent of MSP *men* teachers with wives in professional work were married to teachers

14.9 percent of all MSP *women* teachers with working husbands were married to teachers and three out of five of the remainder were married to husbands in other white-collar occupations

44.1 percent of all MSP *women* teachers with husbands in professional work were married to teachers.

Additional meaning is given to the analysis when teaching couples alone are considered and when the level of school at which the husband and wife teach is taken into account. A little over 90,000 married couples reported a teaching profession for both the husband and wife specifically at the college, secondary-, or elementary-school level; for approximately 7,000 additional couples, both spouses were classified as teaching, but the level for one or both was not reported. After some minor adjustments in the figures to bring those for husbands and wives into closer agreement, the percentage distribution of 93,900 teaching couples in 1960 shown in Table 7.16 was derived.

The table shows that 72 percent of the wives in teaching couples instructed at the elementary-school level and 54 percent of the husbands at the high-school level. The most frequently occurring combination, accounting for 36 percent of all teaching couples, comprised a husband teaching in secondary (junior- or senior-high) school with a wife teaching in elementary school. In another 28 percent, both taught at the elementary level and in 17 percent at the secondary level. Very few men (3 percent) taught in elementary school while their wives taught in secondary school.

Among fully one-half of the teaching couples with the husband at a college or university, the wife was teaching in an elementary school (8 out of 15 percent); perhaps many of these couples included husbands who were teaching assistants while they were attending graduate school, with wives helping to pay their way until they obtained master's or doctor's degrees.[8] Among the other nearly one-half of the teaching couples with the husband at the college level, the wife was somewhat more likely to be teaching at the college level (4 percent) than at the secondary-school level (3 percent). Among four out of five teaching couples with the wife teaching at the college level, the husband was also teaching at the same level.

The foregoing analysis leads to the summary statement that, among teaching couples, one-half of the teaching husbands in 1960 were instructing at the same level as their wives; and nine out of ten of the remaining teaching husbands were instructing at a higher level than their wives. Among only 4 percent of the teaching couples was the wife instructing at a higher level of school than the husband. To what extent, if any, couples are inclined to disrupt their marriage when the wife's teaching status rises above that of the husband is unknown.

For the approximately 12,500 nonwhite teaching couples in 1960, the general relationship between the teaching levels of husbands and wives is similar to that for all such couples. The percentages of wives teaching at each level were the same as those for all couples, but the percentages of husbands teaching at the college and secondary-school levels were lower, and at the elementary-school level considerably higher, than those for white and nonwhite husbands combined.

Among the noteworthy consequences of the downward scaling of the distribution of nonwhite teaching husbands, as compared with all teaching husbands, is the fact that nonwhite teaching couples displayed a smaller percentage of husbands teaching at the college level with wives teaching at the elementary-school level and a considerably larger percentage of husbands and wives both of whom were teaching at the elementary-school level. Moreover, twice as large a proportion of nonwhite teaching couples as compared with teaching couples in general (6 versus 3 percent) consisted of the husband teaching at the elementary-school level and the wife at the secondary-school level.

The findings regarding nonwhite teaching couples are related to the small proportion of nonwhite youths who attend college and hence who, at least in the past, have created demand for nonwhite college faculty members. Evidently nonwhite college-trained men find a much larger proportion of teaching positions available at the elementary-school level than similarly trained white men. In addition, nonwhite MSP men teachers evidently are less inclined than white MSP men teachers to object to teaching at the elementary-school level or to teaching at a level below that of their wife.

Among nonwhite MSP teachers with working spouses, the proportion married to teachers was half again as large as the corresponding figure for MSP teachers in general. This generalization is equally applicable to teaching husbands and teaching wives. The pattern also held for teachers at each of the three levels.

MSP men teachers below the college level with working wives were *more* likely to be married to a teacher than were MSP men teachers at the college level. A contrary situation prevailed among MSP women teachers.

A minority, 35 percent, of the teaching wives (of all races combined) with working husbands were married to men employed as manual, service, or farm workers. Half again as large a proportion of nonwhite as white teaching wives had husbands engaged in manual or service work, whereas about twice as large a proportion of white (8 percent) as nonwhite (4 percent) teaching wives had farm husbands. The proportion with spouses working at manual, service, or farm jobs tended to be highest at the elementary-school level.

A promising area for further research would be the types of work done by working husbands and wives who are engaged in occupations other than teaching. Such research might be expected to confirm the hypothesis that some fields of employment, including farming and certain varieties of retail trade, are likely to have an even higher proportion of husbands and wives in the same line of work than was found for the teaching profession.

Also worthy of mention in this context is the proportion of college enrollees who are married. According to annual data from the Census

Bureau's Current Population Survey, the proportion of college students who were married and living with their spouse has varied around 25 percent for men and 15 percent for women during the 1960's. However, in 1967–68, only 16 percent of the men and 8 percent of the women attending college on a full-time basis were married, spouse present, as compared with 66 percent of the men and 44 percent of the women attending college on a part-time basis.

Group Variations in Income of Married Persons

The emphasis in the present discussion is on persons in the middle years of life; at this period, income relates mainly to earnings. Income is a kind of summary measure which portrays the ultimate consequence of innumerable variables, including the extent of full employment and the level of skill required to be engaged in the occupation involved.

In 1960 nearly all of the husbands (98 percent), but only a little over one-half of the wives (55 percent), had received income during the preceding year (see source of Table 7.17). Even among wives with income, their median receipts were only about 30 percent as large as those of husbands in general, and their earnings constituted only about one-fourth of the entire family income. Hence among married couples, who are featured here, the income of the wife is usually regarded as supplemental to that of the husband. The economic status of the 55 percent of wives with no income depends largely or entirely on the income of the husband; this income must be shared by at least two adults and more often than not by children as well. This interpretation is appropriate for a full understanding of the meaning of the income of wives as compared with "nonwives."

Differences in income by marital status. The figures in Table 7.17 document the relatively high average incomes of "married, spouse present" (MSP) men as compared with divorced and separated men, and the relatively low average incomes of MSP women as compared with divorcees. Women who obtain a divorce no doubt tend to be the ones who are capable of supporting themselves and their children, if any. Also, a substantial proportion of the separated white women are probably in process of obtaining a divorce, whereas a similar proportion of separated nonwhite women probably have been deserted.

Table 7.17. Median income in 1959 of persons with income, by marital status, color, and sex, with data by age for those married, spouse present: United States, 1960

Marital status and age	Median income for men		Median income for women		Median for women as percent of that for men	
	White	Nonwhite	White	Nonwhite	White	Non-white
Total, 14 & over, with income	$4,291	$2,342	$1,569	$ 923	37	39
Marital status:						
Single	1,663	1,202	1,704	893	102	74
Married, spouse present	5,072	2,842	1,528	907	30	32
Married once	5,122	2,933	1,516	921	30	31
Separated	3,139	2,088	1,938	1,283	62	61
Other married, spouse absent	3,116	2,206	1,616	1,226	52	56
Widowed	1,969	1,112	1,232	779	63	70
Divorced	3,416	2,497	2,640	1,681	77	67
Age--for MSP:						
14-24 years	3,539	2,202	1,431	781	40	35
25-34 years	5,329	3,248	1,646	1,077	31	33
35-44 years	5,944	3,506	1,890	1,169	32	33
45-54 years	5,590	3,045	2,160	925	39	30
55-64 years	4,867	2,499	1,396	773	29	31
65 & over	2,301	1,163	640	577	28	50

Source: U.S. Bureau of the Census, U.S. Census of Population: 1960, Subject Reports, Marital Status, Final Report PC(2)-4E, table 6.

Moreover, it may be inferred that women with a relatively low degree of employability are likely to marry sooner than other women and, when married, to remain that way.

If their marriages become broken, women with the greatest earning capacity are probably the least inclined to remarry soon. Among men, on the other hand, those whose marriages become disrupted by divorce tend to have lower incomes than men who remain married; and men who remarry are inclined to have higher incomes than those who do not remarry, as will be shown in Table 7.19 below. Consequently, the ranks of divorced men with relatively high incomes tend to be quickly depleted. These differentials explain partially why the median income of all women who received income was only about three-eighths as large as that for men, whereas the corresponding ratio for divorced women was about three-fourths of that for divorced men.

The incomes of separated persons are uniformly lower than those of divorced persons — a fact which may reflect a heavy weighting of the separated group with persons who have serious marital problems but who cannot afford to resolve them by divorce. Incidentally, the general similarity of income levels of persons classified as separated and of those classified as "other married, spouse absent" suggests that the latter may include a substantial proportion of persons who were already separated but were not so reported or who were in an early stage of becoming separated.

The uniformly low income level for widowed persons as compared with married persons is probably a function not only of their higher average age but also of the likelihood that, at any age, the lower socioeconomic classes are present to a greater extent among the widowed than the married. Also, the greater eligibility for remarriage of those with more substantial incomes may be important, although it is probably impossible to demonstrate the point convincingly with census data. The relatively high ratio of the median income of widows to that of widowers may reflect reluctance, to some extent, on the part of many widows to remarry lest they thereby lose income.

Single men have far lower incomes than married men, but the income level of single women differs from that of married women in a complex pattern. The low average age of single men, the selectively high marriage rates for single men of high income, and the low incomes of single college students and (single) priests probably account for most of the deviation downward in the income of single men. White single women with income have a higher median income than white MSP women with income. Most of the single women probably have a greater need for self-support from full-time employment; many are highly educated and devoting their lives to their professional or clerical careers. Furthermore, single women in the paid labor force are younger and have better educational backgrounds, on the average, and therefore greater earning capacity than married women workers. In fact, white single women of all ages 14 and over combined — and ages 45 to 64 years old in particular — have higher median incomes than white single men of comparable ages. Nonwhite single women with income, by contrast, have about the same income level as nonwhite MSP women with income, perhaps partly because a smaller proportion of nonwhite single than married women are full-year workers.

The distribution of median income by age in Table 7.17 shows that MSP men about 40 years old in 1960 had higher average incomes than those younger or older. However, among white MSP men, the second-highest median income was for those about 50 years old, whereas among nonwhite MSP men the second-highest was for those about 30 years of age. These facts reflect, among other things, differences in the educational and occupational distributions of white and nonwhite husbands by age.

When median incomes are analyzed by age for each educational level separately, the peak tends to occur close to age 45 for men in each educational group with 5 or more years of schooling and close to age 35 for those with less than 5 years.[9] Moreover, when median earnings are analyzed by age for each major occupation group, the peak tends to occur around age 40 for 8 of the 11 occupation groups; of the remaining 3, men in professional or technical and private household work reach their peak at about age 50 and farm laborers at about age 30. The second-highest median earnings are for those 10 years younger than the peak age in the case of professional or technical workers, farmers, and service workers; for all other occupation groups, the second-highest median earnings are for those 10 years older than the peak.[10]

The upgrading of incomes in recent years is especially noteworthy in the context of the foregoing discussion. This process is evidenced by the fact that MSP men in 1960 were earning more by the pre-prime age of 30 than those who were in the still-prime or early post-prime age of 60. Those in their twenties in 1960 were also profiting from the abundance of responsible positions available and the scarcity of young adult men to fill them (as a result of the small birth cohorts of the 1930's). However, in terms of income per family member, husband-wife families with the husband between 55 and 64 years old tended to be the best situated financially, as will be shown later in Table 7.22.

These observations are intended as a caution against an uncritical interpretation of the age pattern of median incomes for MSP men in 1960 as being typical of changes in relative financial status throughout the marital cycle. Moreover, these observations relate only to the incomes of husbands; when the analysis is in terms of family income, the patterns are somewhat different. The employment of wives during the 1940's and 1950's was particularly marked for women at their middle ages and thereby contributed substantially to family income at this stage of the cycle. At any rate, the increase in median family income between 1947 and 1964 in constant 1964 dollars was highest — about 62 percent — where the husbands were 25 to 54 years old, as compared with 50 percent at ages 55 to 64, 47 percent at ages under 25, and 33 percent at ages 65 and over.[11]

For wives with income, the peak level of income occurs about 10 years later for white women than for nonwhite women — between 45 and 50 for white and between 35 and 40 for nonwhite. Overall, the median income of women is nearer that of men for nonwhite than for white couples. White men are more likely to have full-time jobs than are nonwhite men; but nonwhite working women are more likely to have full-time jobs than are white working women. The relationship between the median income for wives and that for husbands varies considerably by age, with peaks for white wives at ages under 25 and 45 to 54, the pre-childrearing and post-childrearing periods.

Table 7.18. Percent distribution by income in 1959 and median income in 1959 for persons 45 to 54 years old married once, spouse present, and for ever-married persons 45 to 54 years old married more than once: United States, 1960

Income	Married once, spouse present				Ever-married, married more than once			
	Men		Women		Men		Women	
	White	Nonwhite	White	Nonwhite	White	Nonwhite	White	Nonwhite
Total	100.0	100.0	100.0	100.0	100.0	100.0	100.0	100.0
With income	98.3	96.5	44.4	52.6	97.4	95.5	59.9	69.4
Without income	1.7	3.5	55.6	47.4	2.6	4.5	40.1	30.6
With income	100.0	100.0	100.0	100.0	100.0	100.0	100.0	100.0
$1-$999 or loss	3.9	15.3	29.5	52.7	5.4	18.3	27.2	53.4
$1,000-$2,999	12.4	33.4	37.3	32.7	14.3	35.1	37.1	34.6
$3,000-$4,999	25.0	32.5	24.8	11.3	25.8	30.5	25.5	9.6
$5,000-$6,999	28.8	14.2	6.1	2.7	27.9	12.7	7.2	2.0
$7,000-$9,999	17.1	3.3	1.5	0.5	15.9	2.5	1.8	0.3
$10,000 & over	12.9	1.2	0.8	0.1	10.6	0.9	1.2	0.1
Median income	$5,613	$3,045	$2,100	$ 949	$5,320	$2,805	$2,228	$ 936

Source: U.S. Bureau of the Census, U.S. Census of Population: 1960, Subject Reports, Marital Status, Final Report PC(2)-4E, table 6.

A closer examination of the incomes of persons married once and of those married more than once who were at or near the prime of life in 1960 can be made by reference to Table 7.18. Nearly all the men who had married were income recipients at this age, but the percent who were not income recipients was somewhat larger for those married more than once than for those still living with their first wife. Moreover, among men, those in unbroken first marriages averaged between $200 and $300 more income than those who had entered remarriages.

The reverse tendencies are apparent for women. Women in first marriages were much less likely to have had any income during the preceding year than those who had remarried. Nonwhite women consistently had higher percentages with income, as expected from their larger percentages in the labor force. On the other hand, the pattern of median incomes of white and nonwhite women by number of times married was not consistent in the way that the pattern for men was. Among white women, the median income of those with income was 6 percent larger for the remarried than for those with intact first marriages, whereas there was little difference between the corresponding two median income figures for nonwhite women.

Income patterns for remarried white and nonwhite men and for remarried white women were intermediate between those for persons still living with their first spouse and those (not shown in the table) with a current marital status of separated, widowed, or divorced. Thus except for nonwhite women, the data suggest that persons whose first marriage is discontinued are more likely to return to the married state if they are men with relatively high incomes or if they are women with relatively low incomes. Evidently widowed and divorced men with low incomes tend either to lose out in seeking another marital partner or voluntarily to drop out of the race, whereas widowed and divorced white women who continue to earn income tend to remain out of the search for another marital partner — especially if their incomes are above $3,000 or $4,000.

Permanence of marriage by social and economic level. The relationship between the tendency to remain married to the original marital partner or to remarry if widowed or divorced, on the one hand, and the amount of education and earnings the man has, on the other hand, is set forth in Table 7.19 for white men at the prime ages 45 to 54 years in each of the major occupation groups. (Corresponding data are not available for other age groups; data for nonwhite men are available from the same sources but are not shown.) The first two and last two columns in the table relate to employed men and the other four columns relate to men with earnings, but the minor differences in coverage are believed to have no significant effect on the patterns discussed.

Positive correlations between the percentage of men still in their first marriage, the extent of their education, and the amount of their earnings become evident by scanning the data in the table by occupation groups. Considering for the moment only nonfarm workers, men in professional and technical occupations registered the highest proportion (84 percent) still living with their first wife; they had by far

Table 7.19. Marital characteristics, education, and earnings of white men 45 to 54 years old, by major occupation group: United States, 1960

| Major occupation group | Men living with first wife | | | | | | Men living with wife in remarriage as percent of all men ever widowed or divorced | |
| | As percent of all men ever married | | Median years of school completed | | Mean money earnings | | | |
	Percent	Index	Median	Index	Mean	Index	Percent	Index
White men 45-54	79.3	100	10.6	100	$6,748	100	74.3	100
Professional, technical	83.8	106	16.2	153	11,308	168	77.2	104
Managers, off'ls., prop'rs.	81.8	103	12.4	117	10,568	157	81.6	110
Clerical workers	80.6	102	12.1	114	5,898	87	70.5	95
Sales workers	79.5	100	12.3	116	7,981	118	78.0	105
Craftsmen, foremen	78.3	99	9.6	91	5,858	87	77.9	105
Operatives	78.2	99	7.9	75	4,992	74	73.2	99
Service workers	72.4	91	9.1	86	4,561	68	67.7	91
Laborers, exc. farm & mine	75.8	96	6.4	60	4,031	60	66.0	89
Farmers, farm managers	90.3	114	7.7	73	3,659	54	72.3	97
Farm laborers & foremen	70.1	88	5.6	53	2,442	36	56.9	77

Source: U.S. Bureau of the Census, U.S. Census of Population: 1960, Subject Reports, Marital Status, Final Report PC(2)-4E, tables 5 and 7; percent living with wife in remarriage derived in part from National Center for Health Statistics, Vital Statistics--Special Reports, Vol. 45, No. 12, table 21.

the largest amount of schooling (more than 16 years); and their earnings, at $11,300 in 1959, topped that of men in all other occupations. Men in managerial occupations ranked next with 82 percent living in first marriages (but they ranked first in percent of eligibles who had remarried, also 82 percent); they ranked nearly as high as the professionals on income, with $10,600 earnings, but they had nearly 4 years less education.

On the basis of earnings and education, sales workers would have been expected to rank above rather than below clerical workers with respect to percentage with first marriages intact among all who had ever married. The data in the source of Table 7.19 show that sales workers are more likely than clerical workers to marry for the first time, are more likely to have had their first marriage dissolved (generally by divorce), and are more likely to have remarried if they had been widowed or divorced. In other words, sales workers showed evidence of a greater tendency than clerical workers to prefer the married state, although they did not necessarily place as high a premium on continuing in their first marriage.

Another example of irregularity in the patterns of data in the table is found in the information on service workers. While they rank substantially above laborers with respect to education and earnings, they rate lower on percentage living with first wife. By way of explanation, laborers probably are more likely to live at home while they work than are service workers, two-thirds of whom at ages 45 to 54 are in food-serving occupations (cooks, waiters, kitchen workers), hairdressing, and caretaking (hospital and institutional attendants and practical nurses). Of additional explanatory value may be the "way-of-life" principle — especially the kinds of personal contacts service workers (and salesmen) make in connection with work experience.

Farm workers are shown separately from nonfarm workers because the level of earnings has a somewhat different meaning for the two broad groups. Farmers and farm managers had very distinctly the highest percentage of middle-aged men still living with their first wife (90 percent), whereas farm laborers and farm foremen had the lowest (70 percent), even when compared with those in nonfarm occupations. Farm laborers likewise had by far the smallest proportion of eligibles who had remarried (57 percent) as well as the poorest educational and earnings levels of all. These observations supplement those made earlier in the chapter to the effect that farm operators tend to place a higher value on constant (or renewed) married life than expected on the basis of the other social and economic characteristics shown here.

Income of wives as a supplement to family income. Most wives below the retirement age who have incomes are workers who earn

Table 7.20. Income in 1959 of husband by income in 1959 of wife, for married couples with wife 25 to 44 years old, by color of husband: United States, 1960

(Numbers in thousands)

Income of husband	White--income of wife						Nonwhite--median income of wives with income
	Total	Wives with no income	$1-$999	Wives with income		Median (wives)	
				$1,000 $2,999	$3,000 & over		
Total married couples with wife 25-44	18,179	10,810	2,650	2,631	2,087	$1,737	$1,089
Percent	100.0	100.0	100.0	100.0	100.0	...	...
With no income	0.9	0.9	0.7	1.3	1.4	2,311	1,194
With income:							
$1-$999 or loss	2.5	2.3	3.1	3.2	2.4	1,600	452
$1,000-$1,999	3.8	3.4	4.3	5.0	3.2	1,569	653
$2,000-$2,999	6.2	5.5	6.9	9.4	5.1	1,698	889
$3,000-$3,999	10.4	9.2	11.0	14.8	10.6	1,833	1,313
$4,000-$4,999	14.8	13.3	15.3	18.2	17.6	1,937	1,796
$5,000-$5,999	18.2	17.5	18.5	18.8	21.3	1,879	2,021
$6,000-$6,999	14.1	14.5	13.8	12.2	15.0	1,748	2,373
$7,000-$9,999	18.7	20.9	17.5	12.4	16.5	1,630	2,407
$10,000-$14,999	6.6	8.1	5.9	3.2	4.6	1,201	2,846
$15,000 & over	3.5	4.3	3.2	0.9	2.4	1,070	2,266
Median (husbands)	$5,644	$5,904	$5,496	$4,933	$5,490	...	...

Source: U.S. Bureau of the Census, U.S. Census of Population: 1960, Subject Reports, Sources and Structure of Family Income, Final Report PC(2)-4C, table 17.

wages or salary. Therefore the distribution of wives with no income according to income of the husband resembles that of wives not in the labor force classified by income of husband. Likewise, the distribution of wives with income by amount of income cross-classified with income of husband bears a close resemblance to the distribution of labor-force-participation rates of wives by education of the wife; that is, the largest average income of wives and the largest labor-force-participation rates are found for those of intermediate status with respect to education and husband's income.

These trends are highlighted in Table 7.20 and Figure 7.2, which are limited to married couples where the wife was 25 to 44 years old at the time of the 1960 census. Most of the husbands of these women were 30 to 50 years old. Fuller detail is shown for white than nonwhite couples, but comparable data are available in the original source for both color groups.

Among the wives of white men, the median income was highest of all for those few whose husbands reported no income, with a secondary

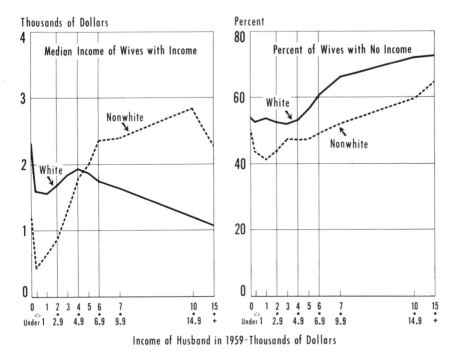

Fig. 7.2. Median income of wife and percent of wives with no income, by income of husband: United States, 1959

Source: Table 7.20.

peak (involving far more women) where the husband's income was a little below average, in the $4,000–$5,000 range. Among the wives of nonwhite men, however, the median-income level was at a maximum for those whose husbands were in next-to-the-highest income class, namely $10,000–$15,000.

Wives of white men had median incomes significantly above the average level of $1,737 where the income of the husbands was in the middle range of $3,000 to $6,000. Wives of nonwhite men, by contrast, had median incomes significantly above the average level of $1,089 where the income of the husbands was in the middle or, especially, in the upper range; however, only 9 percent of the nonwhite husbands (as compared with 43 percent of the white husbands) had incomes in the upper range, defined for present purposes as $6,000 or more.

Further enlightenment on the relationship between husbands' and their wives' incomes can be gained from an examination of the detail on the four broad levels of incomes of white wives. About 59 percent of the white wives 25 to 44 years old reported no income, 15 percent reported $1 to $999, another 14 percent $1,000 to $2,999, and the remaining 11 percent $3,000 and over. The median income of their husbands, as a whole, was $5,644; that of husbands whose wives reported no income was above this overall average; that of husbands whose wives had incomes of an intermediate level was well below this average; and the median incomes of husbands whose wives had incomes in the highest and lowest levels were close to the overall average. Still another way to summarize the relationship between the incomes of the marital partners under examination is given in the following exhibit based on the second to fifth columns of Table 7.20:

White wives 25–44 years old are likely to have —
No income if the husband's income is high ($7,000 and over);
Incomes of $1,000–$3,000 if the husband's income is low (less than $5,000);
Incomes of $3,000 and over if the husband's income is intermediate ($4,000–$7,000).

Family income in relation to family size. If the main purpose of income analysis is to show the economic welfare of the married couple, rather than the economic prestige of the husband, family income is generally a better measure than income of the husband alone. Obviously, family income reveals more clearly the amount of money available to the family for the purchase of consumer goods and services. This is true even if one of the items purchased is service which permits the wife to work outside the home in preference to doing her own housework. Family income includes money received by all related persons who constitute the family and not only by the family head and his wife.

The general relationship between income of husband and income of family at successive ages of the husband is evident from the first three columns of Table 7.21. Family income tends to be about one-

Table 7.21. Median income in 1959 of husband for married couples, and median family income in 1959 for husband-wife families by color of husband, by age of husband: United States, 1960

Age of husband	Median income of husband, for married couples	Median family income, for husband-wife families			Nonwhite	
		Total		White		
		Median family income	As percent of median income of husband		Median for non-whites	As percent of median for whites
Total	$4,862	$5,901	121	$6,102	$3,637	60
Under 25 years	3,409	4,284	126	4,419	2,737	62
25-34 years	5,144	5,838	113	5,980	3,861	65
35-44 years	5,761	6,739	117	6,933	4,286	62
45-54 years	5,383	6,860	127	7,108	3,938	55
55-64 years	4,671	5,915	127	6,015	3,323	55
65 & over	2,231	3,052	137	3,185	1,820	57

Source: U.S. Bureau of the Census, U.S. Census of Population: 1960, Subject Reports, Families, Final Report PC(2)-4A, table 13; Sources and Structure of Family Income, Final Report PC(2)-4C, table 1; and Marital Status, Final Report PC(2)-4E, table 6.

fifth larger than husband's income for all couples combined. The differential is larger than the overall average when the husband is under 25 and the wife is likely to be still childless. It is smallest when the husband is 25 to 44 years old and the wife tends to be preoccupied with childrearing. The difference then rises during the empty-nest period of the family-life cycle, when the likelihood that the wife is in the labor market rises again. At the retirement age of 65 years and over, the ratio of family income to husband's income reaches its peak; this is the situation partly because 65 percent of the wives at this age, as compared with 45 percent of wives at all ages, have money receipts, but more specifically because the incomes of wives more closely approximate those of their husbands at this period of life.

Among all husband-wife families in 1960, 81 percent of aggregate family income was received by the husbands, 12 percent by the wives, and 7 percent by other family members; but among husband-wife families with the head 65 years old and over, only 61 percent of aggregate family income was received by the husband, whereas 12 percent was received by the wife, and 27 percent by other family members.[12] A significant element in this income picture at the older ages is the receipt of social-security benefits by husband and wife.

The median family income of nonwhite husband-wife families was only 60 percent as large as that of white families. Yet this proportion exceeded the corresponding figure, 56 percent, for the ratio of the median income of nonwhite husbands to that of white husbands. The main reasons, of course, are that nonwhite wives are more likely than white wives to be in the paid labor force, to be employed full time, and, if so, to have an income somewhat closer to that of their husbands.

For families with the husband at the younger ages (under 45), the ratio of median income for nonwhite families to that for white families was higher than the ratio for older families. This difference is probably one of the indirect consequences of the greater relative advancement in education of nonwhite persons in the last few decades. The ratio is largest at the peak period for childrearing, when nonwhite wives are more likely than white wives to work for pay outside the home. It is also slightly higher in the oldest age group than in the next two younger groups, perhaps partially as a consequence of the large proportion of income at this age which comes from social-security payments.

Three measures of average family income are presented in Table 7.22 for the purpose of showing that relative economic deprivation or abundance from one stage of the family life cycle to another is subject to substantially differing interpretations, depending on which measure is used. All three measures — median and mean family income, and income per family member — have the same general contour, in the sense that families with heads in the intermediate age range have more income than those with either younger or older heads.

Mean family income is 15 percent larger than median family income, on the average, and the proportion by which it exceeds median income increases steadily with age. This observation is an

Table 7.22. Median and mean family income and income per family member in 1959, for husband-wife families by age of husband: United States, 1960

Age of husband	Measures of family income			Indexes of family income		
	Median family income	Mean family income	Income per family member	Median family income	Mean family income	Income per family member
All husband-wife families	$5,901	$6,813	$1,841	100	100	100
Under 25 years	4,284	4,522	1,454	73	66	79
25-34 years	5,838	6,380	1,526	99	94	83
35-44 years	6,739	7,568	1,667	114	111	91
45-54 years	6,860	7,970	2,154	116	117	117
55-64 years	5,915	7,333	2,564	100	108	139
65-74 years	3,542	5,027	2,003	60	74	109
75 & over	2,206	3,601	1,494	37	53	81

Source: U.S. Bureau of the Census, U.S. Census of Population: 1960, Vol. I, Characteristics of the Population, Part 1, United States Summary, table 224; Subject Reports, Families, Final Report PC(2)-4A, tables 4 and 13; Persons by Family Characteristics, Final Report PC(2)-4B, tables 5 and 12; and Sources and Structure of Family Income, Final Report PC(2)-4C, table 1.

obvious consequence of the increasing proportion of upper-half families with incomes that are far above the median for the age group as heads become successively older. It takes many years, as a rule, for those who become earners at the upper level to reach that level; in the meantime the proportion by which their earnings — augmented increasingly by income from substantial savings — exceed that of the average earner rises continuously. Although the absolute amount of the difference between mean and median income diminishes at the upper ages, the proportional difference does not diminish. The age range when median family income significantly exceeds the overall average (that is, when the head is 35 to 54) is narrower than the age range when mean family income exceeds the average (35 to 64).

The third measure of family income — namely, income per family member — is derived by dividing mean family income by mean size of family, where all family members are included and are given equal weight. This measure shows less relative deprivation of families with the head under 25 and over 75 than either of the other measures, because it takes into account the small average family size at these extreme ages as compared with the overall average. The per-capita measure tellingly reveals, however, the negative effect which the presence of children has on the income available per member during the childrearing period (that is, when the head is under 45). In equal measure, it impressively reveals a relative abundance of family income per member extending into a still older range (45 to 74) than that shown by mean family income. Especially noteworthy is the value of $2,564 income per family member — 39 percent above the average for all families — when the family head is 55 to 64 years old. At this age, the chances that the wife is supplementing the near-peak income of the husband are fairly high, and the chances that some or all of the sons and daughters at home have income are also high.

For each of these three frequently used measures of family income, the values in the last three columns of the table may be considered as showing equivalents for a given age of family head. These values, as well as those in the first three columns of the table, may be used as national standards against which to compare study results for subgroups of the population. To these measures one could readily add others, one of which is income per "ammain," or income per equivalent adult family member. In this concept, different weights are ascribed to the several types of family members; for example, half-weight might be given to each child under a given age. The effect of introducing this variation of income per family member is to produce a measure intermediate between mean income and income per member, but closer to the latter.

Table 7.23 provides further insight into the dispersion of family income at each stage of the cycle of family life for husband-wife families. Each succeeding line of the table (after the total line) relates to the next stage of the cycle as defined in this part of the study.[13]

The values in the table vary widely, ranging from only $622 income for the lowest decile of families with the husband 65 and over, all the way up to $14,235 for the highest decile of families with the husband 45 to 64 years old and with young children still living at home. As the lower half of the table demonstrates, if all the values in the upper half of the table are compared with the median family income $5,901 set equal to 100, then the lowest value in the table is only 11 percent of the median and the highest value is 241 percent of the median.

This table raises the important question as to whether, early in the cycle of family life, the income of the family tends to reach a level, in relation to that of other families, where it varies within a rather narrow range throughout later stages of the cycle. The second

Table 7.23. Dispersion of family income, for husband-wife families, by age of husband and presence of own children under 18 years old: United States, 1960

Age of husband and presence of own children under 18	Percent of all families	Family income				
		Top decile	Top quartile	Median (one-half)	Bottom quartile	Bottom decile
All husband-wife families	100.0	$12,719	$8,535	$5,901	$3,747	$1,904
Under 35: No children	4.9	10,472	8,300	5,767	3,667	2,108
With children	21.8	9,601	7,312	5,496	3,916	2,434
35-44: With children	21.4	13,295	9,298	6,667	4,816	3,067
No children	3.5	13,405	9,598	6,838	4,541	2,605
45-64: With children	15.5	14,235	9,721	6,647	4,328	2,307
No children	20.9	14,040	9,529	6,304	3,939	1,935
65 & over	12.1	9,679	6,569	3,052	1,555	622
Index of family income	...	216	145	100	63	32
Under 35: No children	...	177	141	98	62	36
With children	...	163	124	93	66	41
35-44: With children	...	225	158	113	82	52
No children	...	227	163	116	77	44
45-64: With children	...	241	165	113	73	39
No children	...	238	161	107	67	33
65 & over	...	164	111	52	26	11

Source: U.S. Bureau of the Census, U.S. Census of Population: 1960, Detailed Characteristics, U.S. Summary, Final Report PC(1)-1D, Table 224; Special Reports, Families, Final Report PC(2)-4A, Tables 4 and 13; Persons by Family Characteristics, Final Report PC(2)-4B, Tables 5 and 12; and Sources and Structure of Family Income, Final Report PC(2)-4C, Table 1.

column shows the amount of income, at each cycle stage, received in 1959 by husband-wife families whose income was exceeded by only 10 percent of all husband-wife families. Similarly, the third column shows the amount exceeded by 25 percent of the families at each stage. A comparison of these two columns reveals that the smallest value for the top decile is virtually as high as the highest value for the top quartile. Likewise, there is no overlap of income between family groups in succeeding pairs of columns of the table, except for those with the head 65 and over.[14]

Patterns of change in family income during the first three stages of the family cycle for families in the lower two income levels shown differ from those for families in higher income levels. The income level of the low-income families is still lower during the childless first stage of the cycle of married life than during the second phase when children have arrived, whereas the income level of families in the higher brackets tends to dip somewhat between the first and second stages. Contributing factors are probably lower rates of labor-force participation and higher rates of childbearing during the early years of marriage for women in low-income levels. Moreover, peak family income tends to be reached by the poorer families while the head is 35 to 44 years old, but not before ages 45 to 64 by the more affluent.

Earnings level of husbands by education and occupation. The fore-going analysis of family income level in relation to stage of the life cycle of the family would assume added meaning if education and occupation equivalents to the income levels could be established. This section presents an initial attempt at approximating these equiv-alents, in the hope of stimulating research aimed at refining the first estimates. The proposed equivalents appear in Table 7.25, which is rather complex. The table presents the educational range of husbands at or near the peak of earning capacity (45 to 54 years old) which tends to be associated with a given broad income level, with values shown for husbands in each major occupational group.

The table is designed for various uses, including translation of the broad income levels set forth in the columns of Table 7.23 into "education-by-occupation" equivalents. For this purpose, the admit-tedly rough but practical assumption could be made that changes in family income during the cycle of family life for couples with the hus-band possessing a given combination of educational and occupational characteristics tend to correspond to the changes in income during the cycle stages shown in the most relevant column of Table 7.23. Such a table of equivalents, in combination with Table 7.23, would reveal the approximate amount of money income (in 1959 dollars) which married men who embark on a particular occupational career with a particular amount of education might reasonably expect to have available for the welfare of their families at successive stages of the family cycle.

In developing Table 7.25, several conversions of data were required in order to transpose available statistics into the desired form. Table 7.23 shows percentiles of family income, whereas data from the 1960 census were available in usable form only in terms of mean earnings of the husband. Therefore median family income was converted to equivalent mean family earnings (at each family-income level), and family earnings were converted in turn to equivalent earnings of the husband. The resulting equivalents are presented in Table 7.24.

The first three lines of this table provide three different ways in which to classify husband-wife families according to their income level. The fourth and fifth lines show that mean family earnings and mean earnings of the husband do not bear a linear relationship to median family income. Mean family earnings were estimated as about 91 percent of median family income at the upper end of the continuum, 93 percent at the upper quarter and halfway points, 87 percent at the

Table 7.24. Median family income in 1959, mean family earnings in 1959, and mean earnings of husband in 1959, for husband-wife families, by broad income level: United States, 1960

Measure of income	Broad income level of husband-wife families				
	Top decile	Top quartile	Median	Bottom quartile	Bottom decile
Median family income	$12,719	$8,535	$5,901	$3,747	$1,904
Estimated equivalent:					
Mean family earnings	11,537	7,977	5,503	3,242	1,240
Mean earnings of husband	9,741	6,985	5,012	3,050	1,182
Percent of median family income:					
Mean family earnings	91	93	93	87	65
Mean earnings of husband	77	82	85	81	62
Percent of family earnings earned by husband	85	88	91	93	95

Source: U.S. Bureau of the Census, U.S. Census of Population: 1960, Subject Reports, Sources and Structure of Family Income, Final Report PC(2)-4C, tables 7, 12, and 140.

lower quarter, and 65 percent at the lower end of the continuum. This modified downward slope is the net result of such complex factors as the proportion of income received from investments (high at the upper end) or from unemployment compensation and old-age assistance (high at the lower end), the proportion of families with the wife as earner (highest between the median and top quartile), the proportion of family income earned by wives with earnings (likewise highest near the top quartile, but with a minor mode at the lower end of the range), and the proportion of family income received by persons other than the husband and wife. Moreover, the estimated mean earnings of the husband evidently are a linearly downward proportion of mean family earnings as the income level of the family increases, being about 95 percent at the lower end of the income scale and about 85 percent at the upper end.

Table 7.25 shows the end product toward which the discussion in this section has been directed. Whereas the results are shown for white and nonwhite husbands separately, the five mean earnings levels shown were derived from data on all husbands (white and nonwhite combined) rather than for white distinct from nonwhite. A uniform standard of comparison for both white and nonwhite husbands is thereby provided. The basic tables from which these earnings levels

Table 7.25. Educational level and major occupation group most closely corresponding to broad earnings levels of husbands 45 to 54 years old in first marriages with earnings in 1959, by color of husband: United States, 1960

Major occupation group and color of husband		Earnings level of husband				
		Top decile	Top quartile	Median	Bottom quartile	Bottom decile
Total:	White	College 1+ years	High school 1-4	Below HS		
	Nonwhite		College 4+ years	Coll 1-3, HS 4	Below HS 4	
Professional:	White	College 1+ years	Below college			
	Nonwhite		College 4+ years	Coll 1-3, HS 4	Below HS 4	
Managerial:	White	Coll 1+, HS 1-4	Below HS			
	Nonwhite		Coll 1+, HS 4	Below HS 4		
Clerical:	White		College 1+ years	Below college		
	Nonwhite			Coll 1+, HS 1-4	Below HS	
Sales:	White	College 1+ years	High school 1-4	Below HS		
	Nonwhite			Coll 1+, HS 1-4	Below HS	
Craftsmen:	White	College 4+ years	Coll 1-3, HS 4	Below HS 4		
	Nonwhite			Coll 1+, HS 1-4	Below HS	
Operatives:	White		College 4+ years	Below coll 4		
	Nonwhite			Coll 1+, HS 4	Below HS 4	
Service:	White		College 4+ years	Coll 1-3, HS 1-4	Below HS	
	Nonwhite				All levels	
Laborers:	White			Coll 1+, HS 1-4	Below HS	
	Nonwhite				All levels	
Farmers:	White		College 4+ years	Coll 1-3, HS 4	Below HS 4	
	Nonwhite				HS 1-4	Below HS
Farm laborers:	White			College 1+ years	Below coll	
	Nonwhite				HS 1-4	Below HS

Source: U.S. Bureau of the Census, U.S. Census of Population: 1960, Subject Reports, Sources and Structure of Family Income, Final Report PC(2)-4C, tables 7, 12, and 14; and Marital Status, Final Report PC(2)-4E, table 7.

were derived are available by color, however, so that alternative standards by color could be prepared.

One of the most informative features of the table is the light it throws on differences in amount of education associated with a given level of earnings for husbands in the several occupational groups. White husbands who were managers, officials, and proprietors (except farm) with only a partial or full high-school education had mean earnings nearer to the level of the top decile of earnings for husbands than to any lower earnings level shown. At the same time, professional and technical workers and sales workers had to have at least some college training to rate classification in the top decile, and craftsmen and foremen (except farm) had to have a full college education to be so rated. Otherwise stated, the average man who starts his employment career with a given upper level of educational background may reasonably aspire to achieve a higher earnings level by middle age if he enters and stays in a managerial occupation than if he chooses a professional, technical, or sales position, and a much higher earnings level than if he chooses a position as a craftsman or foreman.

White husbands with a given combination of education and major occupation group were characteristically classified one or two mean earnings levels (as defined here) above nonwhite husbands in the same education and major occupation group. White husbands in four of the ten occupation groups — but nonwhite husbands in none — qualified for classification at the highest earnings level. In other words, no amount of education through college graduation was large enough to bring the average earnings level of nonwhite husbands in any occupation group all the way up to the top decile.

White husbands in four occupation groups — sales workers, craftsmen, service workers, and farmers — were distributed over three mean earnings levels according to how much education they had acquired. Nonwhite husbands who were in these four groups had mean earnings which rose no more than two levels beneath the highest level for white husbands. These are occupations in which Negroes evidently experience great difficulty in their efforts to prosper, regardless of the amount of education they have received. By contrast, white husbands in professional and managerial occupations regardless of educational level had mean earnings in or near the highest or next-to-highest level.

As stated, the listings in Table 7.25 are based on 1960 census data for husbands at or near the peak of their earning careers, 45 to 54 years old; this is the only age group for which the required data were available by marital status. Husbands at this prime period of life in 1960, however, had less education by about 2 years than husbands 25 to 44 years old. As these better-educated young husbands reach 45 to 54 years of age — and as the value of the dollar depreciates — the mean earnings of the younger generation will undoubtedly rise. By that time, men will have to earn larger amounts of money to attain a given position such as the top decile.

Factors other than future increases in education and changes in price levels may also be expected to affect levels of income of white and nonwhite husbands at successive stages of the family-life cycle during future generations. One of the leading additional factors will undoubtedly be the degree to which nonwhite husbands with educational levels literally identical to those of white husbands find opportunities to enter the same kinds of occupations at the same earnings levels as their white counterparts.[15]

8 / GROUP VARIATIONS AMONG SEPARATED AND DIVORCED PERSONS

There are various methods whereby an individual adjusts to marital discord.[1] Divorce and separation are the two about which most is known by means of objective statistics. The other forms of adjustment to an unsatisfactory marital situation are of importance to students of the family, but statistical information is limited. In the treatment of separation and divorce in this text, there is no implication that these conditions cover all, or even most, of the cases of marital difficulty; they cover cases for which demographic data are available.

A great deal more is known about the divorced population than about the separated. "Divorced" is a recognized status following court action, and there is an official record. "Separated" may be an official status duly recorded, but more frequently it is simply a situation where husband and wife are living apart because of marital discord. Thus in the following discussion, the statistical information presented for the separated is limited.

Currently Separated and Divorced Persons

The marital status of the population of the United States is constantly changing. On a given census enumeration date, certain persons will be recorded as divorced or separated; if the enumeration were repeated a day, month, or year later, many of them would be recorded in a different marital status and other persons previously recorded as married would now be recorded as separated or divorced. This cross-sectional feature is relevant to the analysis of census data on the separated and divorced population, on the time factor in changing marital status, and on the age at which persons entered a given marital status.

The numbers of separated and divorced persons in the population are substantial. At the time of the 1960 census, over 2 million were separated and over 3 million were divorced (see Table 8.1). In each category the number of women was substantially larger than the number of men, probably due in part to inaccuracies in the reporting of marital status.[2]

Table 8.1. Separated and divorced persons, by age, color, and sex: United States, 1960

(Numbers in thousands)

Age and sex	Separated persons		Divorced persons		Percent separated		Percent divorced	
	White	Nonwhite	White	Nonwhite	White	Nonwhite	White	Nonwhite
Men, 14 & over	541	337	1,150	154	1.0	5.4	2.1	2.4
Percent	100.0	100.0	100.0	100.0	...	...	...	...
14-24 years	8.7	6.4	4.9	3.2	0.4	1.4	0.5	0.3
25-34 years	18.8	23.0	17.1	19.2	1.0	6.3	2.0	2.4
35-44 years	20.5	27.3	22.7	27.0	1.0	7.8	2.5	3.5
45-54 years	20.3	22.2	23.4	24.9	1.2	7.6	2.9	3.9
55-64 years	16.3	13.4	18.3	15.9	1.3	6.5	3.1	3.5
65-74 years	10.9	5.9	10.1	7.6	1.3	4.8	3.6	2.8
75-84 years	4.0	1.6	3.1	1.9	1.2	3.7	2.0	2.0
85 & over	0.5	0.2	0.4	0.3	1.0	2.7	1.4	1.4
Median age (years)	45.9	42.2	47.2	45.2	...	...	...	...
Women, 14 & over	741	576	1,609	249	1.3	8.4	2.8	3.6
Percent	100.0	100.0	100.0	100.0	...	...	...	...
14-24 years	13.4	11.8	6.7	5.6	0.8	4.0	0.9	0.8
25-34 years	20.5	30.7	17.4	24.0	1.5	12.4	2.7	4.2
35-44 years	22.8	28.0	24.6	30.5	1.5	12.2	3.6	5.7
45-54 years	20.3	17.5	24.2	22.7	1.6	9.7	4.1	5.4
55-64 years	13.7	8.5	16.7	11.6	1.4	6.6	3.6	3.9
65-74 years	7.2	2.9	8.1	4.4	1.0	3.7	2.4	2.4
75-84 years	2.0	0.5	2.1	1.1	0.6	1.9	1.4	1.6
85 & over	0.1	0.1	0.2	0.1	0.2	1.0	0.9	0.7
Median age (years)	41.9	37.3	45.5	41.5	...	...	...	...

Source: U.S. Bureau of the Census, U.S. Census of Population: 1960, Subject Reports, Marital Status, Final Report PC(2)-4E, tables 1 and 4.

Separated persons were considerably younger among nonwhite than among white persons. Nonwhite men were strongly concentrated between ages 25 and 54 years, where over 70 percent were found; their median age was just over 42 years. Among white men there were relatively more in the older ages, and the median age was about 46 years. Nonwhite women were concentrated between 25 and 44 years, where over one-half of them were found; their median age was about 37 years. White separated women were also concentrated in the younger ages, with three-fourths of them being under 55 years of age; their median age was about 42 years.

A substantially higher proportion of nonwhite than of white persons was reported as separated. Among men, only 1 percent of the white but over 5 percent of the nonwhite were separated. Among white men, the highest proportion separated (between 55 and 74 years) was 1.3 percent; among nonwhite men, the highest proportion (between 35 and 54 years) was over 7 percent. For women the disparity between white and nonwhite was even greater, with the proportion reported as separated among nonwhites being six times as high as that of whites. A likely conjecture is that part of the discrepancy between the proportions of white and of nonwhite women reported as separated is related to the far higher illegitimate birth rate of nonwhite than of white women at the younger ages.

Persons reported as divorced in the 1960 census excluded the formerly divorced who had remarried. Those reported as divorced, as with those reported as separated, were younger among nonwhite than among white persons. For men the nonwhites had a median age of about 45 years, while the whites averaged 2 years older. Divorced men, regardless of color, were especially numerous between 35 and 54 years of age. Nonwhite women were also younger than white divorced women, with a median age lower by 4 years. Both groups were strongly concentrated between 35 and 54 years of age, where about one-half of them were found, but there were relatively more nonwhite divorced women in the younger ages.

Relatively more nonwhites than whites were divorced: among nonwhite men, the proportion divorced exceeded the white by a ratio of 8 to 7. The highest proportion of nonwhite men divorced (3.9 percent) was reached at 45 to 54 years old; among white men, the highest proportion (3.6 percent) was reached at 65 to 74. For women, the proportion divorced among the nonwhite exceeded that of the white by a ratio of 5 to 4. The highest proportion of nonwhite women divorced (5.7 percent) was that for the age bracket 35 to 44 years old, where the proportion was one and one-half times that for white women. The highest proportion of white women divorced (4.1 percent) was found at 45 to 54 years old.

Consideration of reasons behind the differential rates of divorce, and especially of separation, for white and nonwhite persons leads into an area where only some of the facts are clear. In the long historical perspective, it is evident that the many years of Negro slavery (and the great majority of nonwhites are Negroes) left its adverse mark on family stability. Although slavery ended more than a century ago, evidently more time must pass before its effects are entirely erased. Up to the present, incomes of most Negro families are substantially lower than those of white families, as documented elsewhere, and this places a greater strain on family stability. During recent decades an extraordinary migration of Negroes has taken place; they have moved from country to city and from one region of the country to another. The family who moved from the rural South to

Table 8.2. Median duration of marriage prior to
separation and divorce for first marriage
and remarriage of husbands and wives:
District of Columbia, 1957

Number of marriage of husband by number of marriage of wife	Median duration in years prior to--	
	Separation	Divorce
First marriage of both	4.9	10.5
First marriage of wife, remarriage of husband	4.4	9.4
First marriage of husband, remarriage of wife	2.7	6.6
Remarriage of both	1.7	5.1

Source: Hugh Carter and William F. Pratt,
"Duration of Marriage Prior to Separation and Divorce:
A Study Based on Vital Records," presented at annual
meeting of American Sociological Society, 1958 (processed).

a crowded slum area of a city in the North faced many problems of
adjustment. Moreover, the discrimination experienced by Negro families in seeking housing and employment, and in other ways, provided
an added strain.

It is not surprising that the average age of separated persons is
below that of the divorced, since marital disruption usually begins
with separation and frequently continues for some years prior to divorce. As shown in Table 8.2, data from the District of Columbia
indicate that first marriages ending in divorce usually lasted almost
5 years before the final separation, but the divorce decree was not
issued until another 5 years had passed. If either husband or wife had
been previously married, the process was shortened. However, even
where both husband and wife had been previously married, there was
an average interval of 3 years between the final separation and the
divorce.

Age at remarriage varies by previous marital status; the previously
divorced are, of course, younger by several years than the previously
widowed. From Table 8.3, which tabulates survey data relating to
the period around 1950, it becomes evident that while the divorced
men (who had not been widowed) had a median age at remarriage of

Table 8.3. Age at first marriage or last marriage, for persons married between January 1947 and June 1954, by previous marital status and sex: United States

Marital status	Age at current marriage					
	Men			Women		
	First quar-tile	Median	Third quar-tile	First quar-tile	Median	Third quar-tile
In first marriage	21.3	23.7	27.0	18.6	20.7	23.6
Remarried[a]	31.0	39.3	50.2	26.7	33.0	42.0
Previously divorced (never widowed)	28.7	34.8	42.8	25.0	30.2	36.9
Previously widowed (never divorced)	40.9	52.4	55+	32.5	42.0	51.5

Source: Hugh Carter, Sarah Lewit, and William Pratt, Socioeconomic Characteristics of Persons Who Married Between January 1947 and June 1954: United States, Vital Statistics - Special Reports, Selected Studies, Vol. 45, No. 12, Sept. 9, 1957, tables 13 and 21.

[a] Includes persons who had been both widowed and divorced, not shown separately because of small number of cases.

35 years, the widowed men (who had not been divorced) had a median age of 52 years. This difference of 17 years is substantially greater than that of 12 years for the comparable group of women, the medians being 30 years and 42 years. For comparative purposes, the median ages at first marriage of men and women (about 23 years and 21 years) from the same survey are shown; these are higher than the medians from more recent surveys. First and third quartiles of age at marriage by previous marital status are also shown.[3]

Age at Separation and Divorce

More detailed and more recent information is available on age at divorce than on age at separation. Probably in many instances husband and wife would disagree on the date when the separation began, hence data on age at separation must be viewed as approximate. One of the 1950 census reports is the only available nationwide source for such information, and in that report data are available only for women. Table 8.4 shows both age at separation and age at divorce from that source.

It is clear that a majority of the 1 million separated women 15 to 59 years old recorded in the 1950 census — and especially the nearly

Table 8.4. Separated and divorced women 15 to 59 years old, by age at separation or divorce and color: United States, 1950

| Age at separation or divorce | Separated women | | | | Divorced women | | | |
| | Total | | Separated less than 2 years | | Total | | Divorced less than 2 years | |
	White	Nonwhite	White	Nonwhite	White	Nonwhite	White	Nonwhite
Total	578,430	464,010	183,480	104,550	1,012,110	142,260	233,070	29,970
Percent	100.0	100.0	100.0	100.0	100.0	100.0	100.0	100.0
14-19 years	10.5	14.3	10.8	14.6	5.8	8.6	6.4	7.5
20-24 years	18.7	23.4	23.6	26.2	17.9	19.8	21.4	24.4
25-29 years	17.2	21.7	18.3	23.3	18.6	21.2	19.5	22.0
30-34 years	15.6	16.0	13.4	12.7	17.6	19.3	13.4	16.1
35-39 years	13.5	11.8	11.1	11.3	14.7	14.1	12.0	14.7
40-44 years	11.3	6.6	10.1	4.9	12.8	9.4	12.4	7.7
45-49 years	7.6	3.9	5.7	3.9	8.4	4.8	8.1	5.7
50-54 years	4.1	1.9	4.2	2.2	3.3	2.2	4.4	1.2
55-59 years	1.5	0.4	2.8	0.9	0.9	0.6	2.4	0.7
Median age	30.6	27.3	28.8	26.5	31.7	29.6	30.5	28.6

Source: U.S. Bureau of the Census, U.S. Census of Population: 1950, Vol. IV, Special Reports, Part 2, Chapter E, Duration of Current Marital Status, tables 16 and 21.

one-half million nonwhite women — were quite young at the time of separation. When the marital break occurred, a majority of the nonwhite women (59 percent) were under 30 years of age, and nearly one-half (46 percent) of the white women were also under 30.

Over one-quarter of a million of these separated women were reported in 1950 as having been separated for less than 2 years. A majority had been separated before reaching 30 years of age and had experienced this marital break, on the average, at a younger age than the women who had been separated for a longer period of time. Of the white women separated less than 2 years, 53 percent were under 30 years of age; the corresponding figure for nonwhite women was 64 percent. Thus in 1950 separations had occurred at an early age and the trend appeared to be toward more of the separations taking place at an early age. In addition, these findings probably reflect rather high divorce and remarriage rates among those who are relatively young at separation.

In 1950 the divorced women 15 to 59 years old totaled approximately 1,150,000, and they had been divorced at an older age (median about 31 years) than the separated women had been separated (median about 29 years). The nonwhite women had divorced at an earlier age (median about 30 years) than had the white women. While divorces occurred at all ages shown, more of the women had been divorced in ages over 35 years than had been separated in these

Table 8.5. Quartile of age at divorce: Divorce
Registration Area and selected states
in the United States, 1960 to 1962

Quartile of age at divorce	Divorce Registration Area			4-state study[a] 1960-1961	Divorce-Census Match[b] 1960
	1960	1961	1962		
Husband					
First quartile	26.9	27.0	27.2	26.5	28.1
Median	34.1	34.0	34.5	33.4	36.2
Third quartile	43.7	43.2	44.1	43.9	47.4
Wife					
First quartile	23.8	23.9	24.1	23.3	25.2
Median	30.9	30.8	31.0	30.0	33.0
Third quartile	39.7	39.6	40.2	39.6	41.5

Source: National Center for Health Statistics, Divorce Statistics Analysis, United States: 1962, Series 21, No. 7, tables 1 and 3; and U.S. Bureau of the Census, unpublished records.

[a]The four states (Hawaii, Iowa, Tennessee, Wisconsin) were studied in detail for use in this monograph because of the excellence of the divorce data. The information from most states regarding age and other characteristics was very incomplete.

[b]The five states (Georgia, Iowa, Ohio, Oregon, Pennsylvania) had adequate address information on their divorce report forms, and all divorces occurring in March 1960 were matched, if this was possible, with the 1960 census records. The 25-percent census sample was used for this purpose.

older ages. Of the women divorced less than 2 years, more of them were in the younger age brackets (median about 30 years at divorce) than those who had been divorced longer (median about 32 years).

More recent information is available on age at divorce for both men and women based on vital records (see Table 8.5). Again, it is clear that divorces were granted to a relatively young group. Of the husbands, around one-quarter were under 27 years of age, one-half were under 34, and three-fourths were under 44 years of age. These figures include divorces following not only the first but also the second and subsequent marriages. The wives, on the average, were some 3 years younger than the husbands at divorce. One-fourth of them were under 24 years of age, one-half were under 31, and three-fourths of them were under 40 years of age at the time of divorce. But obviously there were also many divorces at the older ages; one-fourth of the men were over 44 years of age, and one-fourth of the women were over 40 years of age.

It is noteworthy that the medians and quartiles from the Divorce-Census Match, shown in the fifth column of Table 8.5, are generally 1 to 3 years higher than the figures appearing in the first four columns. In this special study of five states, the approximately 4,500 state divorce records for decrees granted in March 1960 for which there were street addresses were matched with the 25-percent sample of census records, and the ages at divorce were derived from the census records on date of birth.[4] A prime consideration in the selection of states for the study was the existence on report forms of an adequate address for the plaintiff. State divorce forms often lack this essential item for matching with census records. In addition, many of the records from the five selected states could not be matched because the address written on the form was inadequate — or because it was inaccurate, possibly because of change of address by the plaintiff after the decree was granted. The records of 554 persons were matched. The five states, as a group, had a higher-than-average age at divorce.

By contrast, the four-state study shown in the fourth column of Table 8.5 had a bias toward younger ages at divorce, with medians one-half to one year less than the figures for the Divorce Registration Area. Two of the four states (Hawaii and Wisconsin, with less than 5,000 divorces annually) had medians higher than the DRA, and the other two (Iowa and Tennessee with over 13,000 divorces) had medians lower than the DRA. Consequently, the four-state study and the Divorce-Census-Match Study may be discounted in estimating average age at divorce.

As Table 8.6 shows, there were marked variations among states in age at time of divorce. For the 12 states listed, the median age of husbands at divorce was 34.1 years and of wives 30.9 years. The lowest median age of husbands at divorce was that for Tennessee, 32.4 years, and the highest was that for Oregon, 35.9. There was

Table 8.6.   Divorces and annulments, by median and quartile ages
of husband and wife at decree: 12 states of the
Divorce Registration Area, 1961

| | Age at decree | | | | | |
| | Husband | | | Wife | | |
Area	First quartile	Median	Third quartile	First quartile	Median	Third quartile
Total	27.1	34.1	43.3	24.0	30.9	39.7
Hawaii	28.0	34.9	43.3	25.1	31.4	38.5
Idaho	25.5	33.5	43.5	22.8	29.6	39.7
Iowa	26.1	33.2	42.4	22.9	29.5	39.0
Kansas	26.9	33.7	43.0	23.7	30.4	40.3
Maryland	28.1	34.4	43.2	24.5	32.0	39.0
Michigan	26.8	33.2	41.6	24.1	30.0	38.4
Missouri	27.0	35.1	45.2	23.6	31.4	41.0
Oregon	28.3	35.9	44.7	24.8	33.4	41.3
Pennsylvania	27.8	34.9	43.5	25.4	31.9	40.6
Tennessee	26.5	32.4	43.0	23.0	28.8	37.9
Virginia	25.3	34.0	41.9	24.4	31.1	39.0
Wisconsin	28.0	35.3	45.3	24.6	32.2	41.6

Source: National Center for Health Statistics, Vital Statistics
of the United States, 1961, Vol. III, Divorces, tables 3-D and 4-3; and
unpublished data from vital records.

Table 8.7.   Divorces by number of times married, 1952 to 1959, and
median age at divorce by number of times married, 1959:
Selected states

| Number of times married | Divorces, with number of times married reported | | | | Median age at divorce, 10 states, 1959 | |
| | 16 states, 1952 to 1959 | | 10 states, 1959 | | | |
	Husband	Wife	Husband	Wife	Husband	Wife
Total	2,582,930	2,582,061	38,290	38,452	34.0	30.7
Percent	100.0	100.0	100.0	100.0	...	...
Married:						
Once	79.8	78.9	71.3	69.9	31.2	27.8
Twice	17.3	17.9	21.9	22.7	39.9	36.0
Three times	2.5	2.8	5.2	5.8	43.5	40.4
Four or more	0.4	0.4	1.6	1.7	45.4	42.3

Source: National Center for Health Statistics, Vital
Statistics of the United States: 1952 to 1959, Vol. I.

thus a spread of 3.5 years in average age of men at divorce in these 12 states. For women, the lowest was 28.8 years in Tennessee, and the highest was 33.4 years in Oregon, giving a spread of 4.6 years.

In a given year, a substantial majority of the divorces for which data were available represented the legal termination of a first marriage. Information from 16 states, for the eight years 1952–1959, indicated that nearly 8 out of 10 of the decrees ended a first marriage (see Table 8.7). Second marriages were terminated in some 17 to 18 percent of the divorces, third marriages in 2 to 3 percent of the cases, and fourth or higher-order marriages in 0.4 percent of these cases. However, these results differed somewhat from a tabulation

Table 8.8. Number of previous marriages of persons divorced in Iowa in 1966

Number of times married and sex	Divorces		Marriages involved	
	Number	Percent	Number	Percent
Men				
Total	5,516[a]	100.0	7,672	100.0
Married:				
Once	3,929	71.2	3,929	51.2
Twice	1,158	21.0	2,316	30.2
Three times	324	5.9	972	12.7
Four times	74	1.3	296	3.8
Five times	27	0.5	135	1.8
Six times	4	0.1	24	0.3
Women				
Total	5,517[a]	100.0	7,662	100.0
Married:				
Once	3,929	71.2	3,929	51.2
Twice	1,172	21.2	2,344	30.6
Three times	311	5.7	933	12.2
Four times	78	1.4	312	4.1
Five times	18	0.3	90	1.2
Six times	9	0.2	54	0.7

Source: Iowa State Department of Health, Des Moines, Iowa, Annual Report, 1966, table 32.

[a]Total excludes "other" and "not stated."

based on 10 states for 1959, where 7 out of 10 decrees ended first marriages and correspondingly higher proportions than in the 16-state study ended second, third, and higher-order marriages. Available data do not make possible a closer approximation.

Age at divorce rises with the number of previous marriages (see Table 8.7). For husbands ending a first marriage, the median age was 31 years; but for those ending their fourth or subsequent marriage, it was 45 years. For wives, the corresponding medians were 28 and 42 years. The difference between the median ages of husbands and wives at divorce was about 3.3 years.

Although comprehensive national data on the total number of marriages involved during the lifetime of divorced persons are not available, information was compiled for one state, Iowa, on the number of marriages by husband and wife up to the sixth marriage (see Table 8.8). In 1966 about 7 out of 10 divorces ended a first marriage, while a minor fraction of 1 percent ended a sixth marriage. These 5,500 divorces in Iowa in 1966 brought to a legal end that number of marriages; however, since many of these individuals had been married more than once, the total number of marriages involved was considerably higher. In fact, the individuals ending first marriages had experienced only 51 percent of total prior marriages, whereas persons married more than once (sometimes after widowhood) accounted for 49 percent of them.

Among these Iowa divorces the number of previous marriages by women was about equal to the number by men; however, the number of previous divorces was probably substantially higher for men. A

Table 8.9. Percent divorced and married once or more than once, for persons ever married, by selected number of years since first marriage, color, and sex: United States, 1960

Number of years since first marriage	Percent divorced and married only once				Percent divorced and married more than once			
	Men		Women		Men		Women	
	White	Nonwhite	White	Nonwhite	White	Nonwhite	White	Nonwhite
Total	2.1	2.7	2.6	3.5	0.6	0.8	0.8	1.1
Less than 5 years	2.0	1.6	2.0	2.1	0.1	0.1	0.1	0.1
5-9 years	2.5	2.8	2.7	3.9	0.3	0.3	0.4	0.4
10-14 years	2.2	3.6	2.6	4.7	0.5	0.6	0.6	0.9
20-24 years	2.3	3.3	3.1	4.5	0.8	1.1	1.2	1.7
30-34 years	2.3	2.8	3.2	3.5	1.0	1.5	1.3	1.9
40-44 years	1.8	1.9	2.4	2.0	0.9	1.2	1.0	1.6
50-54 years	1.3	1.0	1.5	1.2	0.8	1.2	0.6	1.0
60 & over	0.9	0.5	0.7	0.6	0.6	0.7	0.3	0.2
Median years since first marriage	18.5	17.1	21.2	17.6	26.5	27.5	26.3	25.4

Source: U.S. Bureau of the Census, U.S. Census of Population: 1960, Subject Reports, Marital Status, Final Report PC(2)-4E, table 2.

large number of the previous marriages doubtless were ended by death of the marital partner, and far more women than men become widowed.

Census data for 1960, tabulated in Table 8.9, throw further light on the extent of repeated marriages by the divorced population. Three times as many divorced persons had been married only once as had been married more than once, but as the number of years since the first marriage increased the proportion of the divorced population who had been married only once decreased. Thus if only 5 to 9 years had passed since first marriage, 8 to 10 times as many persons had been married once as had been married more than once; but after 20 to 24 years, only about 3 times as many had been married once.

Data from the 1950 census indicate that a surprisingly large proportion (about one-fifth) of the 1,042,000 separated and 1,154,000 divorced women 15 to 59 years old had been married more than once (see Table 8.10). Even 8 or 9 percent of the teenaged separated or

Table 8.10. Percent of separated women 15 to 59 years old who remarried, by age at separation, and percent of divorced women 15 to 59 years old who remarried, by age at divorce: United States, 1950

Separated women		Divorced women	
Age at separation	Percent remarried	Age at divorce	Percent remarried
Total, 14-59	20.5	Total, 14-59	19.6
14-19 years	9.2	14-19 years	7.9
20-24 years	12.6	20-24 years	12.4
25-29 years	18.9	25-29 years	15.4
30-34 years	21.5	30-34 years	19.0
35-39 years	27.6	35-39 years	22.5
40-44 years	30.5	40-44 years	28.0
45-49 years	31.2	45-49 years	27.8
50-54 years	35.6	50-54 years	40.4
55-59 years	46.1	55-59 years	37.7

Source: U.S. Bureau of the Census, U.S. Census of Population: 1950, Vol. IV, Special Reports, Part 2, Chapter E, Duration of Current Marital Status, tables 16 and 21.

divorced women had already been married more than once. As the age at marital disruption advanced, the proportion of women with at least two marriages increased; nearly one-half of the separated women and more than one-third of the divorced women in their late fifties had been married more than once.

Variations in Permanence of Marriage

Since all marriages must be terminated at some time, it is of interest to note the attrition rate of marriages through the combined effects of divorce and death; also (for the spouses who survive marriage terminations) to note the rate at which new marriages are contracted.

Marital dissolution by age at first marriage. Rates of marital dissolution by age at marriage for white and nonwhite men and women during the first 20 years after first marriage are illustrated in Tables 8.11 and 8.12 and Figure 8.1. Dissolutions began shortly after marriage in a few instances; by early 1960, among the men who married in 1955 to 1957, some 5 percent of the white and 6 percent of the

Table 8.11. Percent of men first married in 1940 to 1957 whose first marriage was dissolved by death of spouse or divorce by 1960, by year of first marriage, color, and age at first marriage: United States, 1960

Year of first marriage and color	Total men	Age at first marriage (years)				
		14-19	20-24	25-29	30-34	35 & over
First marriage dissolved by 1960						
White						
1955-57	5.4	7.9	4.6	3.9	5.4	9.0
1950-54	9.2	14.7	8.5	6.7	8.0	10.8
1945-49	12.3	22.5	11.8	9.4	10.0	14.0
1940-44	16.6	27.9	16.0	13.1	13.8	16.6
Nonwhite						
1955-57	6.0	6.2	4.7	5.4	7.6	11.1
1950-54	12.3	15.2	11.6	10.7	10.4	14.6
1945-49	20.4	26.4	20.1	17.2	18.4	20.3
1940-44	27.8	35.5	27.9	23.6	24.2	25.2

Source: U.S. Bureau of the Census, U.S. Census of Population: 1960, Subject Reports, Age at First Marriage, Final Report PC(2)-4D, table 4.

Table 8.12. Percent of women first married in 1940 to 1957 whose
first marriage was dissolved by death of spouse or
divorce by 1960, by year of first marriage, color, and
age at first marriage: United States, 1960

Year of first marriage and color	Total women	Age at first marriage (years)				
		14-17	18 & 19	20-24	25-29	30 & over
First marriage dissolved by 1960						
White						
1955-57	6.6	10.9	5.9	4.1	5.9	10.4
1950-54	11.0	18.6	11.1	7.4	8.7	14.2
1945-49	14.8	25.8	16.0	10.8	11.2	17.9
1940-44	21.0	32.9	22.9	16.6	16.5	24.1
Nonwhite						
1955-57	8.2	7.4	7.2	6.5	10.4	13.8
1950-54	15.5	16.4	14.6	13.4	16.2	20.3
1945-49	24.3	27.4	23.5	21.4	23.8	28.2
1940-44	33.7	37.0	33.2	30.6	32.4	36.6

Source: U.S. Bureau of the Census, U.S. Census of Population:
1960, Subject Reports, Age at First Marriage, Final Report PC(2)-4D,
table 4.

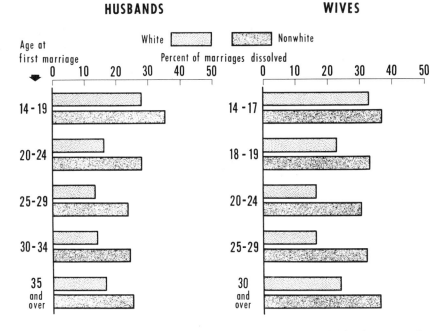

Fig. 8.1. Percent of persons first married in 1940 to 1944 whose marriage
was dissolved by 1960, by age at first marriage: United States, 1960

Source: Tables 8.11 and 8.12.

nonwhite men had experienced a marital dissolution. With the passage of time since first marriage, an increasing proportion of the marriages had been dissolved and the white-nonwhite differential had widened: for men who had married some 15 to 20 years before the census enumeration, about 17 percent of the white and 28 percent of the nonwhite men had experienced a marital dissolution.

It is also evident that the rate of marital dissolution is affected by the age at marriage. The "worst" age for men to marry (in terms of the rate of dissolution) was between 14 and 19 years of age, and the "best" (by the same criterion) was 25 to 29 years of age, followed closely by the next older age group, 30 to 34 years.

Among women, too, marriages of the very young had the highest dissolution rates — led by early teenagers and followed by late teen-

Table 8.13. Percent of persons first married in 1940 to 1957 whose first marriage was dissolved by death of spouse or divorce by 1960, and percent whose first marriage was not intact by 1960, by year of first marriage, color, and sex: United States, 1960

Year of first marriage and sex	White, with first marriage--		Nonwhite, with first marriage--	
	Dissolved by 1960	Not intact	Dissolved by 1960	Not intact
Men				
1955-57	5.4	6.9	6.0	12.9
1950-54	9.2	10.3	12.3	19.9
1945-49	12.3	13.3	20.4	28.1
1940-44	16.6	17.5	27.8	35.1
Women				
1955-57	6.6	8.5	8.2	19.1
1950-54	11.0	12.6	15.5	28.3
1945-49	14.8	16.0	24.3	36.8
1940-44	21.0	22.1	33.7	44.8

Source: U.S. Bureau of the Census, U.S. Census of Population: 1960, Subject Reports, Age at First Marriage, Final Report PC(2)-4D, table 4.

agers. Lowest dissolution rates among white women were for marriages at ages 20 to 29 years and among nonwhite women at ages 20 to 24 years. Again, the differential between white and nonwhite persons in rate of marital dissolution was marked. After 15 to 20 years of marriage, about four-fifths of the white women but only two-thirds of the nonwhite women were still in marriages undissolved by divorce or death of husband.

Before the marriage is dissolved there is frequently a period of separation of the marital partners. "Not-intact" marriages include the separated as well as the dissolved unions, and it is evident that by this measure the rate of attrition is especially high among nonwhite marriages (see Table 8.13). Thus, among white persons almost 18 percent of the men and 22 percent of the women were in "not-intact" marriages after 15 to 20 years, but the corresponding figures for non-

Table 8.14. Percent distribution of persons 20 to 24 years old at first marriage with first marriage between 1935 and 1960, by whether married once or more than once, by marital status and sex: United States, 1960

Year of first marriage and sex	Divorced and separated in 1960			Married (excluding separated) and widowed in 1960		
	Total	Married once	Married more than once	Total	Married once	Married more than once
Men 20 to 24 at first marriage						
Total, 1935-1960	100.0	83.7	16.3	100.0	90.8	9.2
1958-1960	100.0	97.9	2.1	100.0	99.6	0.4
1955-1957	100.0	95.7	4.3	100.0	97.8	2.2
1950-1954	100.0	89.9	10.1	100.0	93.8	6.2
1945-1949	100.0	82.9	17.1	100.0	90.2	9.8
1940-1944	100.0	76.0	24.0	100.0	85.9	14.1
1935-1939	100.0	72.6	27.4	100.0	83.0	17.0
Women 20 to 24 at first marriage						
Total, 1935-1960	100.0	85.5	15.5	100.0	92.2	7.8
1958-1960	100.0	98.0	2.0	100.0	99.0	1.0
1955-1957	100.0	95.7	4.3	100.0	98.1	1.9
1950-1954	100.0	91.0	9.0	100.0	95.3	4.7
1945-1949	100.0	85.1	14.9	100.0	92.6	7.4
1940-1944	100.0	79.8	20.2	100.0	88.3	11.7
1935-1939	100.0	76.2	23.8	100.0	86.8	13.2

Source: U.S. Bureau of the Census, U.S. Census of Population: 1960, Subject Reports, Age at First Marriage, Final Report PC(2)-4D, table 4.

white persons were 35 and 45 percent, respectively. The difference in the proportion of "not-intact" marriages is already apparent in marriages of only 3 to 5 years duration, where the rate for nonwhite persons is twice that of whites.

Remarriages of persons with dissolved marriages. The disruption of marriages by separation and then divorce or the dissolution of marriages by widowhood is often followed by remarriage. One view of this process is afforded by examining the persons who married during the years 1935 to 1960 at the popular ages of 20 to 24 years and observing the changes in marital status that occurred as shown in the 1960 census. Such an analysis is given in Table 8.14.

Of the men and women first married between 1958 and the census date in 1960 — a period of slightly over 2 years at the most — 2 percent reported that they had already been married more than once by 1960. In view of the slow pace frequently seen in divorce courts, it is surprising that even this proportion of young people could arrange to marry, divorce, marry again, and be recorded in the census either as divorced or separated. If these data are to be accepted at face value, they imply that for this group the decision to end the first marriage by divorce must have been taken very shortly after the marriage ceremony. Also, after the divorce became final, a second marriage was contracted quickly; but this marriage too was soon in trouble, since at the time of the census it was recorded as either a separation or a divorce.

Predictably, the number of remarriages was larger for those whose marriages took place in the more distant past; about one-fourth of the persons who first married between 1935 and 1939 (and were divorced or separated in 1960) had married more than once.

Marriages that ended through the death of a marital partner are combined in the right-hand side of Table 8.14 with intact marriages (marriages that had not been disrupted by separation). The remarriage rate in this group was approximately half that of the group who were divorced or separated in 1960. For persons first married immediately before the census (1958 to 1960) only 1 percent or less had been married more than once, and for those who had first married between 1935 and 1939 — some 20 to 25 years before the enumeration — only 13 to 17 percent had married more than once. At each duration but one, remarriages were more numerous among men than women.

Table 8.15. Percent of persons first married in 1940 to 1957 with first marriage dissolved who had remarried by 1960, with those not remarried classified by marital status in 1960, by year of first marriage, color, and sex: United States, 1960

Year of first marriage, color, and sex	Total with first marriage dissolved by 1960	Remarried by 1960	Not remarried by 1960		
			Total	Widowed	Divorced
MEN					
White					
1955-57	100.0	49.3	50.7	5.1	45.6
1950-54	100.0	69.5	30.5	4.0	26.5
1945-49	100.0	77.3	22.7	4.7	18.0
1940-44	100.0	81.5	18.5	5.5	13.0
Nonwhite					
1955-57	100.0	54.5	45.5	12.8	32.7
1950-54	100.0	67.9	32.1	8.6	23.5
1945-49	100.0	73.9	26.1	8.5	17.6
1940-44	100.0	77.7	22.3	9.7	12.6
WOMEN					
White					
1955-57	100.0	53.3	46.7	8.5	38.2
1950-54	100.0	66.8	33.2	9.1	24.1
1945-49	100.0	70.4	29.6	11.7	17.9
1940-44	100.0	71.2	28.8	14.9	13.9
Nonwhite					
1955-57	100.0	48.8	51.2	19.4	31.8
1950-54	100.0	57.6	42.4	17.4	25.0
1945-49	100.0	62.1	37.9	18.3	19.6
1940-44	100.0	63.9	36.1	21.9	14.2

Source: U.S. Bureau of the Census, U.S. Census of Population: 1960, Subject Reports, Age at First Marriage, Final Report PC(2)-4D, table 4.

A related view of marital dissolution and remarriage is shown in Table 8.15 for all first marriages (1940–1957) that were dissolved by 1960. Two questions are answered: What proportion remarried? and What was the marital status of those who did not remarry?

A high proportion of these marital dissolutions was followed by remarriage, and there were variations by sex, color, and date of first marriage. White men whose first marriage occurred at least 15 years before the census had the highest rate of remarriage. Remarriages were reported by more than 4 out of 5 of those first married in the early 1940's who had experienced a marital dissolution. The lowest remarriage rate was experienced by nonwhite women; less than two-thirds of those with first marriages in the early 1940's which had been dissolved had remarried by 1960. White women had distinctly higher remarriage rates than nonwhite women.

A substantial minority of these marital dissolutions had not resulted in a remarriage by 1960; of this minority, substantially more had been divorced than had been widowed. The distribution of the widowed and the divorced varied by sex, color, and years since first marriage. The widowed who had not remarried were more numerous among

Table 8.16. Percent divorced for white and Negro persons of selected ages, by sex: Conterminous United States, 1960, 1930, and 1910

Year and race	Men by age (years)			Women by age (years)		
	20-24	35-44	65 & over	20-24	35-44	65 & over
Percent of whites divorced: 1960	1.0	2.5	2.3	1.8	3.6	2.0
1930	0.4	1.5	1.1	1.0	1.8	0.5
1910	0.1	0.7	0.7	0.4	0.8	0.3
Index: 1960	1000	357	329	450	450	667
1930	400	214	157	250	225	167
1910	100	100	100	100	100	100
Percent of Negroes divorced: 1960	0.7	3.7	2.4	1.7	5.9	2.0
1930	0.9	2.1	1.1	2.3	2.8	0.6
1910	0.4	1.0	0.7	1.1	1.5	0.4
Index: 1960	175	370	343	155	393	500
1930	225	210	157	209	187	150
1910	100	100	100	100	100	100

Source: U.S. Bureau of the Census, U.S. Census of Population: 1960, U.S. Summary, Detailed Characteristics, table 177; Subject Reports, Nonwhite Population by Race, Final Report PC(2)-1C, tables 9 and 19; Fifteenth Census of the United States: 1930, Population, Vol. II, Statistics by Subjects, tables 5 and 6, pages 843 and 844; Negro Population, 1790-1915, table 8, page 241.

women than among men and represented a larger proportion of the nonwhite dissolutions than of the white. Among the dissolutions which followed the most recent first marriages, the great majority were divorced persons, but among women whose marriages had been terminated for more than 15 years the majority were widowed.

Social Characteristics of Divorced Persons

Among the important social characteristics of divorced persons recorded in census reports are race and national origin; nativity, parentage, and residence; living arrangements; children in the family; and educational level. Limited data concerning the separated are also available on some of these topics.

Race and national origin. Over the 50 years from 1910 to 1960 there were marked changes in the percent of the population divorced. A look in Table 8.16 and Figure 8.2 at three age groups of the di-

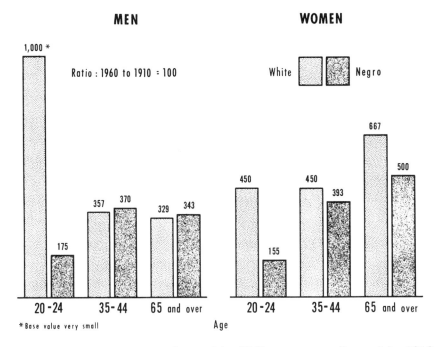

Fig. 8.2. Ratio of percent divorced in 1960 to percent divorced in 1910 times 100, by age: United States

Source: Table 8.16.

vorced — ages 20 to 24 where the remarriage rate is quite high, 35 to 44 where the remarriage rate is moderate, and 65 and over where the remarriage rate is low — shows strikingly that the percent of persons divorced was much higher in 1960 than in 1910 for both the white and Negro population of each sex. For Negroes 20 to 24 years of age, the percent divorced in 1930 was higher than in 1960.

The largest proportional increase, although one of the smallest absolute increases, in the percent of persons divorced was among white men 20 to 24 years old, where the percent for 1960 was ten times that of 1910. Some caution is appropriate here because both values were quite small, but clearly there was a marked increase. The proportion divorced for Negro men in this age group increased only from 0.4 to 0.7 percent. White and Negro men in the two other age groups had an increase to three and one-half times the 1910 level during the 50-year period.

Among white and Negro women at ages 20 to 24 years there was a marked disparity in rate of increase in the percent divorced. For white women, the percent divorced was four and one-half times as large in 1960 as in 1910, while for Negro women the advance was only slightly more than one-half; white women had the higher percent divorced in 1960 but not in 1910. In the age bracket 35 to 44 years, proportions divorced in all years shown were higher for Negroes than for the whites; but Negro women had a slower rate of increase than white women, their index number moving to 393 compared with 450 for white women. In the age group 65 years and over, between 1910 and 1960 there was a rapid increase in the percent divorced among all groups shown; the proportional increase was especially large among the women, partly because their percent divorced was so low in 1910.

Variations noted in the rising percent divorced over recent decades reflect, among other things, the unequal impact of changing attitudes toward divorce among the several social groups in the population. It should also be emphasized that the divorced persons appearing in census reports represent all divorced persons minus the attrition by remarriage or death. Remarriage is negatively correlated with age; the older the divorced person, the smaller the probability of a remarriage. Loss by death, obviously, is positively correlated with age; the older the divorced person, the higher the probability that death will occur. During the 50 years between 1910 and 1960, the increase in life expectancy was one of the many changes that affected the percentages divorced.

Table 8.17.   Percent divorced, for persons 14 years old and over, by race and sex, standardized for age and unstandardized: United States, 1960

Race	Percent divorced, standardized for age[a]		Percent divorced, unstandardized		Difference-- effect of standardization	
	Men	Women	Men	Women	Men	Women
Total, 14 & over[b]	2.1	2.9	2.1	2.9	-	-
White	2.1	2.7	2.1	2.8	0.0	-0.1
Negro	2.6	3.8	2.4	3.7	0.2	0.1
American Indian	3.3	3.2	2.9	3.1	0.4	0.1
Japanese	1.3	1.7	1.2	1.7	0.1	0.0
Chinese	1.4	1.7	1.5	1.6	-0.1	0.1
Filipino	3.8	2.1	4.4	2.0	-0.6	0.1

Source: U.S. Bureau of the Census, U.S. Census of Population: 1960, Detailed Characteristics, United States Summary, Final Report PC(1)-1D, table 176; and Subject Reports, Nonwhite Population by Race, Final Report PC(2)-1C, tables 9-13 and 19-23.

[a]Standardized on the basis of the age distribution for the total population in 1960.

[b]Includes the small number of persons of other nonwhite races, not shown separately.

One consideration in evaluating the extent of divorce in various segments of the population lies in the varying age distributions of these segments. This may be illustrated for important racial groups by examining the percent divorced both standardized for age and unstandardized, as in Table 8.17. The effect of standardization is relatively minor for most of the groups, especially among women. The lowering of the percent divorced among Filipino men through standardization was a consequence of their including a large proportion of old men. On the other hand, standardizing raised the percent divorced for American Indian men because a large proportion of these men were younger than the male adult population in general. Negro males had the percent divorced raised only 0.2 percent by standardization; other males and all the females had changes of 0.1 percent or less.

The percent divorced among foreign-born (first generation) per-

Table 8.18. Percent divorced, for persons 14 years old and over and
45 to 54 years old of foreign stock, by country of origin,
nativity, parentage, and sex: United States, 1960

Country of origin	Percent divorced, 14 years old & over				Percent divorced, 45-54 years old			
	Foreign born		Native of foreign or mixed parentage		Foreign born		Native of foreign or mixed parentage	
	Men	Women	Men	Women	Men	Women	Men	Women
Total	1.9	2.2	2.0	2.6	2.4	3.4	2.5	3.5
Austria	2.0	2.3	1.9	2.8	1.9	3.5	2.4	3.5
Canada	2.4	3.0	2.2	3.0	2.8	4.4	2.9	4.3
Czechoslovakia	1.8	1.8	1.8	2.4	2.1	3.2	2.2	3.1
Germany	1.6	2.3	2.1	2.7	1.9	3.6	2.4	3.7
Ireland	0.8	0.8	1.9	1.8	0.9	1.2	2.6	2.5
Italy	1.3	1.1	1.5	2.0	1.5	1.7	1.9	2.7
Mexico	1.9	3.5	2.0	3.3	2.9	5.4	3.6	5.7
Poland	1.8	1.8	1.8	2.2	1.8	2.6	2.3	2.9
Sweden	2.4	2.5	2.4	3.2	2.9	4.6	2.6	3.9
United Kingdom	1.8	2.3	2.2	3.0	2.2	3.5	2.9	4.2
U.S.S.R.	1.8	2.4	1.7	2.7	2.2	3.5	1.9	3.4
Other & not reported	2.3	2.5	2.2	3.0	3.1	3.9	2.8	3.9

Source: U.S. Bureau of the Census, U.S. Census of Population:
1960, Subject Reports, Nativity and Parentage, Final Report PC(2)-1A,
tables 7, 10, and 13.

sons and among native persons with foreign-born parents (second generation) may be examined in Table 8.18. Because of the distorting effect of the age distribution of the relatively old foreign-born population, and to a lesser degree of persons of foreign or mixed parentage, the age bracket 45 to 54 years is shown. This group is one in which the number of divorced persons is high and in which relatively few remarriages take place. The following discussion relates to those 45 to 54.

Overall, there was a slight increase in the percent divorced among those in the second generation when compared to the first generation of the same age group. However, this overall result grew out of different movements among the various nationality groups. The highest rates in the last two columns were for Mexicans, 3.6 for men and 5.7 for women. This origin group includes many whose ancestors were peasant farmers in Mexico and many who are found in this country among the migratory farm workers and in the central cities of large urban areas. Rates for the second generation of Mexican origin aged 45 to 54 moved toward conformity with prevailing standards.

The lowest rate among second-generation women 45 to 54 was recorded for the Irish (2.5 percent divorced). Yet the proportion divorced for native persons of Irish origin was two to three times that of foreign-born persons of Irish origin. Relating as they do to a country where the divorced are very few in number, these figures illustrate the tendency for the divorce rate in various groups within the nation's population to move toward a common level, as noted in Chapter 2. For the foreign born from Sweden, the percent divorced was relatively high, but for the second generation the rate moved downward. Among native Americans with parents born in Germany, the percent divorced increased markedly for men and slightly for women, bringing both rates close to the average of the total group. Thus as the descendants of the foreign born are less influenced by Old World customs, their divorce rates evidently tend to approximate those of the native stock.

Nativity, parentage, and residence. The divorced population 25 to 64 years of age is shown in Table 8.19 as a percent of the married population, with details on nativity, parentage, and residence; the same information is provided for the separated population in Table 8.20. Most of the divorced and separated are included in this age range; obviously, only married persons are subject to divorce or separation. Type of residence of the divorced and separated adds important information, as does the region of residence.

Among the divorced, the overall differences run in the expected direction, but the magnitudes of the differences may be surprising. Generally, the number divorced per 100 married was higher among women than men; the native white of native parentage, constituting two-thirds of the whole, had essentially the same ratio of divorced to married as the United States total; the foreign white stock, constituting about one-fourth of the whole, had a lower-than-average ratio (except in the South); and the Negroes, constituting almost one-tenth, had a higher-than-average ratio.

By regions, the most frequent order among these groups was for the Northeast to have the lowest ratio and the West the highest. By type of residence, rural ratios were lower than urban and frequently, from lowest to highest, it was rural farm, urban fringe (suburbs of large cities), rural nonfarm, other urban, and the central cities of urbanized areas. However, there were numerous exceptions to these

Table 8.19. Number of divorced persons 25 to 64 years old, per 100 married persons, by sex, residence, nativity, and parentage: United States, by regions, 1960

Area, race, nativity, and parentage	Divorce ratio for men					Divorce ratio for women				
	United States	North-east	North Central	South	West	United States	North-east	North Central	South	West
Total	3.1	2.0	3.1	2.9	5.0	4.5	3.4	4.4	4.4	6.7
Urban	3.4	2.1	3.5	3.4	5.2	5.4	3.7	5.5	5.9	7.7
Urbanized areas	3.4	2.1	3.7	3.6	5.4	5.6	3.6	5.7	6.4	8.2
Central city	4.3	2.6	4.7	4.3	6.8	6.9	4.5	7.3	7.4	9.9
Urban fringe	2.3	1.4	2.1	2.2	4.0	3.8	2.6	3.4	4.2	6.4
Other urban	3.1	2.4	3.0	2.9	4.3	4.9	3.9	4.8	5.0	5.7
Rural nonfarm	2.7	1.8	2.7	2.5	4.7	2.6	2.2	2.5	2.5	3.5
Rural farm	1.6	1.4	1.3	1.7	2.9	1.0	1.0	0.7	1.2	1.3
Native white of native parentage	3.1	2.2	3.0	2.9	5.1	4.5	3.6	4.2	4.2	6.6
Urban	3.5	2.4	3.4	3.3	5.3	5.7	4.2	5.5	5.7	7.8
Urbanized areas	3.7	2.4	3.6	3.6	5.6	6.0	4.1	5.7	6.3	8.4
Central city	4.8	3.2	4.8	4.4	7.2	7.6	5.5	7.6	7.5	10.3
Urban fringe	2.5	1.6	2.1	2.1	4.2	4.2	2.9	3.5	4.2	6.6
Other urban	3.1	2.6	2.9	2.9	4.4	4.9	4.6	4.9	4.7	5.8
Rural nonfarm	2.7	1.9	2.6	2.5	4.6	2.6	2.3	2.6	2.5	3.5
Rural farm	1.7	1.4	1.4	1.8	2.9	1.0	1.0	0.8	1.2	1.2
Foreign white stock	2.5	1.7	2.6	2.5	4.6	3.7	2.8	3.6	4.6	6.2
Negro	4.1	2.9	6.4	3.2	8.1	6.8	5.5	10.1	5.3	13.5
Urban	4.6	2.9	6.3	4.0	8.0	8.0	5.6	10.3	7.1	14.0
Urbanized areas	4.8	2.9	6.3	4.2	8.1	8.3	5.6	10.3	7.3	14.4
Central city	5.0	3.0	6.4	4.4	8.9	8.5	5.7	10.5	7.7	15.2
Urban fringe	3.6	2.5	4.8	3.2	5.4	6.7	5.1	8.5	5.1	11.6
Other urban	3.8	3.5	6.9	3.3	7.4	6.8	4.4	9.8	6.6	8.1
Rural nonfarm	2.8	2.9	9.9	2.2	9.8	2.8	3.8	6.0	2.6	5.0
Rural farm	1.4	2.4	4.7	1.3	4.8	1.2	2.1	1.3	1.2	1.6
Other races	4.0	2.7	5.3	3.8	4.0	3.7	2.3	3.5	4.0	3.9

Source: U.S. Bureau of the Census, U.S. Census of Population: 1960, Subject Reports, Marital Status, Final Report PC(2)-4E, table 3.

patterns. It should be emphasized that the ratios are based on place of residence at the time of the 1960 census and not necessarily the place where the individual lived at the time of divorce. Thus a woman residing on a farm at the time of divorce and lacking financial resources would be likely to move to a different type of area where the labor market would offer improved employment possibilities.[5]

Lowest ratios of divorced to married for a major group were recorded for the foreign white stock. Several factors were probably involved. Lack of familiarity with the legal system of the country and a reluctance to become involved in court actions probably resulted in some marital conditions being tolerated that otherwise would have resulted in divorce. The fact that so many of the foreign white stock reside in the Northeast region, where divorce laws are most restrictive, also tended to curtail the number of divorces. And the customs regarding divorce brought over from the Old Country undoubtedly had a profound effect upon the marital behavior of the foreign born.

The highest ratios of divorced to married were those for the Negroes, especially Negro women in the West. Since one-half of the Negroes in this country reside in the South, the relatively low ratios there keep the nationwide ratios for Negroes smaller than they would otherwise be. For Negro men in the South, the overall ratio — 3.2 divorced per 100 married — is not significantly different from the ratio of 3.1 for men in the country as a whole, and the rural ratios are slightly lower for Negro men than for white men in the South. However, Negroes have been migrating from rural to urban areas throughout the country for many years (typically to central cities), and the urban ratio of 4.0 in the South (including a central-city ratio of 4.4) is one reason for the high overall ratio for Negroes. The ratios of divorced to married for Negro women are substantially higher than those for Negro men (probably in part because the former are more completely reported) and reach their maximum level of 15.2 for Negro women in central cities of the West.[6]

The ratios of separated per 100 married persons, given in Table 8.20, were about one-third lower than the ratios for divorced persons.

Table 8.20. Number of separated persons 25 to 64 years old, per 100 married persons, by sex, residence, nativity, and parentage: United States, by regions, 1960

Area, race, nativity, and parentage	Separation ratio for men					Separation ratio for women				
	United States	North-east	North Central	South	West	United States	North-east	North Central	South	West
Total	2.0	2.3	1.4	2.5	1.7	3.1	3.7	2.0	3.8	2.3
Urban	2.2	2.4	1.8	2.8	1.8	3.6	4.2	2.7	4.8	2.6
Urbanized areas	2.4	2.5	2.0	2.9	1.9	3.8	4.4	3.0	4.8	2.8
Central city	3.2	3.5	2.9	3.6	2.5	5.1	6.1	4.2	6.0	3.5
Urban fringe	1.2	1.4	0.7	1.4	1.3	2.0	2.3	1.2	2.3	2.0
Other urban	1.8	1.9	1.0	2.6	1.4	3.0	3.1	1.5	4.8	2.0
Rural nonfarm	1.6	1.5	0.9	2.2	1.6	1.9	1.7	1.0	2.8	1.4
Rural farm	1.0	1.3	0.4	1.7	0.9	0.9	0.9	0.2	1.6	0.5
Native white of native parentage	1.4	2.0	1.0	1.3	1.5	1.8	2.8	1.2	1.7	1.9
Urban	1.5	2.2	1.1	1.4	1.6	2.2	3.4	1.5	2.1	2.2
Urbanized areas	1.6	2.2	1.3	1.5	1.7	2.3	3.4	1.6	2.2	2.2
Central city	2.1	3.3	1.8	1.7	2.1	3.0	5.1	2.2	2.5	2.7
Urban fringe	1.0	1.4	0.6	0.9	1.2	1.6	2.0	1.0	1.5	1.8
Other urban	1.2	2.0	0.9	1.2	1.4	1.9	3.1	1.3	2.0	1.9
Rural nonfarm	1.2	1.5	0.8	1.3	1.4	1.3	1.6	0.9	1.5	1.3
Rural farm	0.7	1.3	0.3	0.9	0.8	0.4	0.8	0.2	0.7	0.4
Foreign white stock	1.2	1.4	0.8	1.2	1.3	1.9	2.3	1.1	1.9	1.9
Negro	9.5	11.4	10.0	8.8	8.5	15.4	20.7	15.3	14.0	13.6
Urban	10.1	11.4	9.9	10.0	8.3	17.2	21.0	15.4	16.8	14.0
Urbanized areas	10.2	11.5	9.9	10.0	8.2	17.3	21.2	15.7	16.6	14.2
Central city	10.6	12.1	10.2	10.3	8.8	17.9	22.1	16.0	17.0	15.2
Urban fringe	7.6	8.4	6.9	7.8	6.3	13.8	16.5	12.6	13.3	10.7
Other urban	9.8	9.1	9.0	10.0	8.9	16.6	15.7	11.4	17.4	10.1
Rural nonfarm	8.2	12.7	13.7	7.5	11.4	10.5	13.4	12.1	10.4	7.7
Rural farm	5.2	8.5	8.2	5.1	6.7	6.0	6.4	4.4	6.1	3.4
Other races	2.4	5.2	3.1	3.1	1.9	2.3	4.8	3.3	3.9	1.6

Source: U.S. Bureau of the Census, U.S. Census of Population: 1960, Subject Reports, Marital Status, Final Report PC(2)-4E, table 3.

There are both similarities and striking differences in the ratios of divorced and separated to the married population. The patterns are similar in that the rural areas had lower ratios than the urban areas, and the central cities usually had the highest. Ratios of separated were low for the native white of native parents and for the foreign white stock, both of which reported less than 2 separated persons per 100 married. Among the native white of native parents, the lowest ratio of around 1 per 100 was for the North Central states; this group had its highest ratio of about 2 for men and 3 for women in the Northeast. If the Northeast region had not had such extremely restrictive divorce laws, some of the cases of marital discord that were reported as separations might have ended in divorce.

The highest separation ratios by a wide margin were reported for

Table 8.21. Index of percent divorced, for persons 14 years old and over, by size of place, color, and sex: United States, 1960

Size of place	Men		Women	
	White	Nonwhite	White	Nonwhite
Percent divorced	2.1	2.4	2.8	3.6
Index	100	100	100	100
Urban	110	117	118	119
Urbanized areas:				
Central cities	129	125	139	131
Urban fringe	81	96	93	100
Other urban:				
Places of 10,000				
or more	110	104	114	100
2,500 to 10,000	95	87	93	81
Rural	86	62	54	39
Places of 1,000 to 2,500	86	75	75	64
Other rural	86	58	50	36
Rural nonfarm	90	71	64	47
Rural farm	57	33	29	19

Source: U.S. Bureau of the Census, U.S. Census of Population, 1960, Population Characteristics, U.S. Summary, Final Report PC(1)-1B, table 49; and Detailed Characteristics, U.S. Summary, Final Report PC(1)-1D, table 176 (sample data for rural nonfarm and rural farm).

Negroes. The pattern of these ratios for Negroes in the four geographic regions is radically different from that for the divorce ratios, with the separation ratios for Negro women reaching up to 22.1 per 100 married for central cities of the Northeast. Migration is one factor in the numerous separations among Negroes. It frequently separates family members, at least temporarily, and thus tends to loosen family bonds. While major migration of the Negro in recent decades has been from the South to other regions, there has also been extensive migration from the rural to the urban South. Underemployment, a frequent stimulus to migration, is another factor in the numerous separations. A husband may leave home to seek employment in a distant city, intending to save money to send for his family to join him, but for

Table 8.22. Index of percent separated, for persons 14 years old and over, by size of place, color, and sex: United States, 1960

Size of place	Men		Women	
	White	Nonwhite	White	Nonwhite
Percent separated	1.0	5.6	1.3	8.3
Index	100	100	100	100
Urban	110	107	108	114
Urbanized areas:				
Central cities	130	116	131	120
Urban fringe	80	87	85	92
Other urban:				
Places of 10,000				
or more	100	107	108	102
2,500 to 10,000	90	95	92	93
Rural	90	71	62	60
Places of 1,000 to 2,500	80	82	77	82
Other rural	90	71	62	58
Rural nonfarm	90	73	77	65
Rural farm	50	50	31	46

Source: U.S. Bureau of the Census, U.S. Census of Population, 1960, Population Characteristics, U.S. Summary, Final Report PC(1)-1B, table 49; and Detailed Characteristics, U.S. Summary, Final Report PC(1)-1D, table 176 (sample data for rural nonfarm and rural farm).

various reasons this is postponed and a temporary absence becomes a separation.

The foreign white stock, like the Negro, has experienced the shock of migration yet its separation ratio is low. For men it is the lowest reported and for women it is only slightly higher than for native white women. An important difference between the foreign white stock and the Negroes lies in the fact that most of the migration for the former took place in the more distant past. There has been more time to adjust to it. Also, unlike the Negroes migrating to large cities, most of the foreign white stock brought with them traditions of a close-knit family unit.

Index numbers are used in Tables 8.21 and 8.22 to illustrate the percent of the population that is divorced or separated by type of residence. Among divorced men, the nonwhites were considerably more overrepresented in urban areas than were the white (indexes 117 and 110). Correspondingly, nonwhite divorced men were much more underrepresented than whites in the rural areas, most notably on farms where the index fell to 57 for white men and to 33 for nonwhite men. Divorced women presented their most noteworthy difference in the underrepresentation on farms, with the indexes falling to 29 and 19 for white and nonwhite women, respectively.

The relative distributions of the separated populations were generally similar to those of the divorced but with modifications. The concentration in central cities for white persons was similar to the divorced but was less marked for the nonwhite. Separated white men and women on farms showed similar degrees of underrepresentation. But separated women on farms were less markedly underrepresented than divorced women on farms.

Living arrangements. As shown in Table 8.23, the living arrangements of the divorced may be divided into two categories: those living in households and those living in group quarters. Here the real contrast is between men and women, with 97 percent of the divorced women but less than 90 percent of the divorced men residing in households. Nearly four times as many divorced women as men were heads of families, but relatively more men in households were listed as primary individuals (household heads with no relative present) and, especially among nonwhites, as secondary individuals (nonrelatives of household head with no relative present). In group quarters, there were more men than women, largely because of the excess of men

Table 8.23. Percent distribution of divorced persons by family status, color, and sex: United States, 1960

Family status	Men		Women	
	White	Nonwhite	White	Nonwhite
Total, 14 years & over	100.0	100.0	100.0	100.0
In households	86.7	88.2	97.1	97.2
In primary families	38.8	37.7	61.8	65.5
Head of family	9.7	10.8	36.7	40.8
Child of head	17.3	12.6	13.7	11.8
Other relative	11.7	14.3	11.4	12.8
In secondary families	0.2	0.3	0.5	0.7
Primary individual	36.9	32.3	30.2	23.6
Secondary individual	10.8	17.8	4.6	7.4
In group quarters	13.3	11.8	2.9	2.8
Secondary individual	6.3	4.1	1.1	1.4
In rooming house	2.3	1.9	0.5	1.0
In military barracks	2.4	1.4	0.1	0.0
Other	1.5	2.1	0.6	0.5
Inmate of institution	7.0	7.7	1.8	1.3

Source: U.S. Bureau of the Census, U.S. Census of Population: 1960, Subject Reports, Persons by Family Characteristics, Final Report PC(2)-4B, table 2.

living in rooming and boarding houses, in military barracks, and as inmates of institutions. Of the persons residing in group quarters, the proportion of nonwhite men was lower than that of white men in rooming houses or boarding houses and in military barracks but was higher among inmates of institutions.

The residential patterns among divorced persons varied significantly by age (see Table 8.24). For men, at ages 18 to 24 years only about three-fourths resided in households while the other fourth were in group quarters — a majority of them in military barracks. Beginning at age 25, about 85 percent of the divorced men, and still higher percentages of divorced women, were found in households. Family heads were relatively infrequent among divorced men, as compared with divorced women; a quarter of the divorced women under 25 and about one-half of those 25 to 44 years old were heads of families, generally with children present. Thereafter, as the children grew older

Table 8.24. Percent distribution of divorced persons by family status, age, and sex: United States, 1960

Family status	Age (years)					
	18-24	25-34	35-44	45-64	65-74	75 & over
Divorced men	100.0	100.0	100.0	100.0	100.0	100.0
In households	74.4	85.1	87.5	88.5	87.7	85.4
In primary families	55.4	50.0	43.7	33.0	25.2	29.8
Head of family	1.8	6.7	12.0	11.6	7.4	5.9
Child of head	44.1	34.1	22.2	8.5	0.8	-
Other relative	9.6	9.1	9.4	12.8	16.9	23.8
In secondary families	0.2	0.2	0.2	0.2	-	-
Primary individual	10.4	23.3	32.3	43.0	51.0	44.9
Secondary individuals	8.5	11.6	11.3	12.3	11.5	10.7
In group quarters	25.6	14.9	12.5	11.5	12.3	14.6
Secondary individual	19.7	8.0	5.7	4.7	4.1	3.1
In rooming house	1.7	1.8	2.2	2.6	2.7	1.8
In military barracks	16.9	5.3	2.1	0.3	0.0	-
Other	1.1	1.1	1.4	1.7	1.4	1.2
Inmate of institution	5.9	6.9	6.9	6.9	8.2	11.5
Divorced women	100.0	100.0	100.0	100.0	100.0	100.0
In households	97.5	98.0	98.0	96.8	95.3	89.9
In primary families	80.3	78.3	72.8	50.4	40.7	43.2
Head of family	24.3	48.5	53.3	30.2	13.8	8.0
Child of head	46.9	24.2	13.6	5.9	0.8	0.0
Other relative	9.1	5.6	6.0	14.4	26.2	35.1
In secondary families	1.5	1.2	0.5	0.2	0.0	-
Primary individual	10.2	13.7	20.5	40.7	49.7	41.6
Secondary individuals	5.5	4.8	4.1	5.6	4.9	5.1
In group quarters	2.5	2.0	2.0	3.2	4.7	10.1
Secondary individual	1.8	1.2	0.9	1.3	1.0	1.1
In rooming house	0.7	0.7	0.5	0.6	0.6	0.7
In military barracks	0.3	0.1	0.0	0.0	-	-
Other	0.8	0.4	0.3	0.6	0.5	0.4
Inmate of institution	0.7	0.8	1.1	1.9	3.7	9.0

Source: U.S. Bureau of the Census, U.S. Census of Population: 1960, Subject Reports, Persons by Family Characteristics, Final Report PC(2)-4B, table 2.

and left the home, this category of divorced women declined rapidly. As the age of divorced persons rose, the proportion classified as child of the household head declined and the proportion classified as primary individual rose. The sharp increase in the proportion of divorced persons 65 years old and over in institutions was attributable largely to shifts of residence to rest homes.

The family status of separated persons was basically similar to that of divorced persons yet there were differences, perhaps reflecting the fact previously noted that there was a much higher representation of the nonwhite population among the separated than among the divorced. Separated men at ages 18 to 24 years in 1960 showed a much higher proportion in households, whereas relatively more of the younger divorced men were in group quarters; three times as many divorced as separated young men were in military barracks. Inmates in institutions had a slightly larger representation among the divorced than the separated. The proportions of separated women were higher than those of divorced women in the categories of primary family member and family head, with the proportions of divorced women higher in the categories of primary individual and child of family head. However, these differences for women were small.

Children in the family. The number of children involved in the divorces granted in the United States has risen sharply since the early 1950's. In 1962, over 500,000 children under 18 years of age were

Table 8.25. Children under 18 years of age involved in divorces, United States, 1953 to 1962, and percent distribution of divorces by number of children under 18, Divorce Registration Area, 1962

Year	United States: Total children under 18 involved in divorces	Divorce Registration Area, 1962 Number of children under 18	Percent
1962	537,000	Total divorces	100.0
1961	501,000		
1960	463,000	None under 18	39.8
1959	468,000	1 child	23.3
1958	398,000	2 children	18.9
		3 children	10.2
1957	379,000	4 children	4.5
1956	361,000	5 or more	3.3
1955	347,000		
1954	341,000		
1953	330,000		

Source: National Center for Health Statistics, Divorce Statistics Analysis, United States: 1962, Series 21, No. 7, tables 19 and 20.

involved in divorce cases — an increase of 200,000 from the number in 1953 (see Table 8.25). Figures for later years indicate a further rise, with the total passing 650,000 in 1966.[7] The proportion of divorces involving at least one or two children increased markedly.

Table 8.26. Women 15 years old and over in selected marital-status groups, by number of children ever born, age, and color: United States, 1960

(Numbers in thousands)

Marital status and age	White			Nonwhite		
	Women	Children ever born	Children per woman	Women	Children ever born	Children per woman
Divorced						
Total	1,609	3,051	1.9	249	526	2.1
15-19 years	20	17	0.9	2	3	1.3
20-24 years	87	108	1.2	12	27	1.8
25-29 years	121	204	1.7	25	54	2.1
30-34 years	159	295	1.9	35	79	2.3
35-39 years	196	370	1.9	39	84	2.2
40-44 years	200	373	1.9	37	76	2.1
45-49 years	207	383	1.9	32	60	1.9
50 & over	618	1,300	2.1	67	143	2.1
Separated						
Total	741	1,829	2.5	576	1,536	2.7
15-19 years	25	24	0.9	14	19	1.4
20-24 years	72	108	1.5	54	116	2.2
25-29 years	72	151	2.1	82	238	2.9
30-34 years	80	195	2.4	95	282	3.0
35-39 years	86	217	2.5	89	252	2.8
40-44 years	83	213	2.6	72	189	2.6
45-49 years	81	209	2.6	58	147	2.5
50 & over	240	712	3.0	112	293	2.6
Married, husband present						
Total	36,958	88,152	2.4	3,334	9,340	2.8
15-19 years	779	560	0.7	96	120	1.2
20-24 years	3,173	4,386	1.4	329	854	2.0
25-29 years	4,050	8,879	2.2	437	1,230	2.8
30-34 years	4,645	12,060	2.6	474	1,558	3.3
35-39 years	4,926	13,123	2.7	461	1,521	3.3
40-44 years	4,418	11,265	2.6	394	1,245	3.2
45-49 years	4,004	9,516	2.4	348	1,026	3.0
50 & over	10,963	28,353	2.6	795	2,486	3.1

Source: U.S. Bureau of the Census, Census of Population: 1960, Subject Reports, Women by Number of Children Ever Born, Final Report PC(2)-3A, tables 16 and 17.

About 2 out of 5 couples obtaining divorces in 1962 reported no children, about 1 in 4 reported only one child, and about a third reported two or more children. This is not the full measure of children in divorce cases, however, for only children under 18 years of age are reported. Usually, no children are reported for older divorcing couples, and only the children under 18 years of age are reported for middle-aged couples. The figures also exclude all deceased children.

As indicated in Table 8.26, women reported as divorced or separated numbered over 3 million in 1960, and they had borne almost 7 million children. By way of comparison, the 1960 census also reported over 40 million women married with husband present who had borne over 97 million children. The pattern of number of children ever born to divorced and separated women varied by age and color. Among divorced women, the white group averaged 1.9 children per woman and the nonwhite 2.1 children. The principal departures by age groups from these averages were for the younger women.

The separated women included 741,000 white and 576,000 non-white women. It is noteworthy that the average number of children per woman is, at every age but one, higher for the separated than for the divorced; for white separated women the overall average was 2.5 children and for the nonwhite it was 2.7. This higher fertility of separated than divorced women is a reflection, among other things, of the lower average economic level of the former group and the negative relationship between fertility and economic status. Moreover, the divorced women had been living apart from their husbands much longer than the separated women.[8]

Educational level. Additional insight into divorce in different segments of the population may be gained by comparing the educational attainment of white and nonwhite divorced persons who had not remarried. In general, divorced women had advanced further in school than had divorced men. The median years of school completed for divorced white women was 1.5 years higher than that for divorced white men (11.5 versus 10.0 years); corresponding medians for nonwhites were 9.7 and 8.6 years of school. The percent divorced in 1960 for white and nonwhite men and women 14 and over, and corresponding data for persons 45 to 54 years old are shown in Table 8.27. (Similar data for persons 35 to 44 years old in 1960 and changes in the percentages from 1940 to 1950 and from 1950 to 1960 were shown previously in Table 3.17.)

Table 8.27. Percent divorced, for persons 14 years old and over and persons 45 to 54 years old, by years of school completed, color, and sex: United States, 1960

Years of school completed	Percent divorced, 14 years & over				Percent divorced, 45-54 years old			
	Men		Women		Men		Women	
	White	Non-white	White	Non-white	White	Non-white	White	Non-white
Total	2.1	2.4[a]	2.8	3.6[a]	2.9	3.9	4.1	5.4
Elementary:								
0-4 years	2.6	2.3	2.2	2.6	3.2	2.7	3.4	3.8
5-8 years	2.4	2.4	2.6	3.3	3.2	4.0	3.7	4.9
5-7 years	2.5	2.3	2.7	3.1	3.4	3.7	3.8	4.6
8 years	2.3	2.7	2.6	3.6	3.1	4.6	3.7	5.5
High school:								
1-3 years	2.0	2.3	2.8	3.7	3.1	5.0	4.4	6.6
4 years	2.0	2.9	2.8	4.3	2.8	5.6	4.3	7.3
College:								
1-3 years	2.0	3.1	3.1	5.2	2.7	5.4	4.5	8.3
4 or more	1.4	2.3	3.0	5.3	1.8	3.2	4.2	8.9
4 years	1.4	2.5	2.5	4.8	2.0	3.3	3.7	8.1
5 or more	1.4	2.0	4.2	6.5	1.6	3.1	5.2	10.3

Source: U.S. Bureau of the Census, U.S. Census of Population: 1960, Subject Reports, Marital Status, Final Report PC(2)-4E, table 4.

[a]Standardizing marital status of nonwhites by education of whites yields 2.6 percent divorced for nonwhite men and 4.0 percent divorced for nonwhite women.

If the nonwhite population had attained the same level of education as the white population, what effect would this have had on the percent of the nonwhite population divorced? For men 14 and over with less than 8 years of schooling, the percent divorced was higher for whites than nonwhites, but for men and women with 8 years or more of schooling the percent divorced was higher for nonwhites. If the nonwhite population were assumed to have the same level of educational achievement as the white but retained their percentages divorced by educational level, the overall proportion divorced for nonwhite men would be raised from 2.4 to 2.6 percent.

For women, a similar process of standardizing for education would widen the percent divorced considerably more. Before standardization, the proportion divorced for white women (2.8 percent) was 0.8 percentage points below that for nonwhite women (3.6 percent); but after adjusting the nonwhite to the white levels of educational achievement the difference widened to 1.2 percentage points (2.8 vs 4.0 percent).

The relationship between percent divorced and educational level is strikingly different for men than for women. It is also very different for whites and nonwhites. Among white men, the percent divorced tends to diminish as the amount of education increases; however, among nonwhite men, the percent divorced rises irregularly with increasing amounts of education to the level of high-school graduation or entrance into college, depending on the age group, and above that level diminishes. The lack of income to afford a divorce is more likely to be acute among poorly educated nonwhite men. Also, well-educated divorced men, both white and nonwhite, can more readily afford to remarry than the poorly educated.

Among both white and nonwhite women, the percent divorced moves irregularly upward from the lowest educational level up through 1 to 3 years of college; it falls for those with 4 years of college and then makes a sharp rise to a peak level for those with 5 or more years of college. However, the percent divorced rises to a much higher level for nonwhite than white women with a full high-school or some college education. Apparently, the well-educated nonwhite wife has special problems of marital adjustment. Both white and nonwhite women with graduate-school training who become divorced are more likely than less well-educated women to remain divorced and presumably to devote themselves to a working career.

Work Experience and Income

Most of the divorced are involved in earning a livelihood; they are found in all types of occupations, although they are more concentrated in some jobs than in others. A similar observation is probably relevant with regard to separated persons, but less information is available to document it. The incomes of most separated persons tend to be smaller than those of divorced persons, but both groups have incomes which vary over a wide range. Data in this section provide a summary of all these economic aspects of family life for divorced persons and of some of them for separated persons.

Labor-force-participation rates. As will be shown in Table 8.29, 2 percent of the men in the civilian labor force in 1960 were reported as divorced, but for women the proportion was about three times as high, 5.9 percent. This difference emphasizes the disparity of divorced men and women in the labor force and in the marriage market. Men are normally in the labor force, regardless of marital status; if divorced they are likely to continue at the same occupation and are likely to remarry within a short time. On the other hand, women at the time of divorce generally feel economic pressure to enter the labor market if they are not already employed; or they may re-enter the labor market, possibly after an interval of years away from it. In either case, they are likely to face strong competition and to devote extra effort toward making themselves economically independent. This is the case especially for divorced women with small children in their care; these women tend to have little time for social activity where they would meet eligible men. Consequently, the interval between divorce and remarriage is likely to be longer for women than men, and a higher proportion of the divorced women never remarry.

A relatively high proportion of the divorced population participated in the civilian labor force in 1960. About three-fourths of the men and a slightly smaller proportion (about 70 percent) of the divorced women were in the labor force (see Table 8.28). However, participa-

Table 8.28. Labor-force-participation rates of divorced persons, by age, color, and sex: United States, 1960

Age	Labor-force-participation rate				Nonwhite as percent of white		Women as percent of men	
	Men		Women					
	White	Non-white	White	Non-white	Men	Women	White	Non-white
Total divorced	74.0	73.4	71.0	69.4	99.2	97.7	95.9	94.6
14-19 years	72.2	a	57.2	43.6	a	76.2	79.2	a
20-24 years	87.2	78.9	73.4	58.9	90.5	80.2	84.2	74.7
25-29 years	88.6	81.3	77.2	68.7	91.8	89.0	87.1	84.5
30-34 years	87.3	79.6	78.2	72.4	91.2	92.6	89.6	91.0
35-44 years	85.7	81.3	81.6	77.0	94.9	94.4	95.2	94.7
45-54 years	81.5	79.7	79.4	76.4	97.8	96.2	97.4	95.9
55-64 years	69.8	67.1	65.7	60.8	96.1	92.5	94.1	90.6
65 & over	25.6	24.3	23.6	23.4	94.9	99.2	92.2	96.3

Source: U.S. Bureau of the Census, U.S. Census of Population: 1960, Subject Reports, Employment Status and Work Experience, Final Report PC(2)-6A, table 4.

aRate not shown where base is less than 1,000.

tion varied sharply by age. For white men it was over 85 percent between ages 20 and 54 years, thereafter falling to just over 25 percent for those over 65 years old; for nonwhite men it was around 80 percent between 25 and 54 years old, thereafter closely paralleling the white rate. Among white divorced women in 1960, about three-fourths of those between the ages of 20 and 54 years (and about four-fifths of those between 35 and 54 years old) were in the labor force. For nonwhite women, the participation rates were slightly lower. The last four columns of Table 8.28 show remarkably similar levels of participation of divorced men and women, white and nonwhite, in the labor force.

For separated persons, detailed information on labor-force participation is not available in the source cited in Table 8.28, but it may be lower for them than for the divorced population. The related fact will be shown in Table 8.34 that median income is substantially lower for the separated than the divorced among both men and women.

Occupational concentrations. Divorced men and women in 1960 showed marked differences in the major occupational groups in which they were concentrated, as is evident from Table 8.29. These data are examined both from the standpoint of the relative number of divorced persons in major occupational groups and by the proportion of each occupation who were divorced. The total number of divorced men was highest among operatives (over 200,000), followed by craftsmen, service workers (except in private households), and laborers (except on farms); the total number of divorced women was highest among clerical workers (over 350,000), followed by operatives, and service workers. About 60 percent of the divorced men were concentrated in the occupations indicated and about 70 percent of the divorced women in the labor force were located in the four occupations indicated; corresponding proportions of persons other than divorced in these occupations were generally smaller.

The highest proportions divorced for men were found among private household workers (4.2 percent), service workers (except in private households), laborers (except on farms), and operatives. The highest proportions divorced for women were those among managers (except on farms) (7.8 percent), service workers (except private household), craftsmen, clerical workers, and operatives. Those with the lowest proportions divorced for men were farmers, professional workers, managers, and sales workers; among women the lowest proportions were found among farm workers, professional workers,

Table 8.29. Percent of divorced persons in the experienced labor force, by major occupation group and sex: United States, 1960

(Numbers in thousands)

Major occupation group	Men in experienced labor force			Women in experienced labor force		
		Divorced			Divorced	
	Total	By occupation	Percent of total	Total	By occupation	Percent of total
Total	45,713	928	2.0	22,293	1,311	5.9
Percent	100.0	100.0	...	100.0	100.0	...
Prof., tech., and kindred workers	9.9	6.8	1.4	12.5	9.9	4.7
Farmers & farm mgrs.	5.3	2.3	0.9	0.5	0.2	2.5
Mgrs., officials, & proprs. (exc. farm)	10.3	7.3	1.4	3.6	4.7	7.8
Clerical & kindred workers	6.9	6.5	1.9	29.1	29.3	5.9
Sales workers	6.7	5.9	1.8	7.8	6.4	4.8
Craftsmen, foremen, & kindred workers	19.6	19.3	2.0	1.2	1.4	6.8
Operatives & kindred workers	20.2	21.9	2.2	16.2	16.2	5.9
Private household workers	0.2	0.3	4.2	7.9	7.7	5.8
Service workers, exc. private household	6.0	9.2	3.1	13.6	17.3	7.5
Farm laborers & foremen	2.8	2.7	2.0	1.2	0.3	1.3
Laborers, exc. farm	7.4	8.8	2.4	0.6	0.5	5.4
Occupation not reported	4.7	9.0	3.9	5.8	6.1	6.1

Source: U.S. Bureau of the Census, U.S. Census of Population: 1960, Subject Reports, Occupational Characteristics, Final Report PC(2)-7A, table 12.

and sales workers. In most occupational groups more than 5 percent of the women in the labor force were divorced.[9]

The percent divorced in 1960 for men and women in each of selected specific occupations is shown in Table 8.30. All of the professional and technical occupations listed had at least one-tenth larger or smaller percentages divorced than the average for all persons of the same sex in the labor force. Among the men in professional or

Table 8.30. Percent divorced, for persons in the experienced civilian labor force in selected occupations, by sex: United States, 1960

Occupation	Percent divorced		Occupation	Percent divorced	
	Men	Women		Men	Women
Total, all occupations	2.0	5.9	Self-employed managers, offs., & proprietors	1.6	5.6
			Retail eating & drinking		
Total, professional, techn'l. & kindred workers	1.4	4.7	places	2.6	7.8
Accountants & auditors	1.3	9.0			
Artists & art teachers	2.2	7.3	Total, clerical & kindred wkrs.	1.9	5.9
College professors & instructors	0.9	5.3	Bank tellers	1.0	5.1
Editors & reporters	2.2	6.3	Bookkeepers	2.1	6.0
Draftsmen	1.4	9.1	Cashiers	1.7	6.2
Librarians	1.7	4.6	File clerks	1.8	4.8
Musicians & music teachers	3.8	3.8	Office-machine operators	1.3	5.7
Nurses, professional	4.5	5.2	Postal clerks	1.9	5.9
Personnel & labor-relations wkrs.	1.2	9.6	Secretaries	3.6	6.6
Physicians & surgeons	1.1	7.0	Shipping & receiving clerks	1.8	6.1
Teachers, elementary schools	1.5	3.4	Stock clerks & store clerks	1.8	7.3
Teachers, secondary schools	0.9	3.4	Telephone operators	3.3	7.1
Technicians, medical & dental	2.7	6.4			
			Total, service workers, exc. household workers	3.1	7.5
Total, managers, officials, & proprietors, exc. farm	1.4	7.8	Attendants, hospitals & insts.	3.2	6.5
Buyers & department heads, store	1.3	10.1	Bartenders	5.7	12.8
Salaried managers, offs. & propr's:			Charwomen & cleaners	2.6	4.8
Manufacturing	0.9	9.7	Cooks	4.8	6.1
Wholesale trade	1.2	10.4	Counter & fountain workers	2.2	5.1
Eating & drinking places	3.7	13.9	Elevator operators	2.8	8.9
Banking & finance	1.1	7.2	Hairdressers & cosmetologists	4.3	8.0
Insurance & real estate	1.2	9.0	Janitors & sextons	2.7	5.8
Personal services	3.1	12.1	Kitchen workers	3.4	6.1
			Waiters	3.7	9.7

Source: U.S. Bureau of the Census, U.S. Census of Population: 1960, Subject Reports, Occupational Characteristics, Final Report PC(2)-7A, table 12.

technical work, the accountants and auditors, college professors and instructors, draftsmen, personnel and labor-relations workers, physicians and surgeons, and teachers in secondary schools had the lowest percentages divorced. Women in the professional and technical group with especially low percentages divorced were librarians, musicians and music teachers, and teachers in elementary and secondary schools. It is relevant that teaching and work related to the educational process has long been recognized as an established place for single (never-married) women to work, but in recent decades an increasing proportion of teachers have married.

Among the managers, officials, and proprietors the percent divorced for men was relatively low, but for women it was high. Especially low for men were the salaried managers, officials, and proprietors in manufacturing, wholesale trade, banking and finance, and insurance and real estate. Men in these occupations tend to have large incomes and probably not only have low divorce rates but also have high remarriage rates among the few who become divorced. By contrast, the percent divorced among the salaried women classified as managers, officials, and proprietors was especially high in wholesale trade, in eating and drinking establishments, and in personal services.

Most of these women probably had a high potential for being self-supporting and therefore were slow to remarry.

In the occupational group consisting of clerical workers, the proportion divorced was three times as high among the women as among men. Especially low figures were recorded among men bank tellers, cashiers, and office-machine operators. A very similar situation was observed among women employees, because the lowest proportion divorced among clerical workers was found for women in these same occupations. Perhaps the figures are relatively low for these groups because of the strong concentration of young persons in these occupations. For both men and women, relatively high proportions divorced were recorded for secretaries. For stock and store clerks, the divorced were relatively frequent among women but not among men. In general, clerical work is one of the highest-paying types of work for women but not for men.

Service workers (other than household workers) had percentages divorced more than twice as large among women as among men. Both had the highest proportion divorced among bartenders, and

Table 8.31. Employed persons, percent divorced, and percent remarried, for persons 14 years old and over, by major occupation group, color, and sex: United States, 1960

(Numbers in thousands)

Major occupation group and sex	White		Nonwhite		Percent remarried (among the ever married)	
	Number employed	Percent divorced	Number employed	Percent divorced	White	Nonwhite
Employed men, 14 years & over	39,486	1.9	4,005	2.4	11.9	20.1
Profess'l, techn'l. & kind. workers	4,318	1.3	156	2.1	8.6	15.0
Farmers & farm managers	2,216	0.9	177	0.9	7.3	20.2
Mgrs., offs., & propr's. exc. farm	4,537	1.4	91	2.8	12.8	21.1
Clerical & kindred workers	2,821	1.8	206	2.4	10.5	15.9
Sales workers	2,921	1.7	62	1.8	12.7	17.4
Craftsmen, foremen, & kind. workers	8,093	1.8	407	2.6	12.9	20.0
Operatives & kindred workers	7,723	2.0	941	2.2	12.4	19.3
Private household workers	31	3.1	29	5.4	19.3	26.2
Service workers	2,049	2.8	551	3.3	15.7	22.2
Farm laborers & foremen	915	2.1	280	1.2	12.0	25.0
Laborers, except farm & mine	2,211	2.2	772	2.1	12.4	20.8
Employed women, 14 years & over	18,538	5.8	2,618	6.1	15.3	21.8
Profess'l, techn'l. & kind. workers	2,553	4.5	197	6.0	10.2	15.1
Farmers & farm managers	99	2.5	17	2.1	10.5	18.7
Mgrs., offs., & propr's. exc. farm	750	7.8	30	7.9	20.7	29.0
Clerical & kindred workers	6,049	5.8	227	7.3	13.7	15.3
Sales workers	1,614	4.7	46	4.8	15.0	17.9
Craftsmen, foremen, & kind. workers	235	6.7	17	8.8	17.8	21.9
Operatives & kindred workers	2,920	5.9	337	6.0	15.4	18.7
Private household workers	767	5.8	889	5.7	18.5	25.1
Service workers	2,309	7.5	547	7.0	21.5	23.2
Farm laborers & foremen	168	1.1	77	1.1	8.2	21.4
Laborers, except farm & mine	85	5.0	26	6.7	17.8	19.8

Source: U.S. Bureau of the Census, U.S. Census of Population: 1960, Subject Reports, Marital Status, Final Report PC(2)-4E, table 5.

both also had high rates for hairdressers and cosmetologists. The divorced were also relatively frequent among waitresses and elevator operators but relatively infrequent among charwomen and cleaners, counter and fountain workers, and janitors and sextons. Some varieties of service work, such as janitorial work, are frequently performed jointly by husband and wife, and this is probably a factor in producing the lower proportions divorced.

Table 8.31 compares percents divorced for white and nonwhite workers in the same major occupational categories. Perhaps surprisingly, among farm and nonfarm laborers, white men had a higher percent divorced than nonwhite men. Likewise, among women service workers (and the very small number of women farmers), white women had a somewhat larger percent divorced than did the nonwhite women. In all other occupation groups, the percent divorced was as high for nonwhite as white persons, or higher.

Since the percent of the employed persons who were divorced varied markedly by occupation, one may ask what the effect would be upon the percent divorced among nonwhite persons if their employment distribution were exactly the same as that of white employed persons.

Table 8.32. Percent divorced, and percent remarried among persons ever married, for employed persons 14 years old and over, by color and sex, with percent for nonwhite standardized by major occupation group of white: United States, 1960

Color	Percent divorced		Percent remarried, among persons ever married	
	Men	Women	Men	Women
White	1.9	5.8	11.9	15.3
Nonwhite:				
Standardized for occupation	2.2	6.2	18.7	18.4
Unstandardized	2.4	6.1	20.1	21.8

Source: U.S. Bureau of the Census, U.S. Census of Population: 1960, Subject Reports, Marital Status, Final Report PC(2)-4E, table 5.

Standardizing the nonwhite employed persons by major occupation group on the basis of the whites, as in Table 8.32, lowers slightly the proportion divorced for nonwhite men, from 2.4 to 2.2 percent, whereas it increases slightly the corresponding value for nonwhite women, from 6.1 to 6.2 percent. Such standardization by occupation would reduce the percent of the employed nonwhites who were married more than once from 20.1 to 18.7 for men and from 21.8 to 18.4 for women. Thus the percent divorced and the percent married more than once, after standardization for major occupation group, would remain higher for nonwhite persons than for corresponding white persons.

Income levels. Two tables feature the relationship between separation and divorce on the one hand and income on the other. Table 8.33 shows the percent separated or divorced by income level, and Table 8.34 shows the percent of separated and divorced persons in each income level at the time of the 1960 census. These tables bring

Table 8.33.　Percent separated and percent divorced, for persons 14 years old and over by sex, by income in 1959:　United States, 1960

Income	Percent separated		Percent divorced	
	Men	Women	Men	Women
Total, 14 & over	1.4	2.0	2.1	2.9
Without income	1.3	0.8	1.7	0.7
With income	1.4	3.1	2.2	4.7
$1-$999 or loss	2.2	2.6	2.6	2.4
$1,000-$2,999	2.1	4.1	2.8	5.4
$3,000-$4,999	1.5	2.7	2.3	7.3
$5,000-$6,999	0.9	2.0	1.8	8.9
$7,000-$9,999	0.6	1.9	1.4	8.3
$10,000 & over	0.5	1.3	1.2	7.7
Median income	$2,661	$1,637	$3,286	$2,491

Source:　U.S. Bureau of the Census, U.S. Census of Population:　1960, Subject Reports, Marital Status, Final Report PC(2)-4E, table 6.

out the relatively poor economic condition of many of those who were separated or divorced.

The separated had substantially lower incomes, on the average, than the divorced. The median income of separated men with income was $2,661, whereas that of divorced men with income was $3,286. For women, the corresponding values were $1,637 and $2,491. Although this general pattern is the one most worthy of emphasis, an examination of the patterns of percent separated or divorced at the several income levels brings out important additional differences in what marriage means for men as compared with what it means for women under varying economic circumstances.

The percent separated or divorced was only slightly smaller for men without income than for men with income. At the same time, the percent separated was only about one-fourth as high for women without income as for those with income, and the percent divorced was only about one-seventh as high for women without income as for those with income. To an unknown but probably substantial extent, the lower proportion separated or divorced among women without income reflects a tendency for women who are lacking in means of self-support to avoid separation or divorce by remaining married or by remarrying soon after divorce. The results also reflect the greater likelihood that a woman will receive financial support from her estranged husband if she is divorced than if she is separated. Moreover, since separated women have lived apart from their husbands for a shorter time than divorced women, on the average, the results are affected by the smaller proportion of separated women who felt the economic pressure to work throughout the year preceding the census (the period to which the income relates).

In the middle and upper portions of the income distribution — that is, for those with incomes above $5,000 — the percent separated was relatively small, being less than 1 percent for men and 2 percent or less for women. Likewise, the percent divorced for men in this same income range was relatively small, no doubt partly because of low divorce rates and also because of high remarriage rates among men with reasonably good incomes who had been divorced. However, for women, only those with less than $1,000 income (including no income) had lower percentages divorced than women in general. Looked at another way, the percent divorced among women kept rising as income rose until about 8 or 9 percent were divorced among those with incomes of $5,000 or more. Despite this direct correlation between income and percent divorced for women, the fact remains that a large proportion of divorced women are concentrated at the lower end of the income distribution, as will be indicated in the discussion below of Table 8.34.

The percent divorced showed less variation at the several income levels for men than for women. But only 1 percent of the men with incomes of $7,000 or more had been divorced and not remarried; moreover, data in the same source as Table 8.33 show that the smallest proportion remarried was for men with incomes of $7,000 or more. These data give scant support to those who view divorce as especially prevalent among the wealthy. Quite the contrary is true; it is most prevalent among husbands in the moderate- and low-income groups.

The consistently lower incomes of nonwhites than whites who were separated or divorced in 1960 are shown by the data in Table 8.34.

Table 8.34. Percent distribution of separated and divorced persons 14 years of age and over, by color and sex, by income in 1959: United States, 1960

| Income | Separated persons | | | | Divorced persons | | | |
| | Men | | Women | | Men | | Women | |
	White	Nonwhite	White	Nonwhite	White	Nonwhite	White	Nonwhite
Total, 14 & over	100.0	100.0	100.0	100.0	100.0	100.0	100.0	100.0
Without income	8.2	10.4	19.2	15.7	7.9	10.6	10.9	12.1
With income	91.8	89.6	80.8	84.3	92.1	89.4	89.1	87.9
With income	100.0	100.0	100.0	100.0	100.0	100.0	100.0	100.0
$1-$999 or loss	18.7	28.8	29.8	43.6	16.9	24.1	19.2	34.5
$1,000-$2,999	29.5	38.9	43.2	45.1	27.9	34.7	37.5	45.4
$3,000-$4,999	26.0	24.0	21.2	9.7	25.1	27.3	30.4	16.1
$5,000-$6,999	16.2	6.7	4.3	1.3	18.6	11.1	9.3	3.3
$7,000-$9,999	6.2	1.2	1.1	0.3	7.5	2.1	2.4	0.6
$10,000 & over	3.4	0.4	0.4	0.1	4.0	0.7	1.2	0.1
Median income	$3,139	$2,088	$1,938	$1,283	$3,416	$2,497	$2,640	$1,681

Source: U.S. Bureau of the Census, U.S. Census of Population: 1960, Subject Reports, Marital Status, Final Report PC(2)-4E, table 6.

Among the eight groups presented in the table, median incomes were about two-thirds as large for nonwhites as whites and ranged from the extremely low level of $1,283 for separated nonwhite women with income up to a level of $3,416 for white divorced men with income. In addition, about one-sixth of the separated women had no income at all, and yet separated women had more children to care for than divorced women.

White divorced women had more than half again as much income, on the average, as nonwhite divorced women; also, perhaps surprisingly, they had slightly higher incomes than nonwhite divorced *men* and more than one-fourth again as much income as nonwhite separated *men*. Thus, among the eight groups of persons shown in Table 8.34 — all with comparatively low average incomes — white divorced women ranked relatively high; they had the third highest median income and were exceeded in income only by white divorced and separated men.

As pointed out above in the discussion of occupational concentrations, relatively high proportions divorced were found among women in several of the types of work which are interesting and quite remunerative. Evidently many divorced women employed in such lines of work find in their daily routines an inviting alternative to marriage and childrearing. The high rates of remarriage for divorced women below middle age, however, attest in part to the fact that such attractive alternatives are not available to all divorced women and in part to the fact that many divorced women continue their employment after remarriage (and hence become part of the "working-wives" category).

From Marriage Through Marital Disruption to Remarriage

For a considerable number of persons in contemporary American society — and apparently the proportion is rising — there is a marital journey from first marriage through divorce to remarriage. What are the characteristics of these persons at various stages of this journey? Some light is thrown on this question in Table 8.35 by comparing census data for married, separated, and divorced persons with data for recently divorced persons from a special study involving the matching of divorce and census records for persons divorced immediately prior to the 1960 census enumeration.[10]

Men who were living with their (first) wife recorded the highest score on each of three indexes: they had the highest education (46 percent high-school graduates or better), highest proportion employed (91 percent), and highest income (24 percent over $7,000). Incidentally, they also included the lowest proportion nonwhite (8 percent). At the other extreme were the separated men, who were lowest in education (26 percent high-school graduates or better), in employment (69 percent employed), and in income (7 percent over $7,000). Also, the proportion nonwhite was highest for separated men (41 percent).

Table 8.35. Social and economic characteristics of recently divorced persons as compared with married, separated, divorced, and remarried persons, standardized for age: United States, 1960

(Numbers in thousands, except for recently divorced persons)

Subject	Men 14 to 64 years old					Women 14 to 54 years old				
	Married once, wife present	Separated	Recently divorced	Total divorced	Remarried	Married once, husband present	Separated	Recently divorced	Total divorced	Remarried
Total	31,243	769	221[a]	1,132	5,006	28,270	1,077	320[a]	1,379	4,759
Percent	100.0	100.0	100.0	100.0	100.0	100.0	100.0	100.0	100.0	100.0
White	92.4	59.2	85.5	87.7	85.6	91.8	52.9	89.9	85.0	85.7
Nonwhite	7.6	40.8	14.5	12.3	14.4	8.2	47.0	10.1	15.0	14.3
No high school	33.0	52.1	40.4	37.9	38.6	22.8	42.0	19.2	24.0	30.4
High school: 1-3 years	20.7	22.3	22.1	23.8	24.7	22.5	29.5	33.6	27.6	32.0
High school: 4 years	25.5	16.4	26.5	23.3	22.1	38.2	21.4	36.6	33.0	28.0
College: 1 or more	20.8	9.1	11.1	14.9	14.6	16.5	7.1	10.7	15.4	9.6
Employed	90.8	69.2	82.3	69.9	84.0	31.3	58.1	64.7	72.3	33.5
White collar	33.4	12.5	---	19.4	25.4	17.7	16.6	---	38.0	17.3
Blue collar	47.8	44.4	---	40.8	50.9	11.7	36.1	---	29.9	14.4
Farm	6.7	4.2	---	3.3	3.9	0.6	0.8	---	0.3	0.2
Occ. not reported	2.9	8.2	---	6.3	3.7	1.3	4.7	---	4.1	1.6
Not employed	9.2	30.8	17.7	30.1	16.0	68.7	41.8	35.3	27.7	66.5
Under $5,000 or loss	47.7	80.6	64.7	71.1	56.6	97.9	96.6	95.2	90.0	96.5
Without income	1.6	9.0	---	8.1	2.8	57.3	16.5	---	9.9	39.6
$1-$2,999	19.2	46.3	---	37.3	25.9	31.2	65.7	---	52.2	44.0
Under $4,000	---	---	46.7	---	---	---	---	86.4	---	---
$5,000-$6,999	28.1	12.9	25.3	18.3	24.8	1.7	2.5	3.2	7.5	2.7
$7,000 or more	24.2	6.5	10.0	10.5	18.7	0.5	0.8	1.6	2.4	0.9

Source: U.S. Bureau of the Census, U.S. Census of Population: 1960, Subject Reports, Marital Status, Final Report PC(2)-4E, tables 1, 4, 5, and 6; and unpublished records.

[a]Total persons of all ages (not thousands) divorced in Georgia, Iowa, Ohio, Oregon, and Pennsylvania in March 1960 and matched to 25-percent sample of 1960 census.

The divorced men are shown in two groups: those who had become divorced too recently for very many of them to have remarried; and the total of all divorced men, including some who will in time remarry but including the larger number who probably will not, either because their previous marital experience has embittered them or because they have been unable to find a satisfactory matrimonial partner. Although the recently divorced men had about the same proportion as the total divorced who had graduated from high school, the recently divorced had a higher rate of employment and higher income than the total divorced group. Thus the recently divorced men would appear to have a higher potential for remarriage from the standpoint of ability to support a wife.

The remarried men may be contrasted with the divorced, since the great majority of them came from the ranks of the previously divorced rather than the previously widowed. Educationally they were not markedly different from the divorced men, but they definitely had a higher rate of employment and a higher average income, particularly as compared with the total divorced group. The remarried men therefore appear to be more desirable as husbands than those who remained divorced.

Analysis of the data concerning women is complicated by the fact that most married women derive their principal income from their husband, and their own employment depends on such factors as the presence of small children, the husband's income, and their own training. Nevertheless, the data are significant. As in the case of the men, the women who were living with their first spouse had the highest educational achievement (55 percent high-school graduates or better) and the separated women had the lowest educational achievement (29 percent high-school graduates or better). Moreover, for separated women, the proportion nonwhite was extremely high (47 percent).

The recently divorced women had a relatively high proportion with 9 to 12 years of school, whereas the total group of divorced women had a larger proportion who had not gone to high school and also a larger proportion who had gone to college. However, the total group of divorced women showed a greater capacity for self-support by their higher proportion employed and higher income.

The remarried group had less education than either group of divorced women and had a level of employment only slightly higher than that of women living with their first husband. The income of the remarried women was also low, but this does not prove that they tended to have low economic status, since it tells nothing of the husband's income. In fact, the data taken as a whole are consistent with the hypothesis that divorced women tend to have somewhat lower socioeconomic status than married women and that divorced women who are weak on ability to support themselves are the most likely to remarry.

The foregoing discussion of the social and economic characteristics of the separated and divorced population provides important information about marital discord. Obviously, however, these groups do not cover all persons with serious marital difficulties. Even a considerable segment of the population classified as "married, spouse present" may be in serious difficulty, but which members of this group are having trouble and how their characteristics differ from those with no serious marital problems are unknown.

Marriage, as a way of life, is extraordinarily popular in the United States and appears to be growing more so. Only a small fraction of the present high-school graduating class, in all probability, will never marry. So well accepted is marriage as the normal and approved status of maturity and adulthood that it seems probable that a considerable number of individuals who either are temperamentally unsuited to marriage or are incompatible with their prospective marital partners will nonetheless marry because it is "the thing to do." As a result, many of them will become separated for a while, and some of these separated persons will eventually become divorced.

Aid to persons with marital trouble is undertaken by various agencies, as will be discussed in Chapter 12. However, only a small fraction of the couples needing such assistance actually receive it. Thus the prospect for the next several years is for the substantial number of annual divorces to continue.

9 / GROUP VARIATIONS AMONG WIDOWS AND WIDOWERS

Although widowhood and widowerhood are phenomena largely of old age, much of the attention in this chapter is devoted to widowed persons of middle age. Since the monograph is primarily a study of marriage and divorce, the chief purpose of discussing widowed persons is to throw light on the selective ending of marriage through death of one of the spouses and on the selective return of widowed persons to the norm for persons no older than middle age, which is to be married. Only 2 percent of widowed persons are under 35 years old. Accordingly, several of the tables in the chapter present data only for widowed persons between 35 and 54 years old. For present purposes, this period is critical because most of the widowed persons who remarry do so while they are in this age range. Moreover, statistics for persons of this age group on labor-force participation, occupation, and income are not seriously complicated by selective early retirement from the labor market.

Occurrence of Widowhood and Widowerhood

Information about the demographic characteristics of surviving persons as of the time when their spouse dies is seldom if ever available from vital and census statistics. From periodic tabulations of deaths by marital status, the number of married persons who died shows the number of persons of the opposite sex who became widowed. In this respect, vital statistics reports for 1963, 1949–51, and 1940 show the following:[1]

In 1963, about 251,000 men and 592,000 women became widowed;
In 1950, about 219,000 men and 447,000 women became widowed;
In 1940, about 229,000 men and 400,000 women became widowed.

Relating these figures to the numbers of married persons exposed to the risk of becoming widowed at these dates shows the following rates per 1,000 exposed:

In 1963, widowerhood rate, 5.9; and widowhood rate, 13.8;
In 1950, widowerhood rate, 5.9; and widowhood rate, 11.9;
In 1940, widowerhood rate, 7.6; and widowhood rate, 13.3.

These findings reveal an annual widowerhood rate of around 6 to 8 per 1,000 men subject to widowerhood and an annual widowhood rate of around 12 to 14 per 1,000 women subject to widowhood. Thus approximately twice as many persons became widows as became widowers during the period 1940–63, according to these statistics. The complex process necessary to adjust the rates for changes in age composition of the population was not undertaken. The expected effect of the upward trend in the average age of persons most subject to widowhood or widowerhood has been to increase the rates (for persons of all ages combined), but the expected effect of improvements in survival rates has been to lower the rates by extending the period of joint survival of husbands and wives — particularly of those in the middle age range. Which of these offsetting factors predominates is a subject which requires further study.

Differential widowhood rates by educational level, age, and color based on 1950 census data[2] are shown in Table 9.1. The rates were extremely low for white women under 35 years of age who had completed at least 12 years of school. The calculated annual widowhood rate for these women in 1950 was only 1 per 1,000 women subject to widowhood; this was one-half the corresponding nonwhite rate. Likewise, most of the other rates in Table 9.1 are about one-half as

Table 9.1. Widowhood rate per 1,000 women 14 to 54 years old subject to widowhood, by educational level, age, and color: United States, 1948 to 1950

Educational level and color	Widowhood rate				
	Total, 14-54	Age at widowhood (years)			
		14-24	25-34	35-44	45-54
Total	3.6	1.5	1.6	3.5	8.3
Not high-school graduate	4.4	2.0	2.0	3.9	8.9
High-school graduate	2.5	0.9	1.2	2.8	6.9
White	3.3	1.3	1.4	3.0	8.0
Not high-school graduate	4.0	1.6	1.6	5.6	
High-school graduate	2.4	0.9	1.1	4.2	
Nonwhite	5.6	2.2	3.7	8.0	12.2
Not high-school graduate	5.8	2.2	4.1	9.5	
High-school graduate	4.4	2.1	2.2	8.9	

Source: U.S. Bureau of the Census, U.S. Census of Population: 1950, Vol. IV, Special Reports, Part 2, Chapter E, Duration of Current Marital Status, table 29; and Part 5, Chapter B, Education, tables 7 and 8.

large for white women as for their nonwhite counterparts. A complication in interpreting these figures is that the person who died was the husband, whereas the rates of widowhood are for the surviving wife.

Further evidence of the differential occurrence of widowhood among white and nonwhite women during the two years before the 1950 census is provided by Table 9.2. The widows covered by this table had a median age of 45 years; in 1950, about 10 percent of the women 45 years old of all marital-status categories combined were nonwhite.

The average interval between widowhood and remarriage, for those who remarry, is about 3.5 years.[3] The interval is shorter for young widows and longer for the older ones. An effort to determine the approximate magnitude of the movement into and out of the state of widowhood, using available broad age groups, is recorded[4] in Table 9.3.

The findings in the first three columns of the table may be interpreted as showing that about one-half of the widows under 25 years old at the time of the 1950 census became widowed during the two preceding years. For successively older ages the recent accessions to widowhood represent a smaller proportion of all those widowed in the age group.

Table 9.2. Percent nonwhite among recently widowed women, by age at widowhood and educational level: United States, 1948 to 1950

| Age at widowhood | Percent nonwhite | | |
	Total	Not high-school graduate	High-school graduate
Women widowed less than 2 years, at age 14-54	17.5	21.5	7.3
14-24 years	28.2	34.5	11.9
25-34 years	24.2	33.4	8.4
35-54 years	15.4	18.5	6.6

Source: U.S. Bureau of the Census, U.S. Census of Population: 1950, Vol. IV, Special Reports, Part 2, Chapter E, Duration of Current Marital Status, table 29.

The fifth column of the table indicates that about one-half as many widowed women under 55 years old remarried during the year before the 1950 census as the number of married women of that age who became widowed during that year. Moreover, about one-eighth as many widowed women under 55 died during the year as the number who became widowed. The remaining three-eighths of the women who became widowed during the year represented net accessions to

Table 9.3. Percent of widows in 1950 who became widowed during the preceding two years, and widows who remarried or died during the preceding year as percentages of women who became widowed during that year, by age: United States, 1948 to 1950

Age	Percent of widows in 1950 who became widowed during the preceding two years			Women who became widowed in preceding year (percent)	Widowed women who (during the preceding year)--		
	Total	White	Nonwhite		Re-married	Died	Nei-ther
Total, 14-54	14.2	15.0	11.2	100.0	50.2	12.0	37.8
14-24 years	49.9	51.9	45.4	100.0	44.7	1.6	53.7
25-34 years	22.1	23.0	19.6	100.0	63.9	3.7	32.4
35-54 years	12.0	13.5	9.0	100.0	48.1	14.5	37.4
35-44 years	15.6	16.5	---	100.0	55.3	7.9	36.8
45-54 years	11.3	12.4	---	100.0	43.9	18.4	37.7

Source: U.S. Bureau of the Census, U.S. Census of Population: 1950, Vol. IV, Special Reports, Part 2, Chapter E, Duration of Current Marital Status, table 29; also National Center for Health Statistics, Vital Statistics of the United States: 1960, Vol. III, table 2-22, and 1950, Vol. II, table 6; and "Mortality from Selected Causes by Marital Status: United States, 1949-51," Vital Statistics--Special Reports, Vol. 39, No. 7, table 1.

the supply of widowed women under 55 years old. The number of widows remarrying at ages 25 to 34 years was nearly two-thirds as large as the number who became widowed while in that age span — a higher proportion than for any younger or older age group.[5]

Other data from the 1950 study of recently widowed women show that well-educated women of a given, rather young age (35 to 39) have a greater tendency to remarry than those with less education. Moreover, the same source presents data which suggest that widows with three or more children tend to remarry after longer periods of widowhood than those with fewer children.[6]

Table 9.4. Widowers and widows, by age: United States, 1960

(Numbers in thousands)

Age	Widowers		Widows		Widows per 100 widowers
	Number	Percent	Number	Percent	
Total	2,082	100.0	7,862	100.0	378
14-44 years	111	5.3	506	6.4	456
45-64 years	565	27.2	2,728	34.7	483
65-84 years	1,229	59.0	4,203	53.5	342
85 & over	177	8.5	426	5.4	241

Source: U.S. Bureau of the Census, U.S. Census of Population: 1960, Subject Reports, Marital Status, Final Report PC(2)-4E, tables 1 and 4.

Social Characteristics of Widowed Persons

Age distribution. As can be seen from Table 9.4, widows far out-number widowers, nearly 4 to 1. The ratio of widows to widowers is greatest between the ages of 45 and 64, when it approaches a level of nearly 5 to 1; it is almost as high for those below age 45. For those 65 to 84, the ratio drops to about 3.5 to 1 and at 85 and over, to 2.5 to 1. More than one-half of the widowed persons in 1960 were between the ages of 65 and 85, and most of the remainder were between 45 and 65. Only 13 percent of them were either under 45 or 85 and over.

Two underlying factors account largely for the observed differences in the numbers of widowers and widows: (1) the lower death rate among women at all ages, and (2) the older average age of men than women at marriage — especially at remarriage. Although remarriage *rates* are higher among widowers than among widows, the *number* of widows who remarry is larger than the number of widowers who re-marry, as was pointed out in the discussion of Table 3.5 in Chapter 3. A counteracting factor, namely, the excess of men among im-migrants to this country in the early part of the twentieth century, has probably kept the differences between the numbers of widowers and widows from being as large as they might otherwise have been at the older ages. A discussion of differences in the death rates for men and women is presented in Chapter 11; and documentation of differences in previous marital status and in age at marriage of those remarrying was discussed in Chapters 3 and 4.

White widowed persons tend to be about 6 years older than nonwhite widowed persons, and widowers tend to be about 3 years older than widows (see Table 9.5). Higher death rates among young married men than young married women result in a larger number and a larger proportion of young widows than young widowers, a situation particularly marked among nonwhites. The situation is accentuated, rather than counterbalanced, by the higher remarriage rates for widowers than for widows.

Table 9.5. Widowed persons, by age, color, and sex: United States, 1960

(Numbers in thousands)

Age and sex	Widowed persons			Percent widowed		
	Total	White	Nonwhite	Total	White	Nonwhite
Men, 14 & over	2,082	1,795	287	3.4	3.3	4.6
Percent	100.0	100.0	100.0	...	...	...
14-24 years	0.3	0.3	0.6	0.1	0.0	0.1
25-34 years	1.3	1.0	2.8	0.2	0.2	0.7
35-44 years	3.7	3.1	7.4	0.7	0.5	1.8
45-54 years	8.9	8.0	14.8	1.8	1.6	4.3
55-64 years	18.3	17.4	23.8	5.0	4.5	9.8
65-74 years	31.5	31.9	28.8	13.1	12.4	20.0
75-84 years	27.5	29.2	16.8	29.2	28.9	32.1
85 & over	8.5	9.0	5.1	53.0	53.3	50.6
Median age (years)	71.0	71.8	65.2	...	...	...
Women, 14 & over	7,862	6,908	954	12.1	11.9	13.9
Percent	100.0	100.0	100.0	...	...	...
14-24 years	0.3	0.2	0.7	0.2	0.1	0.4
25-34 years	1.4	1.1	3.7	0.9	0.7	2.5
35-44 years	4.7	4.1	9.6	3.0	2.5	6.9
45-54 years	11.7	10.8	17.9	8.8	7.9	16.4
55-64 years	23.0	22.7	25.3	22.3	21.2	32.9
65-74 years	32.2	33.0	26.4	43.4	42.4	55.4
75-84 years	21.3	22.5	12.9	66.1	65.5	74.3
85 & over	5.4	5.7	3.5	81.2	80.9	86.0
Median age (years)	67.8	68.5	62.3	...	...	...

Source: U.S. Bureau of the Census, U.S. Census of Population: 1960, Subject Reports, Marital Status, Final Report PC(2)-4E, tables 1 and 4.

Widowers do not constitute a majority of men until about age 85. For women, however, the corresponding age is much lower. By age 70, one-half of the surviving white women in 1960 were widowed; the corresponding age for nonwhite women was 63. At ages 85 and over, fully 81 percent of the women were widowed; the comparable figure for men was only 53 percent.

During the twentieth century, the reduction in widowerhood and widowhood among older adults has been relatively slow as compared with that among younger adults. This fact is documented in Table 9.6. In fact, between 1900 and 1930, the percent widowed among those 65 years old and over remained unchanged for men and declined

Table 9.6. Percent widowed, for all persons and Negroes 35 years old and over, by age and sex: United States, 1960, 1930, and 1900

Year and race	Men by age (years)				Women by age (years)			
	35-44	45-54	55-64	65 & over	35-44	45-54	55-64	65 & over
PERCENT OF TOTAL WIDOWED								
1960	0.7	1.8	5.0	19.1	3.0	8.8	22.4	52.1
1930	2.5	5.3	10.2	26.6	6.5	14.1	27.8	56.5
1900	3.6	6.8	11.9	26.5	8.6	17.6	32.3	59.5
Index of percent widowed								
1960	19	26	42	72	35	50	69	88
1930	69	78	86	100	76	80	86	95
1900	100	100	100	100	100	100	100	100
PERCENT OF NEGROES WIDOWED								
1960	1.9	6.8		24.6	7.2		23.7	61.7
1930	5.9	11.8		31.0	17.3		33.7	69.5
1900	6.7	12.2		25.0	18.3		33.7	66.0
Index of percent widowed								
1960	28	56		98	39		70	93
1930	88	97		124	95		100	105
1900	100	100		100	100		100	100

Source: U.S. Bureau of the Census, U.S. Census of Population: 1960, Detailed Characteristics, U.S. Summary, Final Report PC(1)-1D, tables 176 and 177; Subject Reports, Nonwhite Population by Race, Final Report PC(2)-1C, tables 9 and 19; Fifteenth Census of the United States: 1930, Population, Vol. II, General Report, Statistics by Subjects, page 844; Negro Population, 1790-1915, page 240.

very little for women; among Negroes the percent widowed in the same age range actually rose during that generation. As the proportion of the population over 65 years of age increased during the following generation, 1930 to 1960, the percent widowed declined substantially among men and moderately among women.

The sharpest decline from 1900 to 1960 occurred in the proportion of widowers among men in the youngest age group for which there are substantial numbers of widowed persons, namely, 35 to 44 years. Here, the 60-year decline in the proportion of widowers among Negroes was so great that the widower rate was only 28 percent as large at the end as at the beginning of the period; for white men it was even lower — less than 19 percent of the original rate. A combination of lower occurrences of widowerhood and widowhood during recent decades, on the one hand, and of higher remarriage rates during the same period, on the other hand, probably account for a large part of the change. Presently available data would probably not permit accurate establishment of the extent to which each of these factors contributed to the decline in the percent widowed.[7]

Duration of marriage. Information on the interval between first marriage and widowhood is given in Table 9.7 for the survivors to the time of the 1960 census of selected first-marriage cohorts. Sepa-

Table 9.7. Percent widowed and married once or more than once, for persons ever married, by selected numbers of years since first marriage, color, and sex: United States, 1960

Number of years since first marriage	Percent widowed and married only once				Percent widowed and married more than once			
	Men		Women		Men		Women	
	White	Non-white	White	Non-white	White	Non-white	White	Non-white
Total	3.7	4.7	12.5	13.0	0.6	1.8	2.1	4.8
0-4 years	0.3	0.7	0.5	1.4	0.0	0.1	0.0	0.1
10-14 years	0.6	1.7	1.7	4.4	0.1	0.2	0.2	0.6
20-24 years	1.5	3.4	5.0	9.8	0.2	0.8	0.8	2.6
30-34 years	3.8	7.0	12.9	18.3	0.7	2.7	2.2	6.5
40-44 years	9.7	12.8	28.7	31.3	1.7	5.8	5.3	13.8
50-54 years	22.8	22.2	50.2	44.5	4.1	9.8	8.9	21.5
60 & over	47.4	32.4	73.5	59.5	9.7	20.6	13.0	28.4

Source: U.S. Bureau of the Census, U.S. Census of Population: 1960, Subject Reports, Marital Status, Final Report PC(2)-4E, table 2.

rate data are shown for those who had been married only once (left half of table) and for those who had been married more than once (right half of table). For example, of all white men who survived to the time of the 1960 census and who entered first marriage 40 to 44 years before the census, 9.7 percent had become widowed from their first wife and had never remarried. At the same time, 28.7 of the white women of comparable age and marital duration had become widowed after their first marriage and had not remarried. On the assumption that relatively few couples of this marital duration had experienced the death of both the husband and wife, the separate experience of husbands and wives can be combined to produce an estimated total of nearly 40 percent of the couples affected by widowhood but not remarriage. Of course, additional husbands and wives had become widowed during those 40 to 44 years but had remarried. These facts are consistent with the values shown in the next-to-last line of Table 6.1, which show the median age of women at widowhood as about 64 years. Moreover, the mean length of widowhood, on the basis of mortality data for 1960, is about 18.5 years and the mean length of widowerhood is about 13.5 years, according to special computations provided to the authors by Robert J. Myers and Francisco Bayo of the Social Security Administration in Washington, D.C.

Ethnic origin. The substantial differences in percentages widowed among adults in various racial and other ethnic groups shown in the following tables reflect complex combinations of demographic, biological, social, and economic characteristics. Essentially, the differences in percent widowed can be ascribed to differing mortality and remarriage rates, but other factors include differences among the groups with respect to economic welfare, religion, immigration histories, and rates of assimilation. These factors affect attitudes toward remarriage in general and attitudes toward remarrying persons who live nearby and who are willing and eligible to marry. In the last analysis, individual widowed persons make decisions as to whether it is better for them to remain widowed or to marry a specific candidate for marriage. Thus the decisions to remarry or not to remarry, which are reflected in the statistics, have their roots in the socioeconomic past of the persons involved. Finally, variations in practices of misreporting marital status by mothers who are unwed is also a possible source of some of the apparent differences in the proportion widowed among women in the several ethnic groups.

Table 9.8. Percent widowed, for persons 14 years old and over, by race and sex, standardized for age and unstandardized: United States, 1960

Race	Percent widowed, standardized for age		Percent widowed, unstandardized		Difference-- effect of standardization	
	Men	Women	Men	Women	Men	Women
Total, 14 & over[a]	3.4	12.2	3.4	12.2	...	...
White	3.2	11.6	3.3	11.9	-0.1	-0.3
Negro	5.4	17.2	4.6	14.3	0.8	2.9
American Indian	5.7	13.2	4.4	9.5	1.3	3.7
Japanese	3.7	13.2	3.1	7.7	0.6	5.5
Chinese	3.9	13.1	3.6	7.0	0.3	6.1
Filipino	3.9	7.9	3.9	2.9	0.0	5.0

Source: U.S. Bureau of the Census, U.S. Census of Population: 1960, Detailed Characteristics, United States Summary, Final Report PC(1)-1D, table 177; and Subject Reports, Nonwhite Population by Race, Final Report PC(2)-1C, tables 9-13.

[a]Includes the small number of persons of other nonwhite races, not shown separately.

As shown in Table 9.8, Negroes had the highest widowhood rates of all racial groups, according to information reported in the 1960 census. "Unstandardized" data show that 4.6 percent of the Negro men and 14.3 percent of the Negro women 14 years old and over were reported as widowed. However, if Negroes had had the same age distribution as the total population (and had retained the same percent widowed in each age group), these figures would have been still higher, 5.4 percent for men and 17.2 percent for women. The effect of similarly standardizing the American Indian population for age was to bring the percent widowed for Indian men up to 5.7 percent — even higher than that for Negro men — and to bring the percent widowed for Indian women above that for white women and about equal to the standardized figures for Japanese and Chinese women.

One effect of standardizing for age was to reduce the percent widowed for white men to the lowest level for any racial group — no doubt reflecting their low death rate and high remarriage rate. Another effect was to reduce the percent widowed for white women to the lowest level for any racial group except Filipino women — again reflecting very low death rates for white women, but extremely high remarriage rates for Filipino women; these women are relatively scarce in the United States at the middle and upper ages as compared with the number of Filipino men of similar age.

Illustrative widowerhood and widowhood statistics for 1960 are presented for persons of foreign stock by country of origin in Table 9.9. The figures on first-generation persons (foreign born) are for

Table 9.9.   Percent widowed, for persons of foreign stock, by country of origin, nativity, parentage, age, and sex: United States, 1960

Country of origin	Men		Women	
	Foreign born, age 45-54	Native of foreign or mixed parentage, age 35-44	Foreign born, age 45-54	Native of foreign or mixed parentage, age 35-44
Total	2.0	0.5	9.7	2.5
Sweden	2.5	0.5	7.5	2.2
Canada	1.6	0.5	7.5	2.6
Italy	1.6	0.5	9.7	2.1
United Kingdom	1.7	0.5	9.0	2.5
U.S.S.R.	1.8	0.4	9.7	2.2
Czechoslovakia	2.0	0.5	9.5	2.5
Germany	1.6	0.6	9.3	2.9
Poland	2.1	0.5	10.1	2.6
Austria	2.1	0.5	9.9	2.7
Ireland	2.9	0.7	10.6	3.2
Mexico	2.9	0.7	12.9	3.5
Other and not reported	2.2	0.5	10.4	2.4

Source: U.S. Bureau of the Census, U.S. Census of Population: 1960, Subject Reports, Nativity and Parentage, Final Report PC(2)-1A, tables 7 and 13.

those 45 to 54 years old, one of the youngest groups with substantial numbers of remarriageable foreign-born persons in the United States; and the figures on second-generation persons are for those 35 to 44 years old, a group which is old enough to include numerous widowed persons but younger than the first-generation group, so as to permit rough comparisons of rankings of origin groups for the older and younger generations with respect to persons of remarriageable ages.

Particularly low percentages widowed were found for first-generation women from Sweden and Canada. Other groups with percentages widowed not exceeding the average for all origin groups combined were those from Italy, the United Kingdom, the U.S.S.R., and Czechoslovakia. On the other hand, both men and women of Irish and Mexican stock showed the highest percentages widowed among those of either first or second generation.

For an understanding of the significance of the findings for these ethnic groups, it would be desirable to gauge the relative importance of death rates among spouses and of remarriage rates among the widowed. For example, it seems safe to infer that women of Swedish stock in 1960 were, in the first place, relatively unlikely to become widowed and, in the second place, relatively likely to remarry if they became widowed. The reverse can probably be safely assumed for both men and women of Mexican stock in 1960.

The foreign stock of Irish origin deserves special comment. Not only was the percent widowed high for both men and women of first- and second-generation Irish foreign stock in 1960, but the percent single was also quite high; consequently, the percent married was quite low — as was also the percent divorced (this being a predominantly Roman Catholic group). Those of Irish foreign stock, who are noted for late marriage, tend to have a low proportion who ever marry and evidently a high proportion who never marry but once.

Living arrangements. Although one-half of the widowers in 1960 were over 71 years old and nearly one-half of the widows were over 68 years old, a majority of widowed persons were heads of their own households (see Table 9.10). Among widowed household heads, only the nonwhite widows more often than not had relatives in their homes and hence were heads of (primary) families; a substantial majority of the other widowed household heads had no relatives in their homes and hence were living as primary individuals. These observations are consistent with the hypothesis that middle- and upper-age Negro widows tend to take the role of family leader among those to whom they are more or less closely related.

About one-fifth of the white widowed persons were living in the home of a son or daughter and hence were the parent or parent-in-law of the household head. The proportion of nonwhite widowed persons similarly living in with their children was smaller — about one-tenth of the widowers and one-sixth of the widows. White widowed persons were somewhat more likely to be a parent-in-law than

Table 9.10. Family status of widowed persons, by color and sex:
United States, 1960

(Numbers in thousands)

Family status	Total		Men		Women	
	Men	Women	White	Nonwhite	White	Nonwhite
Total widowed	2,082	7,862	1,795	287	6,908	954
Percent	...	...	100.0	100.0	100.0	100.0
In households	1,916	7,536	91.8	93.3	95.6	97.6
Head of household	1,234	5,080	59.6	57.2	64.5	65.1
Head of family	456	2,087	21.9	22.0	25.0	37.4
Primary individual	778	2,993	37.7	35.2	39.5	27.7
Parent-in-law of head	201	793	10.5	4.6	10.6	6.5
Parent of head	177	820	8.9	5.9	10.5	9.6
Lodger of head	128	191	5.1	12.7	2.2	4.3
"Other relative"	68	217	2.9	5.2	2.5	4.4
Brother or sister	44	186	2.0	3.0	2.3	3.1
Child of head	35	113	1.5	2.8	1.3	2.3
Bro.- or sister-in-law	26	70	1.2	1.7	0.9	1.1
Resident employee	3	67	0.1	0.4	0.8	1.1
In group quarters	166	326	8.2	6.7	4.4	2.4
In rooming house	27	34	1.3	1.6	0.4	0.7
In home for aged	77	191	4.1	1.3	2.7	0.6
In mental hospital	21	54	1.0	1.0	0.7	0.7
In other institution	23	13	0.9	2.1	0.2	0.2
In other group qtrs.	18	34	0.8	0.6	0.5	0.2

Source: U.S. Bureau of the Census, U.S. Census of Population:
1960, Subject Reports, Persons by Family Characteristics, Final Report
PC(2)-4B, table 2; and Inmates of Institutions, Final Report PC(2)-8A,
tables 17, 26, and 28.

a parent of the household head, whereas the reverse was clearly the case for nonwhite widowed persons. In view of this fact, plus the fact that there was a much larger proportion of female heads of households among nonwhites than among whites, the results for both white and nonwhite widowed persons could very well indicate a preference for living with a daughter rather than a son. Those who lived in with various other types of relatives constituted only about one-eighth to one-twelfth of the widowed persons in the four groups by color and sex. About 3 to 13 percent lived in households of nonrelatives, the largest proportion being nonwhite widowers living as lodgers.

Approximately 500,000 of the nearly 10,000,000 widowed persons in 1960 lived in group quarters and hence were not residents of private households. Over one-half of these persons were living in homes for the aged and dependent, including nursing homes. Somewhat over-represented in these homes were white widowed persons. About 15 percent of the widowed persons in group quarters were in mental hospitals.

Nonwhite widowers had a particularly large proportion in living quarters apart from all relatives. Not only were they by far the most likely to be living in private homes as nonrelatives of the head but also the most likely to be living in large rooming houses. About one-third of the nonwhite widowers in institutions were in prisons, jails, or other correctional institutions; the corresponding proportion for white widowers was one-tenth.

As the age of widowed persons advanced, the proportion who were heads of families in 1960 decreased and, up to about age 75, the proportion who were primary individuals increased (see Table 9.11).

Table 9.11. Family status of widowed persons 35 years old and over, by age and sex: United States, 1960

(Numbers in thousands)

Family status	Men by age (years)				Women by age (years)			
	35-44	45-64	65-74	75 & over	35-44	45-64	65-74	75 & over
Total widowed	77	565	656	749	372	2,728	2,529	2,100
Percent	100.0	100.0	100.0	100.0	100.0	100.0	100.0	100.0
In households	91.0	93.9	94.2	89.3	98.4	98.1	97.1	90.8
Head of household	61.3	68.5	63.5	49.5	80.7	74.3	65.3	48.3
Head of family	37.9	29.6	19.9	16.3	65.3	35.0	19.9	14.8
Primary individual	23.4	38.9	43.6	33.2	15.4	39.3	45.4	33.5
Child of head	12.2	2.6	0.3	0.0	7.5	2.0	0.3	-
Parent-in-law of head	0.5	4.2	10.2	14.7	0.9	6.3	11.4	15.7
Parent of head	0.5	3.3	8.0	14.1	1.0	6.3	11.3	17.0
Other relative of head	8.6	7.3	6.0	6.1	5.1	5.6	5.7	6.9
Nonrelative of head	7.9	7.8	6.2	5.0	3.1	3.7	3.0	3.0
In group quarters	9.0	6.1	5.8	10.7	1.6	1.9	2.9	9.2
In rooming house	2.1	1.6	1.2	1.1	0.5	0.4	0.4	0.5
In home for aged	0.4	1.1	2.5	7.2	0.2	0.4	1.5	6.8
In mental hospital	1.0	1.0	0.9	1.1	0.5	0.5	0.6	1.0
In other institution	3.9	1.4	0.6	0.6	0.2	0.1	0.1	0.3
In other group quarters	1.6	1.0	0.6	0.7	0.2	0.5	0.3	0.6

Source: U.S. Bureau of the Census, U.S. Census of Population: 1960, Subject Reports, Persons by Family Characteristics, Final Report PC(2)-4B, table 2; and Inmates of Institutions, Final Report PC(2)-8A, tables 17, 26, and 28.

Above age 75, about one-half of the widowed persons still maintained their own home, but about 2 out of 3 of those who did so lived alone or with nonrelatives only.

Also, as the age of widowed persons advanced, the proportion who lived in with their parents dropped sharply. Perhaps surprisingly, however, within most age groups a larger proportion of widowed sons than widowed daughters lived in with their parents. This may simply reflect the greater longevity of mothers than fathers and the tendency for widowed sons to live in with their widowed mothers, but this hypothesis cannot be verified from available data.

At the same time, the proportion of widowed persons living in with their children increased, as age advanced, to the point where about 3 out of every 10 were doing so at age 75 and over. Another 15 percent of these aged widowed persons shared their homes with relatives present, with themselves as the titular head of the family. About 7 percent of the widowed men and women 75 and over lived in a nursing home or other home for the aged, 1 percent were in a mental hospital, and 4 percent lived as lodgers (mostly in private homes).

Widowers at each age, but especially at ages under 75, were more likely to live apart from relatives than were widows. Of the 40 percent of widowers 35 to 44 years old living away from relatives, about one-half lived as primary individuals, one-fourth as lodgers (mostly in private homes), and one-tenth as inmates of correctional institutions.

Children in the family. Among both white and nonwhite children, more were living with widowed parents in 1960 than with divorced parents; but among nonwhite children, far more were living with a parent reported as separated than with widowed and divorced parents combined (see Table 9.12). Although 93 percent of all white sons

Table 9.12. Children under 18 years old living with one or both parents, by marital status, color, and sex of parent: United States, 1960

(Numbers in thousands)

Marital status of parents	All children under 18 living with one or both parents		Living with father only		Living with mother only	
	White	Nonwhite	White	Nonwhite	White	Nonwhite
Total	54,412	7,709	555	172	3,382	1,723
Percent	100.0	100.0	100.0	100.0	100.0	100.0
Married, spouse present	92.8	75.4	...	...	...	...
Married, spouse absent	3.0	14.1	45.9	54.2	40.4	57.8
Separated	1.4	10.8	12.4	27.9	21.1	45.6
Other	1.5	3.3	33.4	26.2	19.3	12.2
Widowed	2.1	5.2	31.8	30.5	28.5	20.1
Divorced	2.0	2.9	20.1	10.0	29.6	12.1
Single	0.1	2.4	2.2	5.4	1.4	10.0

Source: U.S. Bureau of the Census, U.S. Census of Population: 1960, Detailed Characteristics, U.S. Summary, Final Report PC(1)-1D, table 185.

and daughters under 18 years old living with either parent were with both parents, only 75 percent of the young nonwhite children were similarly living with both parents. For white children, the next most frequent detailed category of their parents' marital status was widowed (2.1 percent), but for nonwhite children it was separated (10.8 percent).[8] In third place was divorced for whites (2.0 percent) and widowed for nonwhites (5.2 percent).

Urban and rural residence. As indicated in Table 9.13, the proportions widowed for persons in villages and small cities in 1960 were larger than those for either suburbs of large cities or farms. This generalization confirms commonly held impressions about favorite retirement sites of older persons (many of whom are widowed) and the relatively recent expansion of suburban areas through the in-movement of preponderantly young and middle-aged married couples and their children.

White widowed persons were more likely than the nonwhite to be overrepresented in the central cities of metropolitan areas, whereas

Table 9.13. Index of percent widowed, by size of place, by color and sex: United States, 1960

	Men			Women		
	Total	White	Nonwhite	Total	White	Nonwhite
Percent widowed	3.6	3.5	4.9	12.2	12.0	14.0
Index	100	100	100	100	100	100
Urban	100	100	102	106	106	101
Urbanized areas:						
Central cities	114	114	100	114	117	97
Urban fringe	78	80	84	84	85	86
Other urban:						
Places of 10,000						
or more	100	97	116	112	111	124
2,500 to 10,000	108	106	124	119	117	130
Rural	100	97	100	86	85	96
Places of 1,000 to 2,500	117	117	124	122	122	129
Other rural	97	94	98	81	79	93
Rural nonfarm	100	100	106	91	90	105
Rural farm	94	97	90	66	65	69

Source: U.S. Bureau of the Census, U.S. Census of Population: 1960, General Population Characteristics, U.S. Summary, Final Report PC(1)-1B, table 49 (complete-count data); and Detailed Characteristics, U.S. Summary, Final Report PC(1)-1D, table 176 (sample data for rural nonfarm and rural farm).

the reverse was true for smaller cities and other nonfarm areas. This difference probably reflects, among other things, differences in age distributions of whites and nonwhites in cities. White immigrants, who account for a substantial proportion of those who moved into the central cities decades ago, have largely reached the age of widowhood, whereas the more recent mass movement of Negroes from farms, villages, and towns into the large industrial centers has produced a relatively young average age of nonwhite adults in these centers.

White widowers, at the same time, were much less likely than nonwhite widowers to be underrepresented among those living on farms. This fact may reflect a larger proportion of white than nonwhite widowers who continue to receive an income from farm management after the retirement age. Probably also because of differences in the economic status of white and nonwhite widowed persons with a farm background, a larger proportion of white than nonwhite widowers remain on a farm, but a larger proportion of white than nonwhite widows manage to leave the farm. The conclusion that many women who become widowed while living on a farm leave the farm soon thereafter can be inferred from the following information derived from the 1950 census report on *Duration of Current Marital Status,* Table 26 (with "recently" meaning less than two years before the census):

16 percent of the white and nonwhite *farm* widows had become widowed recently; and

13 percent of the *nonfarm* widows had become widowed recently — 14 percent for white and 10 percent for nonwhite nonfarm widows.

The particularly low proportion of nonwhite nonfarm widows who had become widowed "recently" may reflect not only less speedy movement from the farm but also a lower remarriage rate for nonwhite than white nonfarm widows.

Educational level. The percent widowed has a high negative correlation with amount of education, as may be seen in Table 9.14 and Figure 9.1 for those 35 to 54 years old in 1960. In each category by color and sex, this percentage was consistently highest for those with the least education and lowest for those with the most. For those 45 to 54 years old, the percent widowed was twice as high for functional

Table 9.14. Percent widowed, for persons 35 to 44 and 45 to 54 years old, by years of school completed, color, and sex: United States, 1960, and change, 1950 to 1960 and 1940 to 1950

Year or period and years of school completed	Percent widowed, 35-44 years old				Percent widowed, 45-54 years old			
	Men		Women		Men		Women	
	White	Nonwhite	White	Nonwhite	White	Nonwhite	White	Nonwhite
Total, 1960	0.5	1.8	2.5	6.9	1.6	4.3	7.9	16.4
Elementary: 0-4 years	1.1	2.3	4.7	10.8	2.4	5.1	12.2	21.3
5-8 years	0.7	2.0	3.3	7.9	1.8	4.3	8.9	17.1
High school: 1-3 years	0.5	1.4	2.7	6.3	1.5	4.0	7.9	13.4
4 years	0.4	1.5	2.1	4.6	1.3	3.0	6.8	12.4
College: 1-3 years	0.4	1.6	2.3	4.2	1.3	4.1	7.2	11.1
4 or more	0.3	0.8	1.9	3.5	1.0	2.4	6.3	10.4
Change, 1950 to 1960[a]	-0.3	-0.6	-0.6	-2.6	-0.9	-2.0	-2.0	-6.2
Elementary: 0-4 years	-0.4	-0.3	-0.3	-1.1	-1.5	-1.4	-1.1	-4.1
5-8 years	-0.2	-0.6	-0.2	-1.8	-0.9	-1.9	-1.2	-5.5
High school: 1-3 years	-0.2	-0.3	-0.3	-2.2	-0.5	-2.1	-1.5	-5.7
4 years	-0.2	-0.1	-0.5	-2.5	-0.8	-1.3	-2.3	-5.7
College: 1-3 years	-0.1	-0.3	-0.3	-1.9	-0.2	-1.1	-1.7	-6.0
4 or more	-0.1	-0.5	-0.4	-1.0	-0.4	-2.7	-1.4	-2.5
Change, 1940 to 1950[a]	-0.7	-1.5	-1.7	-5.8	-1.2	-2.0	-1.8	-4.6
Elementary: 0-4 years	-1.0	-1.4	-2.7	-5.4	-1.3	-2.4	-2.0	-3.9
5-8 years	-0.8	-1.4	-1.6	-5.3	-1.3	-1.7	-1.6	-3.5
High school: 1-3 years	-0.5	-2.2	-1.6	-4.7	-1.0	-1.1	-2.0	-5.4
4 years	-0.6	-2.2	-1.5	-4.7	-1.0	-1.9	-1.8	-3.7
College: 1-3 years	-0.5	-0.3	-1.5	-6.2	-1.0	-2.3	-1.9	-8.2
4 or more	-0.4	-0.6	-1.1	-4.5	-0.7	-1.4	-1.4	-5.0

Source: U.S. Bureau of the Census, U.S. Census of Population: 1960, Subject Reports, Marital Status, Final Report PC(2)-4E, table 4; U.S. Census of Population: 1950, Vol. IV, Special Reports, Part 5, Chapter B, Education, tables 7 and 8; and Sixteenth Census of the United States: 1940, Educational Attainment by Economic Characteristics and Marital Status, tables 37 and 40.

[a]For 1950 and 1940, data are for conterminous United States. For 1940, data are for native white and Negro population.

illiterates (those with less than 5 years of schooling) as for college graduates; and for those 35 to 44 years old, the percent widowed for the lower education group was approximately three times as high. The degree to which a good education was related to a low percentage widowed was greatest for white men, least for white women, and intermediate for nonwhite men and women. This finding probably reflects, among other things, a strong tendency for white widowers with a college degree to remarry and a weaker tendency for white widows with a college degree to do so.

At the college-graduate level, however, the relationship between age and being widowed was virtually the same for whites and nonwhites. Thus, the percentages widowed for college graduates 45 to 54 years old were quite uniformly about three times as high, among the four categories by color and sex, as the percentages for those 35 to 44 years old. Within the framework of this uniform ratio stands the fact that, at the college-graduate level, the percent widowed for nonwhite men was about two and one-half times that for white men and the percent widowed for nonwhite women was about one and one-

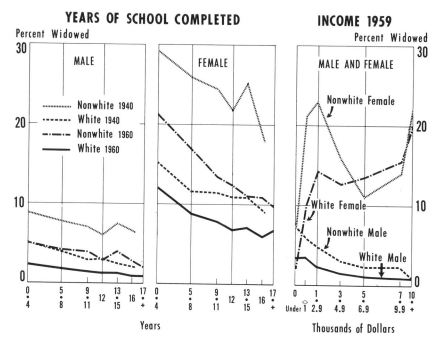

Fig. 9.1. Percent widowed, for persons 45 to 54 years old, by years of school completed, 1960 and 1940, and income in 1959: United States

Source: Table 9.14 and same source as Table 9.18.

half times that for white women. Even so, these differentials by color at the college-graduate level were consistently lower than those for persons with less education.

Decreases in the percent widowed were larger during the 1940's than the 1950's and also larger for the nonwhites than the whites in this 20-year span. However, they were quite unevenly distributed among those of different educational levels and did not eliminate the differences by education, color, and sex. For the 20-year period as a whole, the *absolute* decline in percent widowed was considerably greater among poorly educated persons 35 to 44 years old in each category by color and sex than among their well-educated counterparts.

Perhaps even more significant, in this connection, is the fact that the *relative* decline in percent widowed was much larger for well-educated persons than for the poorly educated. For instance, the decline in percent widowed between 1940 and 1960 as a proportion of the percent widowed in 1940 was about one and one-half times as large for college graduates, on the average, as for persons with less than 5 years of schooling. Thus, the *rate* of decline in percent widowed over the 20 years was more rapid, in general, among the well educated than among those with little education.

Work Experience and Income of Widowed Persons

Labor-force-participation rates. Widowers were much less likely than married men of the same age to be in the labor market in 1960 (see Table 9.15 and source of Table 7.1). This fact reflects in part

Table 9.15. Labor-force-participation rates of widowed persons, by age, color, and sex: United States, 1960

| Age | Labor-force-participation rate | | | | Nonwhite as percent of white | |
| | Men | | Women | | | |
	White	Nonwhite	White	Nonwhite	Men	Women
Total widowed	35.3	44.4	26.9	35.5	126	132
14-34 years	79.9	71.3	52.9	54.5	89	103
35-44 years	86.2	76.8	65.3	63.3	89	97
45-54 years	84.0	78.1	66.4	61.6	93	93
55-64 years	70.2	62.3	45.4	43.3	89	95
65-74 years	26.8	25.8	15.1	16.4	96	109
65-69 years	33.8	30.9	20.0	20.3	91	102
70-74 years	21.3	20.2	10.3	11.5	95	112
75 & over	10.7	11.4	3.7	4.6	107	124

Source: U.S. Bureau of the Census, U.S. Census of Population: 1960, Subject Reports, Employment Status and Work Experience, Final Report PC(2)-6A, table 4.

a relatively high mortality rate for the wives of men of working age who do not work regularly and in part a relatively low remarriage rate for such husbands. The worker rates were higher for white widowers than nonwhite widowers at every age group below 75 years; this is a net difference remaining even after the higher remarriage rates for white widowers have selectively drawn off those most likely to be working.[9]

Widows, on the other hand, had a much higher labor-force-participation rate than married women of comparable age. As pointed out before, women with the most education are the most likely to remain single; and single women are most likely to be members of the labor force. At the same time, well-educated women who marry and become widowed are apparently somewhat less likely to remarry than the corresponding group of widowers — no doubt in large measure because of differences in the availability of persons eligible for a remarriage. Regardless of the motivation for remaining widowed, the fact remains that a substantial majority of widows in the main working ages are found to be working at paying jobs.

White widows in 1960 had virtually the same labor-force-participation rates as nonwhite widows of the same age group, whereas white married women had much lower worker rates than nonwhite married women of comparable age. The white widow who contemplates remarriage may therefore have more reason than the nonwhite widow to expect that she can give up working if she follows through and marries again. To some extent, however, these comparisons may reflect such other factors as a difference in the proportion of white and nonwhite widows who find more personal satisfaction in their work than they would expect to find in remarriage — taking into account available eligibles.

Even at the peak ages for employment of widows, one-third of them were not in the labor market. Some of these had been recently widowed and had not had enough time to prepare for and obtain employment, but this number was undoubtedly a small proportion of the nonworkers. Consequently, at least one-fourth of those who had been widowed for a longer period must have been dependent completely on income from such sources (other than earnings) as insurance payments, savings, inheritances, or contributions by relatives or public agencies. Moreover, a substantial proportion of those who worked must not have had enough income from their jobs to meet all their expenses.

Occupational concentrations. Men in the white-collar, skilled, and semi-skilled occupations in 1960 included smaller percentages of widowers than those in service, unskilled, and farm occupations (see Table 9.16). A particularly low percentage widowed was found for men who were professional and technical workers. Men in this occupation group are being recruited at a rapid rate and hence include a large proportion of younger men; even the older professional workers have many attributes associated with above-average longevity and a high income level. For such reasons, the percentage married is quite high and the percent widowed quite small for this group. Lower recruitment rates during recent decades among younger men

Table 9.16. Percent widowed, for employed persons, by major occupation group and sex, and percent distribution of widowed employed persons 45 to 54 years old by major occupation group, by color and sex: United States, 1960

Major occupation group	Percent widowed		Percent distribution of widowed persons			
			Men, 45-54		Women, 45-54	
	Men	Women	White	Non-white	White	Non-white
Employed persons	1.6	9.8	100.0	100.0	100.0	100.0
Professional, tech. workers	0.9	7.0	6.6	1.9	11.3	4.1
Mgrs., off'ls., proprietors	1.4	15.1	10.2	1.9	6.6	1.4
Clerical, kindred workers	1.4	6.3	7.2	3.0	26.2	2.5
Sales workers	1.4	10.4	5.7	0.8	9.4	0.9
Craftsmen, foremen	1.4	10.4	20.0	9.3	1.5	0.6
Operatives, kindred workers	1.3	9.1	21.0	19.8	17.2	10.7
Private household workers	10.8	20.5	0.4	3.4	5.5	48.1
Service workers, other	2.9	12.8	7.0	14.3	15.6	20.8
Laborers, exc. farm & mine	2.1	8.9	6.7	22.9	0.4	2.6
Farmers, farm managers	2.5	25.0	5.1	3.4	1.1	0.7
Farm laborers & foremen	2.4	5.3	3.0	8.3	0.3	2.6
Occupation not reported	2.7	10.2	7.1	11.0	4.9	5.0

Source: U.S. Bureau of the Census, U.S. Census of Population: 1960, Subject Reports, Marital Status, Final Report PC(2)-4E, table 5.

and other characteristics associated with low marriage rates help to explain the high widowerhood percentages for men in service, unskilled, and farm occupations.

Well-above-average percentages widowed were found among women employed in the service trades and in the managerial and proprietary occupations, including farming. Many of the jobs in the service field are filled by widows without enough skill to perform in better-paying positions, whereas many of the managerial and proprietary positions filled by widows are in retail stores which were formerly managed by their husbands before they died. Low percentages widowed were found among women in jobs in professional, clerical, and factory (operative and laborer) work. Relatively young, recently educated women have no doubt been filling most of the newly available positions in professional and clerical categories, and young women evidently are at a premium in factory jobs.

For widowed persons 45 to 54 years old, separate distributions by major occupation groups are shown for white and nonwhite men and women in Table 9.16. These distributions permit group comparisons for persons in an age range which is old enough to include many widowed persons and young enough for remarriage to be quite common.

One-half the employed white widows 45 to 54 years old were earning salaries in white-collar positions, whereas nearly one-half the employed nonwhite widows were earning wages for doing private household work. Judging from the types of work performed by white and nonwhite widows, the inference seems to be warranted that a larger proportion of the former probably tend to be positively attracted to the type of work they are doing, whereas more of the latter perform work because of economic pressure.

Detailed occupation. More specific detail is given in Table 9.17 on kinds of occupations in which a disproportionately large number of widowed persons were engaged in 1960. The occupations listed were selected from those with at least 50,000 men, or at least 5,000 women, 14 years old and over in the experienced civilian labor force in 1960, where the proportion widowed was at least 2.0 percent for men and at least 12.0 percent for women. Although these detailed occupations were not classified by age, there is an obvious tendency for the occupations listed to be typical of those in which middle-aged and older persons are found.

Relatively high percentages widowed among men in the professions of law, dentistry, and pharmacy, and also public officials may suggest that men in these types of positions tend to be relatively conservative about remarrying. However, men in the occupations cited often work farther into old age than professional or managerial men in general, and hence the evidence is less clear-cut than suggestive. The same age factor applies to many, if not most, of the remaining occupations listed. Above-average percentages widowed (that is, above 1.6 percent widowed) were found in occupations such as cabinetmakers, locomotive engineers, chauffeurs, and farmers, which tend to be declining in numerical importance in the national economy. The long list of service and unskilled laboring jobs with high percentages widowed may be a reflection of the fact that these positions are being filled in large part by older, less vigorous men, while younger men with higher employment potential move into tasks which are more demanding from the standpoint of education and physical agility.

The unique qualities of widowers in the occupations listed are that they are still in the labor force and that they have not remarried;

Table 9.17. Percent widowed, for experienced civilian labor force in selected occupations, by sex: United States, 1960

Occupation and sex	Percent widowed	Occupation and sex	Percent widowed
MEN		**MEN (contd.)**	
Dentists	2.0	Laborers:	
Lawyers & judges	2.0	Gardeners	4.0
Pharmacists	2.1	Longshoremen	2.6
Public-admin. off'ls.	2.2	Railroads	2.7
Self-empl. mgrs., proprs.:		Personal service	6.1
Food & dairy stores	2.1	Public administration	2.4
Eating & drinking places	2.1		
Hardware stores	2.2	**WOMEN**	
Bookkeepers	2.0	Building superintendents	27.3
Messengers, office boys	2.1	Insurance agents	15.4
Real-estate agents	2.8	Sales--apparel, accessories	13.2
Cabinetmakers	2.0	Bakers	14.3
Locomotive engineers	2.6	Tailors	22.3
Painters--constr., maint.	2.2	Dressmakers	26.1
Laundry operatives	2.6	Laundry operatives	12.6
Taxi drivers, chauffeurs	2.3	Confectionery operatives	12.3
Attendants, hosp. & inst.	2.0	Housekeepers, priv. hsld.	33.6
Barbers	2.9	Lodging-house keepers	26.9
Bartenders	2.7	Charwomen	19.5
Cooks, exc. priv. hsld.	2.8	Cooks, exc. priv. hsld.	16.0
Elevator operators	4.6	Elevator operators	12.3
Janitors & sextons	3.8	Housekeepers, exc. priv.hsld	25.6
Guards, watchmen	4.1	Practical nurses	21.5

Source: U.S. Bureau of the Census, U.S. Census of Population: 1960, Subject Reports, Occupational Characteristics, Final Report PC(2)-7A, table 12.

what remains for additional study is the extent to which these unique qualities can be accounted for by the simple variable of age. Actually, of course, explaining the phenomenon on the basis of age alone clarifies but does not eliminate it.

The criterion for listing occupations for women removed all professional occupations. Among the occupations listed, however, are many that are commonly associated with the activities of women in the middle and upper ages: owning and operating or being entrusted to manage apartment buildings and lodging houses, selling insurance or women's apparel, being a skilled dressmaker, working in a laundry or candy store, keeping house for a private family, cooking, cleaning, and being a practical nurse.

These are the types of work performed in 1960 by women who were most prone to be widowed. Some of the women had remained widowed because they considered themselves too old to remarry, and others did so because they had not found a suitable marriage partner or for some other reason. An increasing proportion of widows of marriageable age are becoming quite eligible for entering or remaining in employment through rising educational background and work experience; also, the ratio of eligible marriage partners in that age range is far smaller for widows than for widowers. Hence both choice and necessity tend to encourage most preretirement widows to work.

Income levels. The percent widowed in 1959 was inversely related to income for men but not for women, as demonstrated in Table 9.18 and Figure 9.1. Men in the upper income levels had not only low proportions widowed but also low proportions divorced; in addition, they had the highest proportion remarried among those who had ever been widowed or divorced (refer to Table 8.35).

Table 9.18. Percent widowed, for persons 14 years old and over and 45 to 54 years old by sex, and percent distribution of widowed persons 45 to 54 years old by color and sex, by income in 1959: United States, 1960

| Income in 1959 | Percent widowed | | | | Percent distribution of widowed persons | | | |
| | 14 years & over | | 45-54 years | | Men, 45-54 | | Women, 45-54 | |
	Men	Women	Men	Women	White	Nonwhite	White	Nonwhite
Total	3.4	12.1	1.8	8.8	100.0	100.0	100.0	100.0
Without income	3.3	4.6	4.0	2.4	6.7	10.7	11.7	14.7
With income	3.4	18.4	1.7	13.6	93.3	89.3	88.3	85.3
With income	...	...	...	...	100.0	100.0	100.0	100.0
$1-$999 or loss	7.7	21.0	4.2	12.5	13.3	27.6	20.2	49.9
$1,000-$2,999	5.8	19.3	2.8	15.3	21.9	39.9	40.3	40.4
$3,000-$4,999	2.0	11.2	1.7	12.9	26.0	23.8	26.2	8.0
$5,000-$6,999	1.3	15.2	1.3	13.5	22.5	7.0	8.8	1.2
$7,000-$9,999	1.1	19.7	0.9	15.5	9.7	1.5	2.9	0.3
$10,000 & over	1.4	30.8	0.8	20.1	6.6	0.2	1.7	0.1
Median income	$1,865	$1,110	$3,600	$2,213	$4,138	$2,123	$2,479	$1,007

Source: U.S. Bureau of the Census, U.S. Census of Population: 1960, Subject Reports, Marital Status, Final Report PC(2)-4E, table 6.

For women, the relationship between income and marital status was much more complex. The percent widowed for women with no income at all was uniformly small for women in every age group. Women without income were considerably more likely than women with income to be married and still living with their first husband; they had the smallest percentages widowed or divorced and the smallest percentages of those ever widowed or ever divorced who had not re-married.

Women of every age group with minimal incomes for self-support — $1,000 to $2,999 — had higher percentages widowed than women with incomes in either the next smaller or the next larger income group.[10] In 1960, women 45 to 64 years old with high incomes ($10,000 or more) had about one-fourth of their income from non-earnings such as investments[11] and were considerably more likely than those of intermediate income ($5,000 to $10,000) to remain wid-owed. To what extent those in a given income group who had remar-ried were previously widowed (or divorced) is not available from the 1960 census records; however, a comparison of marital-status distribu-tions for women 45 to 64 years old with high income and those with intermediate income suggests strongly that women in the upper income bracket were much more likely to have remarried if they had been divorced than if they had been widowed. A relevant hypothesis in this connection is that divorced women are more likely than widows to receive their income mainly from earnings rather than from sources provided by their former husband.

The median income of middle-aged widowers was only about three-fourths as high as that of married men of comparable age (see source of Table 9.18). On the other hand, the median income of middle-aged widows with income was around 10 to 20 percent higher than that of married women of comparable age with income; moreover, a larger proportion of the middle-aged widows than married women who worked did so full-time during the work week and full-time during the year. The observation concerning widowers provides further evidence of the negative relationship between income and the occur-rence of widowerhood, on the one hand, and the positive relationship between income and the remarriage of widowers, on the other. At the same time, the findings concerning widows reflect the greater necessity for widows than married women to support themselves and their immediate family members, if any.

White widows 45 to 54 years old with income not only averaged two and one-half times as much income as nonwhite widows of com-parable age but they also had more than 10 percent larger incomes than nonwhite widowers, on the average. Among those 45 to 54 years old, the modal income range for white widowers was $3,000 to $4,999, for nonwhite widowers and white widows it was $1,000 to $2,999, and for nonwhite widows it was $1 to $999. It should not be surprising, in light of these findings, that ever-married nonwhite women in this age-and-income group had the highest percentage who had remarried.

The foregoing analysis shows that much is now known about the social and economic characteristics of widowed persons, but a far more informative study could be made if data were available which permitted the distinction between remarried persons who were previously widowed and those previously divorced. Especially enlightening in the study of widowhood would be knowledge of longitudinal changes in the working patterns and incomes of specific women of different educational levels covering the time before their husband died through the period of widowhood and on into remarriage. Such information would place the work experience of widows in much clearer perspective in relation to that of married women. Similar longitudinal data for women who experience separation and divorce would be equally useful. Along with such information for analysis, data on work experience of women in the state of spinsterhood could be added, so as to encompass the entire range of variation in marital status for women of quite mature adult ages.[12]

10 / GROUP VARIATIONS AMONG BACHELORS AND SPINSTERS

This chapter extends the discussion of marriage to a demographic analysis of persons who marry relatively late in life or never. In accordance with common parlance, these persons who deviate from the social norm of becoming married during young adulthood are referred to as bachelors or spinsters. For present purposes, bachelors are defined as men 35 years old and over who have never married, and spinsters as women 30 years old and over who have never married. About 2.7 million men in 1967 were bachelors and 2.8 million women were spinsters.[1] These numbers are sharply lower than those featured in this chapter for 1960, as in Table 10.1. About 3 out of 5 of those

Table 10.1. Bachelors and spinsters by age and color: United States, 1960

(Numbers in thousands)

Age and sex	Single persons			Percent distribution		
	Total	White	Nonwhite	Total	White	Nonwhite
Bachelors						
Total, 35 & over	2,876	2,553	324	100.0	100.0	100.0
35-44 years	947	815	132	32.9	31.9	40.7
45-54 years	755	667	88	26.3	26.1	27.0
55-64 years	608	542	66	21.1	21.2	20.3
65 years & over	567	528	39	19.7	20.7	11.9
Median age (years)	51.5	51.9	48.4	...	...	...
Spinsters						
Total, 30 & over	3,309	3,016	293	100.0	100.0	100.0
30-34 years	419	349	70	12.7	11.6	23.8
35-44 years	750	657	93	22.7	21.8	31.6
45-54 years	734	674	60	22.2	22.3	20.4
55-64 years	650	605	44	19.6	20.1	15.1
65 years & over	757	730	27	22.9	24.2	9.1
Median age (years)	51.6	52.4	43.3	...	...	...

Source: U.S. Bureau of the Census, U.S. Census of Population: 1960, Subject Reports, Marital Status, Final Report PC(2)-4E, tables 1 and 4.

who enter bachelorhood or spinsterhood eventually will marry, but one-half of the bachelors (and spinsters) who ever marry do so in the first 10 years of bachelorhood (or spinsterhood).[2]

Some bachelors and spinsters deliberately choose to remain single, but they are very likely in the minority. Among those who so choose are persons in convents and monasteries. Many of those who remain single involuntarily reside in hospitals for the mentally ill and defective and in correctional institutions. The great majority of those who remain single, however, are not residing in institutionalized quarters, as will be seen below, but are devoting their time to career activities or otherwise filling a place in the world of work.

The findings in this chapter confirm the fundamental fact that more women than men who never marry are capable of maintaining themselves in comfort through their work at responsible positions, although many thousands of bachelors do so also. Perhaps the cultural imperatives which place the initiative for courtship in the hands of men cause some kinds of women more than others to be bypassed in mate selection. Perhaps, also, the greater pressure on upper-class women than on upper-class men to avoid "marrying down" causes more of the former than of the latter to remain unmarried.[3] There is a general tolerance for men from upper-class families to marry women from lower social levels, particularly when beauty, charm, wit, and other nondemographic assets serve as substitutes for education and affluence as factors in mate selection. The end effect is to leave a larger proportion of women than men of favorable social and economic status among the ranks of the middle-aged single.

The vanishing "maiden aunt" in the home is one of the examples of persons discussed in this chapter. Some information on the numbers of these memorable persons — who are influencing the home life of a diminishing proportion of American youth — is presented in the section below on living arrangements of those who never marry.

Social Characteristics of Bachelors and Spinsters

Age distribution. Half of the bachelors and spinsters in 1960 were less than 52 years old and half were 52 or older. About one-third of them were under 45 years old, and about one-fifth were 65 or older. White bachelors had a median age 3.5 years above that of nonwhite bachelors, and white spinsters about 9 years above that of nonwhite spinsters. These and other demographic facets of bachelors and spinsters by age are given in Table 10.1. When this table is studied in the light of the changes between 1940 and 1960 in the percent single as shown in Table 10.2, some dynamic aspects of the subject emerge.

The expected trend in percent single as the population passes from

Table 10.2. Percent single, for persons 30 to 59 years old, by age, color, and sex: United States, 1940 to 1960

Year, color, and sex	Age (years)					
	30-34	35-39	40-44	45-49	50-54	55-59
White men						
1960	11.3	8.3	7.1	7.0	7.5	8.0
1950	13.1	10.1	9.0	8.8	8.5	8.4
1940	20.7	15.1	12.5	11.2	11.1	10.9
Nonwhite men						
1960	17.1	12.6	9.6	8.5	8.9	10.4
1950	14.4	10.4	9.0	8.3	7.0	6.2
1940	21.3	16.9	13.9	11.3	10.1	9.0
White women						
1960	6.6	5.9	6.0	6.6	7.8	8.4
1950	9.3	8.5	8.6	8.2	8.1	8.0
1940	15.0	11.5	9.8	8.9	9.0	9.0
Nonwhite women						
1960	9.6	7.6	6.4	5.9	6.2	6.9
1950	8.9	6.9	5.7	4.9	4.1	4.2
1940	12.6	8.8	6.8	5.5	4.9	4.4

Source: U.S. Bureau of the Census, U.S. Census of Population: 1960, Detailed Characteristics, Final Report PC(1)-1D, table 177.

age 30 to age 60 is downward, because of successive attrition from the single to the married state. Although this pattern held true almost without exception for 1940 and 1950 among the four groups shown in Table 10.2, the pattern for 1960 invariably showed increases in the percent single for those in their fifties as compared with those in their forties. The main reason for the change was the sharp increase in percent married among those in their twenties during the 1940's, which was discussed more fully in Chapter 3. Those who were in their thirties in 1940 (and in their fifties in 1960) had gone through the depression years of the 1930's at the height of the marriageable ages and had not compensated for the "postponement" of marriage when they reached the period of bachelorhood or spinsterhood.

Moreover, the trend from 1940 to 1960 in the percent single was consistently downward in each age group for white persons between the ages of 30 and 54, whereas the trend for nonwhite persons was consistently downward during the 1940's but upward during the 1950's. Nonwhite men 30 to 49 years old by 1960 had considerably increased their excess in percent single over that for white men, and

nonwhite women 30 to 44 years old had changed from a deficit in percent single as compared with that for white women in 1940 to an
excess in 1960. These facts provide further evidence, in addition to
that presented in Chapters 3 and 4, that conjugal life deteriorated
among nonwhite persons during the 1950's and that nonwhite persons
are more likely than white persons to postpone marriage until the age
of bachelorhood or spinsterhood.[4]

Attrition from bachelorhood or spinsterhood. Information from the
1960 census on age at entrance into first marriage was converted, in
Table 10.3, into information on continuation in bachelorhood or spin-

Table 10.3. Percent of persons who remained, or were
expected to remain, single up to specified
ages, for white persons 30, 35, 40, and 50
years old at census date, by sex:
United States, 1960 and projections

Age at census date and sex	Percent of persons who remained, or were expected to remain, single up to age--			
	29 years	34 years	39 years	49 years
White men				
30 years	14.0	8.4[a]	5.9[a]	4.0[a]
35 years	15.8	9.5	6.6[a]	4.5[a]
40 years	16.9	8.9	6.2	4.2[a]
50 years	23.1	15.9	10.2	6.9
White women				
30 years	8.0	5.4[a]	4.4[a]	3.5[a]
35 years	9.7	6.5	5.3[a]	4.2[a]
40 years	11.7	7.7	6.3	5.0[a]
50 years	19.6	13.0	9.9	7.9

Source: U.S. Bureau of the Census, U.S. Census of
Population: 1960, Detailed Characteristics, U.S. Summary,
Final Report PC(1)-1D, table 157; and Subject Reports, Age
at First Marriage, Final Report PC(2)-4D, table 2.

[a]Projected beyond 1960 by using rate of change for
next older age group.

sterhood up to stated ages. The same source material was used earlier in another way to produce Table 3.3. Projections were introduced for the younger groups whose experience up to certain ages had not been completed by the date of the census. The age groups at census date, shown in the stub of Table 10.3, reflect successively the deterrent effect on marriage resulting from depression (age 50 at census) and war (ages 40 and 35 at census), as compared with the accentuating effect of postwar prosperity (age 30 at census).

Perhaps some of the delay in marriage for those age 50 at the census date can be properly attributed to traditionally higher ages at marriage before the postwar period. The consistently high percentages single for this oldest cohort imply that the persons in it spent much less of their adult life in the "ever-married" state than any of the younger cohorts will spend. By contrast, the youngest cohort clearly trails the rest in percent single and seems likely to continue to do so.

Only one-half as large a proportion of the white men 30 years old in 1960 as of those 50 years old had reached, or were expected to reach, the threshold of bachelorhood without having married. Thus, 8 percent of those 30 years old but 16 percent of those 50 years old are shown as remaining single until the age of 34. Corresponding percentages for white women who approached spinsterhood changed even more drastically, down to 8 percent from an earlier 20 percent.

Only 3 or 4 percent of the youngest cohort of white persons seem likely never to marry, according to the figures projected forward to age 49. This level stands in contrast with the 7 or 8 percent already experienced by those 50 years old at the time of the 1960 census. The corresponding levels for the two intermediate cohorts expected by age 49 come close to the expected terminal level for the youngest cohort despite their relatively slow start into marriage on account of the war. Even though the war and early postwar marriage cohorts may eventually almost catch up with the late postwar marriage cohort with respect to the percent who ever marry, the former cohorts will have "forever lost" far less marriage experience overall than the depression marriage cohort.

Ethnic origin. Bachelorhood and spinsterhood rates among ethnic groups in the United States differ considerably as a consequence of demonstrable demographic factors such as variations in period of immigration, age composition, and sex ratios. Other factors of a cultural or economic nature, such as attitudes toward early marriage and opportunities for gainful employment among those approaching the age of marriage, are less tangible yet may be equally relevant as explanatory variables.

Table 10.4. Percent single by race, for persons 14 years old and over standardized for age and unstandardized, and persons 35 to 44 and 45 to 64, by sex: United States, 1960

Race	Percent single, standardized for age		Percent single, unstandardized		Percent single, 35-44 years old		Percent single, 45-64 years old	
	Men	Women	Men	Women	Men	Women	Men	Women
Total[a]	24.9	19.0	24.9	19.0	8.1	6.1	7.6	7.5
White	24.7	18.9	24.3	18.6	7.7	6.0	7.5	7.6
Negro	26.4	19.3	29.6	21.7	10.9	7.0	7.9	5.6
American Indian	33.6	23.5	40.3	29.1	13.7	7.5	25.9	22.0
Japanese	33.4	21.0	34.2	21.1	14.2	7.7	8.2	4.8
Chinese	38.5	21.2	35.1	22.0	16.1	5.6	16.8	4.1
Filipino	42.4	20.8	40.3	27.7	18.6	5.5	33.7	6.1

Source: U.S. Bureau of the Census, U.S. Census of Population: 1960, Detailed Characteristics, United States Summary, Final Report PC(1)-1D, table 177; and Subject Reports, Nonwhite Population by Race, Final Report PC(2)-1C, tables 9-13.

[a]Includes the small number of persons of other nonwhite races, not shown separately.

The percent single is shown in Table 10.4 for persons 14 years old and over by race with and without standardization for age. The rank-order position of some of the racial groups, notably the American Indians, is very considerably modified by the adjustment for age. Yet both the standardized and unstandardized percentages single are lowest for white men and women.

The values in the table for persons 35 to 44 years old — after which age only a very small proportion of persons ever enter first marriage — provide another kind of statistical control on the age factor in relation to percent single. The listing of racial groups in the table is according to the order of the percent single for men in this age group. The rate for white men is at the lower extreme; the rate for Filipino men, at the upper extreme, is some two and one-half times as high. The low percentages of women single at ages 35 to 64 for the Chinese and Filipinos are traceable to large excesses of men of these racial groups; for those 45 to 64 years old, there were seven Filipino men reported to one Filipino woman of all marital categories combined. The sex ratio as a factor in mate selection was treated further in Chapter 5.

The exceptionally high rates of bachelorhood and spinsterhood among middle-aged American Indians occurred despite almost evenly balanced numbers of Indian men and women in this age range. The percentages for these older Indian men and women could have been a consequence, therefore, of tribal "nonmarriage" customs observed by this age group, which were not followed by the next younger age group.

Countries of origin for persons of foreign stock are listed in Table 10.5 in the sequence of diminishing size of the percent single among foreign-born women 45 to 54 years old. This sequence corresponds fairly closely to the inverse sequence of the difference between the older first generation and the younger second generation with respect to percent single.

The first group of three countries of origin — Ireland, United Kingdom, and Canada — had relatively high percentages single or small differences between the rates of single status for successive generations, or both, for men as well as women. Especially noteworthy is

Table 10.5. Percent single, for persons of foreign stock, by country of origin, nativity, parentage, age, and sex: United States, 1960

Country of origin	Men			Women		
	Foreign born, 45-54	Native of foreign or mixed parentage, 35-44	Differ- ence	Foreign born, 45-54	Native of foreign or mixed parentage, 35-44	Differ- ence
Total	8.3	9.9	1.6	6.7	8.3	1.6
Ireland	15.6	15.3	-0.3	13.3	15.2	1.9
United Kingdom	7.1	7.3	0.2	8.6	7.6	-1.0
Canada	6.2	8.1	1.9	7.4	7.4	0.0
Mexico	7.3	8.8	1.5	6.6	7.0	0.4
Sweden	8.3	8.7	0.4	6.2	6.7	0.5
U.S.S.R.	7.4	8.6	1.2	6.2	6.6	0.4
Germany	6.0	8.3	2.3	6.2	7.3	1.1
Austria	7.3	11.5	4.2	5.8	8.7	2.9
Czechoslovakia	7.4	11.7	4.3	5.0	8.9	3.9
Poland	8.2	12.0	3.8	4.9	7.9	3.0
Italy	5.7	8.8	3.1	4.8	9.3	4.5
Other & not reported	11.4	10.5	-0.9	6.5	7.8	1.3

Source: U.S. Bureau of the Census, U.S. Census of Population: 1960, Subject Reports, Nativity and Parentage, Final Report PC(2)-1A, tables 7 and 13.

the consistently very high percent single for the Irish who came to America themselves or whose parents did so. They apparently brought with them the Irish pattern of late marriage, pointed out in Chapter 4, which has extended into a tendency for many of their group never to marry at all. Moreover, a substantial proportion of (unmarried) Catholic priests and nuns are of Irish descent. The small percentages single for men from the United Kingdom and Canada and the small differences between the rates for women from these countries are probably reflections of the ease with which second-generation stock from these closely allied, English-speaking countries assimilate with other elements in the population of the United States.

Both the first and second groups of countries listed show relatively small differences between the generations with respect to percent single, whereas the third group shows consistently large differences. The third group also tends to have below-average percentages single for the older generation but above-average percentages single for the younger generation. By way of interpretation of these patterns, it seems relevant to observe that the third group and Germany (from the second group) include countries with which the United States was involved during World War II and from which many refugees came to the United States during the 1930's and 1940's. The data are consistent with the hypothesis that the immigrant generation shown here tended to come to the United States as young married persons, hence to have a small percent single in 1960. Those of the second generation shown here were 15 to 24 years old in 1940 and so were at the height of the period for marriage during and soon after World War II; conceivably, the stresses growing out of the war may have been a factor contributing to their relatively large percent single, including some reluctance for persons in the United States of other origins to intermarry with persons of second-generation stock from these countries or vice versa.

Among the foreign stock 45 years old and over, those from the U.S.S.R. had the most consistently small proportions single for both men and women of first and second generation, according to data from the same source as Table 10.5. This fact provides evidence that family life has held a strong position among the values of these persons, who are predominantly Jewish.

Living arrangements. Almost one-fourth of the bachelors and spinsters 35 years old and over in 1960 maintained a household apart from

Table 10.6. Family status of single persons 35 years old and over, by color and sex: United States, 1960

(Numbers in thousands)

Family status	Total		Men		Women	
	Men	Women	White	Nonwhite	White	Nonwhite
Total single, 35 & over	2,876	2,890	2,553	324	2,667	224
Percent	...	...	100.0	100.0	100.0	100.0
In households	2,439	2,552	85.0	83.3	87.9	92.9
Head of household	1,141	1,169	40.6	32.5	40.4	41.1
Head of family	337	373	12.4	6.4	12.4	18.9
Primary individual	803	796	28.2	26.1	28.0	22.3
Child of head	548	534	19.7	13.7	18.7	15.9
Brother or sister	234	389	8.3	6.7	13.8	9.7
Bro.- or sister-in-law	97	106	3.4	3.0	3.7	3.4
Other relative	126	142	3.8	8.7	4.5	10.1
Lodger	278	164	8.6	18.4	5.3	9.7
Resident employee	15	49	0.5	0.4	1.6	3.0
In group quarters	438	339	15.0	16.7	12.1	7.1
Secondary individual	149	161	5.1	5.5	5.9	2.1
In rooming house	68	26	2.2	3.3	0.9	1.2
In religious gr.qtrs.	20	84	0.8	0.0	3.1	0.2
In instit. (staff)	9	22	0.3	0.1	0.8	0.3
Other	52	29	1.7	2.0	1.1	0.4
Inmate of institution	289	178	9.9	11.2	6.3	5.0

Source: U.S. Bureau of the Census, U.S. Census of Population: 1960, Subject Reports, Persons by Family Characteristics, Final Report PC(2)-4B, table 2.

relatives as "primary individuals" (see Table 10.6). In all, about 40 percent of the bachelors and spinsters were heads of households. Nonwhite spinsters were the most likely to be the head of a family, inasmuch as they most often had one or more of their own children living with them.[5] Nearly one-fifth of the white bachelors and spinsters lived with one or both of their parents; for nonwhites, the proportion was less than one-sixth. Table 10.7 shows that among single persons 35 to 44 years old, the most frequent place to live was in the home of parents.

"Maiden aunts" were among the 17.5 percent of white spinsters and 13.1 percent of nonwhite spinsters who were living with relatives as a sister or sister-in-law of the head of the household. There were nearly one-half million of these women 35 years old and over in 1960, and it seems probable that most of them had been living in these

Table 10.7. Family status of single persons 35 years old and over, by age and sex: United States, 1960

(Numbers in thousands)

Family status	Men by age (years)				Women by age (years)			
	35-44	45-64	65-74	75 & over	35-44	45-64	65-74	75 & over
Total single	947	1,363	392	175	750	1,383	476	281
Percent	100.0	100.0	100.0	100.0	100.0	100.0	100.0	100.0
In households	86.9	85.1	82.7	75.8	90.4	89.4	87.9	77.7
Head of household	30.6	41.9	51.1	45.6	30.4	42.1	49.9	42.7
Head of family	10.2	13.0	11.8	10.0	10.5	13.7	14.6	12.3
Primary individual	20.4	28.9	39.3	35.6	19.9	28.4	35.3	30.4
Child of head	36.2	14.8	0.8	0.0	39.5	16.7	1.3	-
Brother or sister	5.3	9.6	9.8	8.2	7.1	14.1	19.9	16.3
Other relative	5.9	8.7	10.7	10.1	6.1	9.0	9.4	12.0
Nonrelative	8.9	10.1	12.7	11.9	7.3	7.5	7.4	6.7
In group quarters	13.1	14.9	17.3	24.2	9.6	10.6	12.1	22.3
In rooming house	1.9	2.4	2.9	3.0	0.8	0.9	1.0	1.2
In religious gr. qtrs.	0.8	0.7	0.5	0.5	2.8	3.1	2.9	2.3
In mental institution	4.1	5.6	6.0	6.0	2.6	3.0	3.0	3.5
In correctional inst.	1.9	1.0	0.3	0.1	0.1	0.0	0.0	0.0
In home for aged	0.5	1.3	4.3	11.7	0.5	0.6	2.7	12.5
In other institution	1.3	1.5	1.4	1.7	1.4	1.1	0.7	1.0
In other group qtrs.	2.4	2.2	1.6	1.4	1.6	1.8	1.6	1.8

Source: U.S. Bureau of the Census, U.S. Census of Population: 1960, Subject Reports, Persons by Family Characteristics, Final Report PC(2)-4B, table 2; and Inmates of Institutions, Final Report PC(2)-8A, tables 4, 7, 17, 25, 26, and 28.

homes when some of their nephews and nieces were growing up. Many must have helped with domestic work, baby-sitting, and nursing care while the lady of the house engaged in employment, civic, or social activities outside the home. Others must have been themselves employed outside the home as schoolteachers, clerks, stenographers, librarians, or domestic workers but lived with a married (or unmarried) sibling for companionship.

Evidence of the decline in the number of maiden aunts living in the home of a brother or sister is presented in Table 10.7, and the following exhibit (based on the same source) shows that the decline has been greater among white than nonwhite single women living in the home of a brother or sister:

Color	Number (000's)		Percent of all women	
	35–44	45–64	35–44	45–64
Total	85	265	0.69	1.43
White	75	250	0.68	1.49
Nonwhite	10	15	0.77	0.82

Twice as large a proportion of older women (1.4 percent) as of younger women (0.7 percent) were living as spinster sisters or sisters-in-law of the household head. Formerly, this was much more a phenomenon of white than nonwhite women; among the older women, almost twice as large a proportion of white (1.5 percent) as of nonwhite (0.8 percent) women were in this category. Nearly all the decline in maiden aunts, however, has occurred among white women; in fact, the rank order of the proportions has reversed, so that among younger women the maiden-aunt rate is actually slightly higher for nonwhite than white women.

Bachelors and spinsters living as "other relatives" of the household head were considerably more likely to be found in nonwhite than white homes, as seen from Table 10.6. Many of these were uncles, aunts, and other fairly close relatives, but many others were "cousins" or other peripheral relatives not much closer than lodgers.[6] The relatively large proportion of such household members among nonwhites may be related to a practice of granting shelter to relatives who were little more than casual acquaintances, which grew among nonwhite migrants who had moved to the large cities in all regions of the country during the 1940's and 1950's and had found difficulty in obtaining either jobs or places to live.

Transiency of residence or relative isolation marks the living quarters of many other older single persons. Fully 18 percent of the nonwhite bachelors were living in private homes as lodgers and an additional 3 percent in rooming houses. At the same time, 3 percent of the spinsters were living in convents and other quarters for religious workers; most of the 84,000 women 35 and over in such quarters were well-educated white Catholic nuns engaged in teaching school. Other quarters included workers' dormitories (for ranch hands, lumbermen, etc.), hospital and institutional staff quarters, and institutions.

Bachelors — especially nonwhite bachelors — were much more likely than spinsters to be inmates of institutions. As will be shown in Chapter 11, the main reason for the difference is the much larger proportion of bachelors than spinsters, and of nonwhites than whites, in mental hospitals and correctional institutions.

Urban and rural residence. The greatest residential concentration in 1960 of bachelors and spinsters 35 to 54 years old, both numerically and as a proportion of the total population, was in cities of 50,000 or more (see Table 10.8). Over 40 percent of all single per-

Table 10.8. Percent distribution of single persons by type of
residence and percent single by type of residence,
for persons 35 to 54 years old by age and sex:
United States, 1960

(Numbers in thousands)

Type of residence	Single persons				Percent single			
	Men		Women		Men		Women	
	35-44	45-54	35-44	45-54	35-44	45-54	35-44	45-54
Total	947	755	750	734	8.1	7.4	6.1	7.0
Percent	100.0	100.0	100.0	100.0	...	...	...	...
Central cities of urbanized areas	42.9	40.6	48.2	46.3	10.8	9.1	8.8	9.2
Urban fringe	15.9	14.3	19.3	18.5	5.3	5.0	4.9	6.3
Other urban	13.1	13.8	14.7	16.4	6.8	6.6	5.7	7.1
Rural nonfarm	19.3	20.8	13.9	14.2	7.2	7.2	4.1	5.0
Rural farm	8.8	10.5	3.9	4.5	10.3	8.7	3.5	4.0

Source: U.S. Bureau of the Census, U.S. Census of Population:
1960, Subject Reports, Marital Status, Final Report PC(2)-4E, tables 1
and 4.

sons in this age range — as compared with about 30 percent of the
corresponding population ever married — lived in these large cities.
Here the extremes of talent tend to congregate, ranging from the
strictly career-oriented professionals to the homeless men on skid row.

Roughly one-tenth of the middle-aged population in the large cities
in 1960 had never married.[7] Urban fringes of metropolitan centers,
as expected, had the lowest percentages of bachelors and below-
average percentages of spinsters. These are generally residential areas
for married men who commute to the city to work.

In places smaller than urbanized areas, the percent single for men
35 to 54 went up as the size of the place decreased, whereas the percent single for women of this age range went down as size of place
decreased. Thus bachelors constituted a relatively large proportion
(roughly one-tenth) of the men in this age range who were living on
farms, whereas spinsters constituted less than half as large a proportion of those on farms. This situation no doubt arises from numerous
factors, perhaps most important of which are the types of work available in various sizes of places for unmarried persons and the qualifications of these persons for nonfarm employment.

For example, spinsters outside urbanized areas who were still of
marriageable age in 1960 included a disproportionately large share

of women with less than 5 years of schooling. However, spinsters in such areas also included nearly as large a share of women college graduates as did the spinsters in urbanized areas. Evidently many of the well-educated (single) women remain in, or are attracted to, the smaller places to teach in their schools.

Educational level. One of the most noteworthy demographic generalizations about persons who never marry is that they tend to include the highest percentages of people in the lower and upper extremes of the educational distribution. In 1960, as shown in Table 10.9 and Figure 10.1, above-average single rates were consistently observed among those with less than 5 years of education. And, significantly, this lowest education group — the functional illiterates — recorded the largest (and among whites the only) increases in percent single between 1950 and 1960 — thereby reversing a generally downward trend.

The selective process of mate selection, during the high-marriage-

Table 10.9. Percent single, for persons 35 to 44 and 45 to 54 years old, by years of school completed, color, and sex: United States, 1960, and change, 1950 to 1960 and 1940 to 1950

Year or period and years of school completed	Percent single, 35-44 years old				Percent single, 45-54 years old			
	Men		Women		Men		Women	
	White	Nonwhite	White	Nonwhite	White	Nonwhite	White	Nonwhite
Total, 1960	7.7	11.2	6.0	7.0	7.3	8.9	7.1	5.8
Elementary: 0-4 years	19.4	12.9	15.1	9.0	13.9	10.5	10.4	6.8
5-8 years	9.1	10.8	5.1	6.6	8.2	8.4	5.2	4.8
High school: 1-3 years	6.5	10.7	3.9	5.9	6.0	8.5	5.1	5.1
4 years	6.7	10.9	5.4	6.7	6.1	8.3	7.3	7.4
College: 1-3 years	6.0	10.4	6.5	7.3	5.4	6.1	8.1	6.6
4 or more	7.8	11.6	14.3	11.8	6.9	6.8	19.1	10.6
4 years	6.9	11.7	9.9	10.3	5.6	8.7	13.4	10.7
5 or more	8.9	11.4	24.9	14.2	8.2	4.9	30.1	10.3
Change, 1950-1960[a]	-1.8	1.7	-2.4	0.8	-1.3	0.9	-1.0	1.3
Elementary: 0-4 years	4.1	3.3	4.5	2.4	1.8	2.3	4.6	2.4
5-8 years	-1.5	2.0	-0.9	1.2	-0.8	1.4	-0.3	1.3
High school: 1-3 years	-1.0	1.8	-1.5	0.6	-0.9	0.6	-1.3	0.2
4 years	-1.8	1.5	-3.7	-0.1	-0.8	-0.2	-2.3	0.9
College: 1-3 years	-1.0	0.3	-3.4	-1.2	-0.2	0.2	-2.7	-0.3
4 or more	-0.9	1.5	-6.9	-1.7	0.0	-0.4	-5.5	-1.5
Change, 1940-1950[a]	-4.1	-4.6	-2.7	-1.5	-2.0	-1.7	-1.9	-0.7
Elementary: 0-4 years	-1.6	-3.6	0.6	-0.7	-0.7	-0.9	-1.3	-0.6
5-8 years	-3.5	-5.4	-1.6	-1.6	-2.1	-3.2	-1.7	-1.1
High school: 1-3 years	-3.8	-5.0	-3.5	-2.4	-2.1	-1.3	-2.6	-0.1
4 years	-4.6	-6.5	-4.9	-3.6	-1.5	-0.1	-3.2	-0.5
College: 1-3 years	-4.0	-4.8	-5.8	-5.4	-2.2	-1.9	-5.3	-0.6
4 or more	-3.9	-2.7	-9.7	-7.1	-1.5	-0.8	-5.6	-2.4

Source: U.S. Bureau of the Census, U.S. Census of Population: 1960, Subject Reports, Marital Status, Final Report PC(2)-4E, table 4; U.S. Census of Population: 1950, Vol. IV, Special Reports, Part 5, Chapter B, Education, tables 7 and 8; and Sixteenth Census of the United States: 1940, Educational Attainment by Economic Characteristics and Marital Status, tables 37 and 40.

[a]For 1950 and 1940, data are for conterminous United States. For 1940, data are for native white and Negro population.

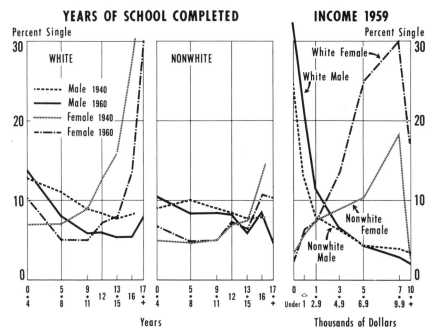

Fig. 10.1. Percent single, for persons 45 to 54 years old, by years of school completed, 1960 and 1940, and income in 1959: United States

Source: Table 10.9 and same source as Table 10.13.

rate era of the 1940's especially, is interpreted as tending to deplete the ranks of the poorly educated single population by drawing off those who had qualifications other than education which made them attractive as potential marriage partners. To the extent that this interpretation is correct, the functional illiterates apparently consist increasingly of a hard core of unmarriageable — as well as largely uneducable — persons.

At the upper part of the educational scale, spinsterhood rates have been outstandingly high but have been falling rapidly, in particular for white women who have attended graduate school. According to data in the 1960 census report cited in Table 10.9, the percent single for white women with 5 or more years of college or university training had dropped from a high level of 46 percent for those 65 years old and over in 1960 to a low level of 25 percent for those 35 to 44 years old.

Perhaps one of the main reasons why the proportion of highly educated women over 30 who do not marry has fallen so sharply is the increasing ease with which most of these women can find employment after marriage. As time goes on, the thinning ranks of the highly educated as well as of the very poorly educated spinsters may consist increasingly of women who would be very unlikely to make a success of marriage.

In 1960, there were a quarter of a million spinsters between 35 and 54 years old with college degrees and two-thirds that many bachelors. Nearly 50,000 single women of this age group (and about one-fourth that number of single men) were in "religious group quarters." The other approximately 200,000 "eligible" spinsters and 150,000 "eligible" bachelors with college degrees provide a rough measure of highly educated persons who will probably never perform the roles of spouse or parent — some of them through choice, but perhaps more of them because of unsurmounted obstacles to marriage (including physical handicaps, frustrated courtships, other emotional problems, and social pressures against women college graduates marrying men with less education. This phenomenon occurred at about twice the rate among white as nonwhite women 45 to 54 years old in 1960; but the difference was much smaller among those 35 to 44 years old, mainly because of a sharp reduction in percent single among the younger as compared with the older group of white women college graduates.

Uniformly low percentages single for men 35 to 54 years old were found among those who had attended but not completed a college education. This educational group of men must include a large proportion who discontinued college attendance because they married and had to support their new family. White men with exactly 4 years of college had below-average percentages single, whereas white men with 5 or more years of college had above-average percentages single. Thus, although bachelors in general tend to have very little education, there is a secondary tendency for white bachelors to have very much education. A part of this latter tendency can be explained by the fact that men in Catholic religious orders include a large proportion with graduate-school training. Further discussion of these men is found in the section below on occupational concentrations.

Uniformly low percentages single were found for women 35 to 54 years old among high-school dropouts. Also those with 5 to 8 years of school had consistently below-average percentages single. Many of these poorly educated women find difficulty in obtaining employment but have the ability to attract men to marry them (see further discussion of education and marriage in Chapters 3 and 4).

Work Experience and Income of Single Persons

Labor-force-participation rates. Age by age, single men below retirement age had lower rates of labor-force participation in 1960 than married men, and yet single women 18 years old and over had consistently much higher rates of labor-force participation than married women (see source of Table 10.10). Marriage is again shown to be selective, on the average, of men who succeed in obtaining regular work and of women who evidently prefer home and family to working outside the home and who are willing to rely on a husband for their livelihood.

Table 10.10. Labor-force-participation rates of single persons 25 years old and over, by age, color, and sex: United States, 1960

| Age | Labor-force-participation rate | | | | Nonwhite as percent of white | |
| | Men | | Women | | | |
	White	Nonwhite	White	Nonwhite	Men	Women
Single, 25 & over	72.3	69.3	65.1	62.7	96	96
25-34 years	85.4	75.4	81.8	67.6	88	83
35-44 years	81.6	72.6	79.6	68.4	89	86
45-54 years	76.6	70.6	77.0	66.2	92	86
55-64 years	65.6	62.3	65.9	49.7	95	75
65-74 years	28.9	28.1	30.6	27.8	97	91
75 & over	14.2	14.5	10.1	14.3	102	142

Source: U.S. Bureau of the Census, U.S. Census of Population: 1960, Subject Reports, Employment Status and Work Experience, Final Report PC(2)-6A, table 4.

Although worker rates tend to be much higher for men than women, as seen from Table 10.10, it is quite noteworthy that at ages 25 to 74 the labor-force-participation rates of white single women were almost as high as — and for some subgroups even higher than — those of white single men. For persons 25 to 54 years old, in whom there is the most interest here, over 3 out of every 4 single persons, women as well as men, were in the labor force. However, nonwhite single women had rates of labor-force participation which fell consistently below those for nonwhite single men in each age group. A relevant observation in this connection is the fact that nonwhite spinsters generally did not have much more education than nonwhite bachelors, whereas white spinsters generally had considerably more education than white bachelors of comparable age.

Occupational concentrations. The kinds of work which bachelors and spinsters perform during the height of their working years throw light on the nature of marriage selection with respect to personality structure and economic status. Table 10.11 shows that among middle-

Table 10.11. Percent single, for employed persons 45 to 54 years old by major occupation group by sex, and percent distribution of single employed persons 45 to 54 years old by major occupation group by color and sex: United States, 1960

Major occupation group	Percent single, 45-54		Percent distribution of single persons			
			Men, 45-54		Women, 45-54	
	Men	Women	White	Non-white	White	Non-white
Employed persons	5.8	11.5	100.0	100.0	100.0	100.0
Professional, tech. workers	6.1	20.8	9.9	2.0	26.3	9.2
Mgrs., off'ls., proprietors	2.6	10.7	6.7	1.9	5.1	0.9
Clerical, kindred workers	8.1	14.5	9.0	3.2	32.6	5.8
Sales workers	3.7	5.3	4.3	0.7	4.5	1.0
Craftsmen, foremen	3.4	10.2	13.3	7.3	1.3	0.6
Operatives, kindred workers	4.8	7.9	16.1	14.6	11.6	11.2
Private household workers	14.8	9.9	0.2	1.7	4.2	37.3
Service workers, other	8.5	5.6	7.4	17.9	6.0	17.0
Laborers, exc. farm & mine	8.9	9.1	8.1	18.4	0.3	1.3
Farmers, farm managers	7.8	10.0	9.6	3.0	0.5	0.8
Farm laborers & foremen	15.3	4.9	4.5	9.5	0.4	1.7
Occupation not reported	...	...	10.9	19.8	7.2	13.2

Source: U.S. Bureau of the Census, U.S. Census of Population: 1960, Subject Reports, Marital Status, Final Report PC(2)-4E, table 5.

aged white women who were in better-paying jobs, the percent single was especially high in 1960 for clerical workers (a category selective of persons who find satisfaction in working on detailed and precise written material) but low for sales workers (a category selective of "outgoing" persons who cumulate knowledge about sales items and enjoy imparting it to customers). Nearly three-fifths of the employed white single women 45 to 54 years old in 1960 were professional or clerical workers; for nonwhite women the comparable figure was less than one-sixth.

Again, among blue-collar workers, the percent single was much higher for middle-aged men in the occupation groups for which average income is relatively low than in those for which it is relatively high. White bachelors were about evenly divided between those in the blue-collar groups with low incomes (service, laboring, and farm workers) and those with higher incomes (craftsmen and operatives). More than two-thirds of the nonwhite bachelors in blue-collar occupations, however, were congregated in the groups with low incomes; difficulty is often experienced even by qualified persons of certain nonwhite races in attempts to enter some of the better-paying occupations. Moreover, no occupation was reported for nearly twice as large a proportion of nonwhite as white employed bachelors (20 versus 11 percent). Differences in the distribution of spinsters by blue-collar groupings were in the same direction but even more marked.

The list of detailed occupations in Table 10.12 sheds additional light on the qualitative aspects of the demography of bachelorhood and spinsterhood. This table includes selected occupations for which there were at least 15,000 single men or 15,000 single women 14 years old and over in the experienced civilian labor force in 1960, where the proportion single was 20.0 percent or more for men and 30.0 percent or more for women, and where the median age of persons of the specified sex in the occupation was 30.0 years or older. The list, therefore, shows occupations with disproportionately large numbers of persons who tend either to delay marriage or never to marry at all.

Far more of the qualifying occupations for single women than for single men were in the professional and technical fields, as might have been expected from differences in educational distributions of bachelors and spinsters. In addition, more extremely high percentages single were found among professional women than professional men. Particularly noteworthy are the values in the range of 55 to 65 percent single for women religious workers and private-school teachers, in which categories about 125,000 (nearly all white) single women, probably mostly Roman Catholic nuns, were classified in 1960. The

Table 10.12. Percent single, for experienced civilian labor force
in selected occupations, with median age 30 years old
and over, by sex: United States, 1960

Occupation and sex	Percent single	Occupation and sex	Percent single
MEN		WOMEN	
Clergymen	22.2	Artists, art teachers	32.4
Draftsmen	21.2	College professors	50.3
Musicians, music teachers	27.5	Librarians	40.1
Medical technicians	21.3	Recreation, group workers	48.0
Bookkeepers	22.4	Religious workers	64.3
Shipping clerks	21.0	Social-welfare workers	32.1
Stock clerks	31.6	Social scientists	38.8
Finance clerks	33.1	Sports instructors	43.5
		School teachers:	
Retail salesmen	24.6	Private elementary	54.8
Deliverymen	23.0	Public secondary	30.3
Laundry operatives	20.3	Private secondary	65.7
Sailors	25.7	Technicians	38.2
Cooks	22.0	Library attendants	49.2
Elevator operators	21.5	Office-machine operators	30.8
Porters	22.7	Secretaries	32.8
Waiters	42.0	Stenographers	35.7
		Limited-price variety	
Gardeners	33.6	retail saleswomen	37.9
Lumbermen	23.4	Housekeepers living in	32.6
Construction laborers	21.0	Other workers living in	49.2
Personal-service laborers	46.3	Nonmfg. laborers	31.1

Source: U.S. Bureau of the Census, U.S. Census of Population:
1960, Subject Reports, Occupational Characteristics, Final Report
PC(2)-7A, table 12.

70,000 single men classified as clergymen, religious workers, and private-school teachers must have likewise included a substantial proportion who were Roman Catholic priests. Many other celibates of the Roman Catholic church must have been among the 25,000 single men and 20,000 (nearly all white) single women classified as college administrators and faculty members.

Several of the occupations on the list call for rendering service with considerable skill and with a degree of compassion that would appeal to persons motivated to sublimate as a compensation for the absence of conjugal living. Several others call for such qualities as quiet work, neatness, and precision. Still others would appear to attract persons with qualities incompatible with the attitude of "give-and-take" sharing which is generally essential for partners in a successful marriage.

Finally, the list contains types of work which are suitable to persons who, because of physical, mental, or emotional limitations, lack the efficiency and effectiveness to command a responsible position. The occupations on the list therefore seem to include a relatively large proportion that demand either extreme devotion to the job or very little devotion.

The list of occupations for women with a high percent single hardly overlaps with a corresponding list of occupations for women with a high percent divorced (Table 8.30). Artists and art teachers are exceptions, with high spinster and divorcee rates. For men, however, the two lists overlap extensively. Occupations with high percentages of single and divorced men include actors (relatively small number), musicians and music teachers, medical and dental technicians, and several types of service workers. Not overlapping are the following occupations with high percentages single only: clergymen, draftsmen, the several types of clerical and sales workers, deliverymen, and lumbermen. Some of the occupations which overlap tend to involve frequent personal and social contacts with other persons; some of the other occupations require the persons to spend more of their working time in almost complete isolation.

Additional occupations with relatively large numbers and proportions of divorced men but not large proportions of single men include: salaried and self-employed managers of eating and drinking establishments; motor-vehicle-accessory salesmen; painters (construction and maintenance); roofers and slaters; structural metal workers; filers, grinders, and polishers; taxicab drivers and chauffeurs; private household workers; various service workers, excluding barbers, firemen, policemen, and detectives; longshoremen; railroad laborers; and public-administration laborers. (Most of these are not listed in Table 8.30 but could have been.) These occupations include several which are tedious, some involving regular confrontation of men with women in commercial relations, and still others which require work that is so lacking in close contacts with women that the employer would be unlikely to have any concern about the man's personal life so long as he did his work well on the job.

Additional occupations in which divorced women, but not single women, tend to abound include the following: actresses (relatively small number); entertainers; buyers and department-store heads; other salaried managers; other managerial agents; ticket, station, and express agents; insurance agents and brokers; real-estate agents; bookbinders; photographic-process workers; welders and flame-cutters; workers in factories manufacturing glass products, motor-vehicle equipment, aircraft equipment, bakery products, paperboard boxes, and rubber products; housekeepers living in; bartenders; elevator operators; hairdressers and cosmetologists; practical nurses; policewomen and detectives; and waitresses. Several of these occupations probably appeal to women workers with an unusual amount of concern about their own personal appearance or about being identified with the production or distribution of a high-quality product. Frequent and close personal contact with men is involved in some of these jobs. Most of the occupations either involve the handling of money or regular reminders of the importance of things money can buy.

This exploration provides clues to underlying differences between those who become bachelors or spinsters and those who become (and may remain) divorced.

Income levels. Further evidence of the critical importance of amount of income in the marital experience may be found in Table 10.13 (see also Figure 10.1). For men, the proportion who remain single

Table 10.13. Percent single, by income in 1959 and sex, and percent distribution of single persons by income in 1959, color, and sex, for persons 45 to 54 years old: United States, 1960

| Income in 1959 | Percent single, 45-54 years | | Percent distribution of single persons | | | |
| | | | Men, 45-54 | | Women, 45-54 | |
	Men	Women	White	Nonwhite	White	Nonwhite
Total	7.4	7.0	100.0	100.0	100.0	100.0
Without income	31.0	2.7	14.1	17.3	16.8	19.9
With income	6.6	10.2	85.9	82.7	83.2	80.1
With income	...	...	100.0	100.0	100.0	100.0
$1-$999 or loss	19.7	6.2	19.2	30.9	14.7	41.3
$1,000-$2,999	10.8	7.5	25.0	36.0	24.9	40.5
$3,000-$4,999	6.7	13.3	26.4	24.5	33.1	13.6
$5,000-$6,999	4.3	24.4	18.5	6.9	19.0	3.4
$7,000-$9,999	2.8	29.9	6.9	1.4	6.7	1.3
$10,000 & over	2.2	17.0	4.0	0.4	1.7	0.0
Median income	$3,250	$3,452	$3,440	$2,062	$3,632	$1,431

Source: U.S. Bureau of the Census, U.S. Census of Population: 1960, Subject Reports, Marital Status, Final Report PC(2)-4E, table 6.

diminishes sharply as income increases until virtually none in the highest bracket fails to marry. For women, the proportion who remain single until middle age is highest among those with incomes of $5,000 to $10,000. Half of the women who were 45 to 54 years old in 1960 had entered spinsterhood during the 1940's when it was becoming easier for a married woman to enter or remain in a position which afforded a high salary. These women did not marry; instead, they retained their good-paying positions in the world of work. The proportion of white single women 45 to 54 who received incomes of $5,000 to $10,000 (26 percent) was as high as that for white single men in the same age group. The corresponding comparison for nonwhite single persons, however, was less favorable to the women.

In the light of observations previously made, it should not be surprising that middle-aged bachelors tend to occupy the lowest position on the income scale for men and that middle-aged spinsters tend to occupy the highest position for women. Yet it will come as a surprise to some, no doubt, that at ages 45 years and over the median income of single women exceeded that of single men, according to data from the 1960 census in the source cited in Table 10.13. These overall generalizations tend to hold for white men and women and for nonwhite men; but for nonwhite women, the median income of divorced women ranked first in each age group and that of single women ranked second.

From this analysis it seems plausible to infer that single and divorced women would be expected to rate higher on an objective test of aggressiveness toward work for pay or profit than either the separated or the widowed of comparable age. The low incomes of married women, however, do not necessarily suggest a corresponding degree of nonaggressiveness toward work, because the economic status of married women is generally determined largely by the income of the husband. At the same time, available evidence suggests strongly that women who are relatively unemployable are the most likely to marry or to remarry. The situation is changing rapidly, however, in the direction of an increasing proportion of the more employable women who marry.

In various parts of this monograph, allusion has been made to the somewhat blurred line between the reporting of single and the reporting of separated as marital-status categories. In this context, the following observations seem relevant. On the one hand, separated persons had consistently smaller median incomes than divorced persons and, for those 25 to 64 years old, separated persons had below-average median incomes for both white and nonwhite men and for white women; this much of the picture tends to confirm the assertion that separation is often the poor man's divorce. On the other hand, median incomes for separated nonwhite women 25 and over were actually above the average for all nonwhite women. Lest this superficial evidence be cited to prove that the typical separated nonwhite woman is able to live a life of comfort, however, the fact from the 1960 census should simultaneously be noted that in no age group did the median income for separated nonwhite women rise above the very low level of $1,550. Perhaps the main reason why the incomes of nonwhite separated women of mature years were "above average" for all nonwhite women was the fact that the incomes of nonwhite single women of comparable ages were — quite unlike those of white single women — so very low that they brought down the average.

The foregoing discussion of the relationship between marital status and income level demonstrates the point which is most relevant to this chapter, namely, that the hierarchical ranking of single persons with respect to income differs from one group to another by color and sex but tends to be relatively high for single women and relatively low for single men of mature age.

Late Marriage versus Nonmarriage

Do persons who are relatively old at first marriage tend to resemble closely those who never marry at all? This question is posed as a prelude to testing the hypothesis that selective factors at work in the year-after-year screening of persons eligible for first marriage may reach the point where those in their thirties or forties who continue to remain unmarried differ little from those who enter marriage at this period of life. The evidence from the 1960 census provides an unqualified negative reply to the question for white men but a qualified positive reply for white women. (See source of Table 10.14; a corresponding analysis of nonwhite persons could be made from the data given therein.)

The uppermost socioeconomic groups of white men tend to enter first marriage during the second half of their twenties, but the range varies according to which index of status is used (see Table 10.14 and Figure 10.2). Those who first married between the ages of 23 and 29 had higher median educational levels than those who entered

Table 10.14. Indexes of socioeconomic status for white men 21 to 44 years old who first married in 1958 or 1959 and for those who remained single, by age: United States, 1960

Age of white men in 1958 and 1959	Median years of school completed			Percent of employed men in professional and managerial occupations			Median income in 1959		
	Married in the period	Re-mained single	Married as per-cent of single	Married in the period	Re-mained single	Married as per-cent of single	Married in the period	Re-mained single	Married as per-cent of single
21 years	12.4	12.6	98	12.2	10.2	120	$3,344	$2,318	144
22 years	12.5	12.6	99	15.5	11.5	135	3,447	2,462	140
23 years	12.6	12.6	100	17.1	13.6	126	3,602	2,744	131
24 years	12.6	12.6	100	19.3	15.8	122	3,972	3,206	124
25-26 years	12.7	12.5	102	22.7	18.3	124	4,318	3,614	119
27-29 years	12.7	12.4	102	26.7	19.0	141	4,731	3,930	120
30-34 years	12.4	12.1	102	24.3	16.7	146	5,054	4,075	124
35-39 years	12.2	11.7	104	19.7	13.8	143	4,880	3,984	122
40-44 years	11.6	10.4	112	14.1	11.8	119	4,619	3,717	124

Source: U.S. Bureau of the Census, U.S. Census of Population: 1960, Subject Reports, Age at First Marriage, Final Report PC(2)-4D, table 17.

first marriage at either younger or older ages. However, those who first married between 25 and 34 had the highest percent of employed men in professional or managerial occupations. Moreover, those who

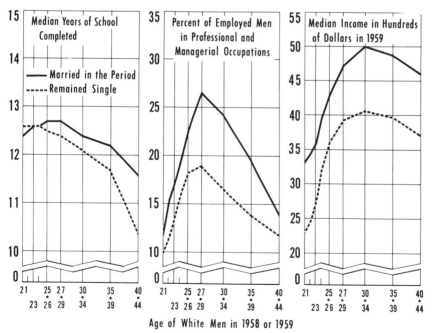

Fig. 10.2. Indexes of socioeconomic status for white men who first married in 1958 or 1959 and for those who remained single, by age: United States

Source: Table 10.14.

first married between 27 and 39 had the highest median income *during the year before marriage;* however, interestingly enough, men who had married a few years earlier had still higher median incomes by the time they were 27 to 39 years old. As age advanced beyond these respective ages, the several indexes showed downward changes for both recently married and single men. Still, they remained substantially higher for those who married than for those of the same age who continued to be single.

These findings lead to the conclusion that, for white men, the process of positive socioeconomic selection continues to operate even at the upper portion of the range of age at first marriage; that is, up to the mid-forties. Hence, even though the average status of white bachelors declines with age, those among them who are of higher status are more likely to enter marriage than those of lower status.

For white women, the situation is quite different (see source of Table 10.14). The median educational attainment of single women throughout the age range from 21 to 44 years was almost identical for those who did and those who did not enter first marriage in 1958 or 1959 (and was above that of the general population). Moreover, the first-marriage rate for women throughout this age range was rather consistently about three times as high for those not employed as for the employed, with some peaking of the ratio between the ages of 25 and 39. Among women with incomes, those who remained single had consistently about 20 percent higher median incomes than those who married. However, the women who married in this two-year period had been married, on the average, for a little over one year as of the date of the 1960 census (April); some of the difference between their employment rate and income, on the one hand, and that of women who remained single, on the other, could have occurred because some of the working wives quit their jobs in the meantime, perhaps generally on account of pregnancy.

The findings for white women suggest that spinsters who marry at ages up to the middle forties have about the same average status as those who remain single but have more of a tendency not to be employed. These and other facts brought out earlier suggest that socioeconomic status, as measured by available census data for persons and their families, may not be as much of a contributing factor in determining whether spinsters marry as it is in determining whether bachelors marry. For both bachelors and spinsters, demographic factors may be less discriminating between those who marry late and those who stay single than certain nondemographic values, such as beauty, common sense, and so on, which cut across socioeconomic levels.

The patterns of marriage rates for white women appear to reflect considerable reluctance on the part of many spinsters to marry available bachelors of similar age (because the men tend to be of lower status) or to marry widowers or divorced men even if they are of comparable or higher status, on the grounds that they (the spinsters) "could be worse off married." A similar statement could be made about bachelors, but the supporting evidence is less substantial. No doubt many of the bachelors and spinsters who become well adjusted in their single state decide not to risk maladjustment in marriage. Census data provide few clues as to how many bachelors and spinsters choose to remain single for such reasons. Nor do they show how many would gladly marry if they had better means of locating and meeting acceptable unmarried persons of the opposite sex who were likewise interested in becoming married.[8] With prospects already pointing to a mere 3 or 4 percent of persons who never marry, the main issue regarding bachelors and spinsters becomes increasingly one of when, rather than whether, they will eventually marry.[9]

11 / MARITAL STATUS AND HEALTH

Differences between married and unmarried adults below old age with respect to morbidity, medical care, hospital care, and mortality are discussed in this chapter. Inasmuch as the great majority of such adults are married, the focus here is on the extent to which the unmarried deviate from the norms set by the married in these areas. The findings in earlier chapters about differences in the socioeconomic levels which tend to characterize the various categories of unmarried men and women are drawn upon to enhance the analysis.

The unique findings in this chapter in turn throw light on the health problems of those who do not marry at all, those who do not remain married, and those who do not remarry. Thus most of the data presented here pertain to negative aspects of the relationship between health and marriage. This material tends to support the thesis that a relatively large proportion of people who have serious trouble with their health are likely to have serious trouble in becoming married, maintaining a viable marriage, or becoming remarried. Moreover, these troubles tend to be compounded by unfavorable socioeconomic adjustment.

In this context, the proposal explored in this chapter is that marked problems in marital adjustment are frequently associated with physical- or mental-health problems and that difficulties in any one of the three aspects of life — health, socioeconomic adjustment, and marriage — have a likelihood of accentuating difficulties which arise in either of the other two.

Firm conclusions are not always feasible in this chapter, because the data on relationships between the health and marriage variables are so often subject to serious limitations. Most of these limitations are discussed in the sources cited in the tables and in the notes; some of them are mentioned in the text of the chapter. In several sections of the chapter suggestions are made regarding more definitive research that is needed.

Perhaps the most beneficial further research would be large-scale longitudinal studies in which personal and family histories would be gathered and analyzed on the whole gamut of variables involved. Ideally, these studies would follow the subjects from childhood through middle age and would show how successive changes in marital status could be better understood through knowledge of past, current, and prospective changes in health, social, and economic adjustment.

In the absence of such ambitious, time-consuming, and costly studies, the author of the present chapter has attempted to summarize the substantial body of demographic data on marital status and health which became available from the 1960 census and several other contemporaneous sources. A digest of these data should at least help to sharpen the issues which would be faced in setting up more definitive studies.

Morbidity

Most of the data discussed here on morbidity by marital status consist of nationwide information on chronic health conditions collected in the Health Interview Survey. This material was gathered by the U.S. Bureau of the Census for the National Center for Health Statistics through interviews with respondents in households. Near the end of this section, the summary of the very limited data on heart conditions and syphilis is based on findings from actual physical examinations in the Health Examination Survey.

Chronic health conditions. One or more "chronic conditions" were reported in the period from mid-1961 to mid-1963 by 54 percent of the civilian noninstitutional population 17 to 64 years old; the proportion was lower than the overall average (48 percent) for those aged 17 to 44, and higher (64 percent) for those aged 45 to 64 (see source for Table 11.2). Among conditions considered chronic are physical or mental impairments and illnesses lasting more than three months. Most of those with chronic conditions (three out of four) usually experienced no limitation of activity thereby. The group of major interest here is the 9 percent of all persons 17 to 64 who found that these conditions limited the amount or kind of their usual major activity (ability to work, keep house, attend school); about 1 out of 7 of these (1.4 percent) was so limited by his health conditions that he was unable to carry on his usual major activity. As family income increased, the proportion of persons with conditions which limited activity decreased.

Persons who had not married were substantially less likely to have any chronic condition than were those who had married (see Table 11.1). However, 15 percent of the single men as compared with 10

Table 11.1. Percent with specified degree of limitation of activity from chronic conditions, for the civilian noninstitutional population 17 to 64 years old, by marital status and sex, standardized for age: United States, July 1962 to June 1963

(Numbers in thousands)

Degree of limitation of activity from chronic condition	Men 17-64 years old				Women 17-64 years old			
	Married	Widowed	Divorced	Single	Married	Widowed	Divorced	Single
Total population	37,269	563	1,061	9,208	40,193	3,277	1,820	7,525
Percent	100.0	100.0	100.0	100.0	100.0	100.0	100.0	100.0
With no chronic conditions	45.8	48.1	39.6	53.4	42.7	39.4	40.4	55.3
With 1 or more	54.2	51.9	60.4	46.6	57.3	60.6	59.6	44.7
No limitation of activity	41.1	34.9	38.9	31.8	44.7	43.0	44.3	35.2
With limitation	13.1	17.0	21.5	14.8	12.6	17.6	15.3	9.5
Total with 1 or more chronic conditions	20,230	340	654	3,480	23,031	2,204	1,102	3,038
Percent	100.0	100.0	100.0	100.0	100.0	100.0	100.0	100.0
No limitation of activity	75.9	67.2	64.4	68.3	78.0	71.0	74.3	78.8
With limitation	24.1	32.8	35.6	31.7	22.0	29.0	25.7	21.2
Not in major activity[a]	6.7	4.5	5.5	5.7	8.8	9.0	9.8	7.5
In amount or kind of major activity	13.7	17.9	21.5	17.8	12.3	17.0	14.5	9.4
Unable to carry on major activity	3.6	10.4	8.6	8.1	0.8	3.0	1.5	4.4

Source: National Center for Health Statistics, unpublished data from Health Interview Survey based on civilian noninstitutional population. Similar data (not by sex but for single and ever-married persons in the age groups 17-44, 45-64, and 65 & over) were published in table 19 of the same source as the following table, 11.2.

[a]Major activity refers to ability to work, keep house, or go to school (according to the person's age-sex group).

percent of the single women reported chronic conditions which limited their activity. Those men who had chronically limited activity probably tended to have lower earning capacity than those with no such limitation and hence diminished ability to succeed in becoming married.

Married men had lower *limiting*-chronic-condition rates than unmarried (widowed, divorced, or single) men. Among those with one or more chronic conditions, married men had especially low rates of those types of chronic conditions that were serious enough to make them report that they were unable to work. Married women likewise had lower limiting-chronic-condition rates than widows or divorced women. Of those with chronic conditions, married women also had the lowest rates of the most severe types, that is, the types which prevent women from carrying on their major activity.

These observations suggest (but do not prove) that married men and women and also adult single women tend to minimize their health problems because they are generally preoccupied with the performance of their major activity. At the same time, it may be inferred that these groups are among those most likely to acknowledge the existence of health problems which they think are really serious and to take steps to cure them by self-treatment or by seeking medical advice.

Type of chronic condition. For several types of limiting conditions which tend to reflect nervous strain and tension, smaller proportions among those with chronic conditions were reported by young married persons (under age 45) than by single adults (over 4 out of 5 of whom are 17 to 44); however, larger proportions of the younger than

Table 11.2. Percent with selected limiting chronic conditions, for the civilian noninstitutional population 17 years old and over with limiting chronic conditions, by marital status and age: United States, July 1961 to June 1963

Type of chronic condition (with some persons reporting more than one condition)	Total, 17 years old & over	Ever married			Single, 17 years old & over
		17 & over	17-44 years	45 & over	
Lower percent for young persons ever married than for the single					
Hypertension without heart involvement	6.4	6.6	3.1	7.6	4.1
Mental & nervous conditions	7.9	7.7	9.6	7.2	10.1
Heart conditions	16.7	17.3	6.6	20.5	11.1
Arthritis & rheumatism	15.8	16.5	6.6	19.4	8.8
Visual impairments	5.6	5.7	2.1	6.7	5.6
Hearing impairments	2.1	2.0	1.3	2.2	2.8
Paralysis, complete or partial	3.8	3.3	2.7	3.5	8.3
Higher percent for young persons ever married than for the single					
Varicose veins	2.5	2.6	2.5	2.7	1.6
Peptic ulcer	2.6	2.7	3.3	2.5	1.6
Conditions of genito-urinary system	5.2	5.4	7.1	4.9	2.9
Diseases (except arthritis & rheumatism) of muscles, bones, & joints	3.7	3.8	6.9	2.9	2.6
Impairments (except paralysis) of back or spine	7.8	7.9	14.0	6.2	6.9

Source: National Center for Health Statistics, Vital and Health Statistics, Series 10, No. 17, "Chronic Conditions and Activity Limitation, United States, July 1961-June 1963," table 21.

of the older married persons with limiting chronic conditions reported chronic mental or nervous conditions (see Table 11.2, the source of which did not include data by sex or data for single adults by age).

The frequency of limitation of activity due to arthritis and rheumatism tended to be relatively *higher* among single adults than among young married persons; limitation of this kind was also relatively frequent for persons from families with low incomes and with housekeeping as their major activity. By contrast, the frequency of limitation caused by other diseases of muscles, bones, and joints tended to be relatively *low* for single persons, nonwhite persons, and persons from families with low incomes. Some of the difference in these rates may have arisen because upper-class white persons are more likely to visit a physician in connection with an illness and therefore to report an accurate diagnosis (see page 7 in the source of Table 11.2).

Some types of impairments evidently reduce substantially the chances of marriage. The three conditions of visual impairments, hearing impairments, and paralysis, taken as a group, were responsible for one-sixth of the limitations due to chronic conditions reported by single persons (mostly under 45 years old) but for only one-sixteenth of the limitations reported by ever-married persons under 45 years of age.

Other types of impairments, such as those of the back or spine, were twice as common as causes of activity limitation among young married persons as among single adults. Back and spine ailments are more frequently found among men, and among those usually at work. These facts support the hypothesis that smaller proportions of single adults (including college students, women who work in offices or stores, etc.) than of young married persons engage in heavy manual work which cripples the back.

Genitourinary conditions and varicose veins, typical of mothers, caused chronic activity limitation among a higher proportion of persons who had married than of those who had remained single. Peptic ulcers, which are more common among men than among women, were reported as limiting by relatively small numbers of persons, but conditions of this kind accounted for a larger proportion of those chronically limited among the ever-married than among single adults.

Heart conditions. In the following brief presentation of results from the Health Examination Survey, definite evidence of coronary heart disease, myocardial infarction, and angina pectoris is referred to simply as coronary heart disease, and definite hypertension and definite hypertensive heart disease are referred to simply as hypertension.

Divorced men had lower rates of coronary heart disease and of hypertension than expected on the basis of their proportion among all men of like ages in the United States. Divorced men also had much lower rates for these conditions than separated men.[1] Since divorced men tend to have a higher socioeconomic level than separated men, this finding conforms to the observation that persons with relatively high incomes have a lower prevalence of cardiovascular disease than those with lower incomes.

Syphilis. White adult single women had very much lower rates of infection by syphilis (past or present, as shown by detected reactions to the Kolmer Reiter Protein test) than would have been expected if they had the rates of all persons in the United States of like age, race, and sex.[2] The actual rate for white single women was only 0.1 percent, as compared with the expected rate of 1.3 percent and as compared with the actual rate of 7.0 percent for nonwhite single women. Notwithstanding the sampling variability of the results, it still is worth noting that, for the other marital-status categories, rates for nonwhite persons were 6 to 12 times as high as those for comparable white persons.

Of interest in interpreting these results is the fact that 4.0 percent of the adults tested were found to have had syphilis; that is, they were reactive to the KRP test, indicating probable infection at some time in their life. Positive reactions were higher for men than for women, both white and nonwhite, but with a larger sex difference for the nonwhites. The rate was found to reach a peak for men at around age 40 and for women at around age 60. These findings may be interpreted as reflecting differences in the rates of syphilitic infection. However, early and effective treatment tends to obscure the traces of the disease. To the extent that early and effective treatment is more likely to have been obtained (1) by women than men, (2) by white than nonwhite persons, and (3) by those who have married than those who remained single, the test findings may exaggerate the observed differences by sex, color, and marital status. No statistically significant differences on a cell-by-cell comparison were found in the tables on syphilis rates by amount of schooling or by family income; but the pattern of the data showed consistently smaller rates for persons in the higher levels of education and income.

Medical Care

The Health Interview Survey provides comparisons of persons in the several marital-status groups with respect to hospital- and surgical-insurance coverage and visits to physicians and dentists. In the interpretation of statistics in the preceding section on reported health conditions, in the present section on visits to a doctor, and in the next section on care in a hospital, the financial ability of the person or his family to provide care for his ailments stands out as an important contributing factor. Using this financial ability to provide hospital and surgical insurance makes it easier, in turn, for the person to take care of certain health needs.

In the absence of data controlled by income level, many of the differences from one marital status to another in the data presented on morbidity, medical care, and hospital care can be interpreted at least in part as reflections of differences in average income of persons or of their families. Other differences in health measures by marital status arise out of extreme contrasts in the age distribution of the single and the widowed populations. Insofar as possible, therefore, data shown

Table 11.3. Percent with hospital and surgical-insurance coverage, for the civilian noninstitutional population 17 to 64 years old, by marital status, standardized for age: United States, July 1962 to June 1963

(Numbers in thousands)

Marital status	Persons 17 to 64 years old	Percent with hospital insurance		Percent with surgical insurance	
		Percent	Index	Percent	Index
Married	75,826	77.8	100	72.9	100
Single	16,746	63.7	82	57.3	79
Divorced	2,892	58.9	76	55.2	76
Widowed	3,784	55.8	72	50.9	70
Separated	2,022	45.5	58	40.5	56

Source: National Center for Health Statistics, Vital and Health Statistics, Series 10, No. 11, "Health Insurance Coverage: United States, July 1962-June 1963," table 11. Not published by sex.

here are limited to those 17 to 64 years old and are standardized for age so as to minimize age differences as an element affecting the comparisons. Because of the fact that this monograph features data on married persons, the standard used in several tables for adjusting the data was the age distribution of married persons.

Health-insurance coverage. Insurance in the form of hospital or surgical coverage was held by about three-fourths of all married persons and by considerably smaller proportions of other persons, as shown in Table 11.3. Next highest coverage was that of single persons, with about three-fifths, followed by the divorced and widowed, and finally the separated, with only about two-fifths insured. Surgical insurance was 3 to 6 percentage points below the level of hospital insurance for each marital status.

Physician visits. A large proportion of married adults in the nationwide household sample made one or more visits to a physician within a year before the survey — 72 percent of the wives and 60 percent of the husbands (see Table 11.4). The difference between these percentages was largely at ages under 45 years and undoubtedly reflected, at least in part, visits by women associated with childbearing. Despite the relatively high rate of health-insurance coverage by single adults, their rate of physician visits (standardized for age) was clearly the lowest, averaging about one-sixth below that for married persons.

Table 11.4. Percent with last physician visit within a year, for the civilian noninstitutional population 17 to 64 years old, by marital status and sex, standardized for age: United States, July 1963 to June 1964

Marital status	Total		Men		Women		Rate for women as percent of rate for men
	Percent with physician visit	Index	Percent with physician visit	Index	Percent with physician visit	Index	
Married	66.3	100	59.8	100	72.4	100	121
Widowed	65.0	98	59.9	100	68.7	95	115
Divorced	64.5	97	50.7	85	71.2	98	140
Separated	61.3	92	52.6	88	66.5	92	126
Single	55.4	84	48.1	80	62.5	86	130

Source: National Center for Health Statistics, *Vital and Health Statistics*, Series 10, No. 19, "Physician Visits: Interval of Visits and Children's Routine Checkup, United States, July 1963-June 1964," table 29.

Evidently the reputation adult single men have for engaging in hazardous work and recreation is not reflected in high rates of visits to physicians; their low visit rate seems less likely to imply that adult single men actually have a low disability rate than that they have a tendency to neglect personal health. Less surprising, perhaps, is the low visit rate for adult single women, who include only a small minority who make physician visits associated with childbirth.

Visits to a physician by widowed, separated, and divorced persons tend to be of intermediate frequency in general, but quite different for men than for women. The rate of physician visits for divorced women was 40 percent higher than that for divorced men and was almost as high as that for married women. This finding is consistent with the fact that women who remain divorced tend to have relatively high socioeconomic status and corresponding likelihood to afford physician visits, whereas divorced men tend to have the reverse socioeconomic situation and probably much more of a tendency to neglect their health needs. The higher rate for separated women than separated men may reflect the high proportion of "separated" women who are believed to be actually unwed mothers; many of these women require visits to the physician within a given year in connection with childbearing.

Dental visits. As seen in Table 11.5, single women below age 65 were more likely than married women to have visited a dentist during the preceding year. They were even more likely to have sought dental service than were single or married men. The least likely were widowed, divorced, and separated men. Single men and women under 25 years old were one-third more likely to visit a dentist during the year than were married persons under 25. Also, women who remained single into middle age were one-fourth again as likely to visit a dentist as married women of the same age, whereas middle-aged single men were one-fourth less likely to visit a dentist. These differences no doubt reflect a direct correlation between socioeconomic status and attention paid to dental needs.

Hospital Care

In both the 1950 and 1960 censuses, 1.3 percent of the males and 0.8 percent of the females in the United States were in institutions; that is, they were living in such places as hospitals for patients requir-

Table 11.5. Percent with one or more dental visits in the past year, for the civilian noninstitutional population 17 to 64 years old, by marital status and sex, standardized for age: United States, July 1963 to June 1964

Marital status	Total		Men		Women		Rate for women as percent of rate for men
	Percent with dental visit	Index	Percent with dental visit	Index	Percent with dental visit	Index	
Married[a]	45.2	100	42.3	100	47.9	100	113
Single	46.5	103	38.8	92	54.0	113	139
Other[b]	34.9	77	28.6	68	37.5	78	131

Source: National Center for Health Statistics, Vital and Health Statistics, Series 10, No. 29, "Dental Visits: Time Interval Since Last Visit, United States, July 1963-June 1964," table 11.

[a]Married, except separated.

[b]Widowed, divorced, and separated.

ing long-term care, or were under custody for correctional treatment following conviction for a serious legal offense. These inmates of institutions totaled 1.6 million in 1950 and 1.9 million persons in 1960.

Regardless of the type of institution in which inmates reside, the very fact of being voluntarily or involuntarily isolated from the usual social relationships provided in most homes tends to have a bearing on the mental and physical health of such residents. It is in this context that the discussion here relates to all inmates rather than only to those hospitalized because of a health condition. However, attention is focused largely on persons receiving long-term hospital care.

If an actual or potential inmate of an institution has a spouse from whom he or she is not estranged and who can be counted on to promote recovery or rehabilitation of the person, the fact is usually taken into account in determining whether the person should be committed and, if committed, how long the stay will last. Such an inference seems warranted on the basis of the statistics on residents of institutions when classified according to marital status. Although the cause-and-effect relationships regarding the variables are complex, a close association between satisfactory adjustment in marriage and remaining free from residence in an institution seems apparent.

Specifically, in 1960 fully 68 percent of the men 14 years old and

Table 11.6. Institutional-residence rate per 10,000 population 45 to
64 years old, by type of institution, marital status, and
sex: United States, 1960

Type of institution and sex	All inmates, 45-64	Married, except separated	Widowed	Divorced	Separated	Single
Men						
In all institutions	152	45	340	676	589	935
Mental hospitals	75	22	97	237	215	550
State and local	63	18	76	183	189	472
Federal	11	3	16	48	23	72
Private	1	1	5	6	3	7
Correctional institutions	31	12	84	215	186	103
Homes for aged and needy:						
Known to have nursing care	7	1	38	29	30	40
Not known to have such care	16	3	68	103	64	91
Tuberculosis hospitals	12	6	35	62	63	36
Chronic hospitals (except tuberculosis and mental)	5	1	16	26	27	24
Institutions (mostly) for juveniles	7	0	2	4	4	89
Women						
In all institutions	90	37	99	193	247	475
Mental hospitals	62	31	51	150	193	297
State and local	60	30	48	144	187	286
Federal	1	1	1	3	5	4
Private	2	1	2	3	2	7
Correctional institutions	1	1	2	5	9	2
Homes for aged and needy:						
Known to have nursing care	6	1	16	10	10	26
Not known to have such care	8	1	21	17	12	38
Tuberculosis hospitals	3	2	4	5	10	6
Chronic hospitals (except tuberculosis and mental)	2	1	4	4	9	8
Institutions (mostly) for juveniles	8	0	1	2	4	97

Source: U.S. Bureau of the Census, U.S. Census of Population:
1960, Subject Reports, Inmates of Institutions, Final Report PC(2)-8A,
tables 17 and 25-30; and Marital Status, Final Report PC(2)-4E, tables
1 and 4.

over were married, yet only 22 percent of the inmates of institutions were in this marital class. Likewise, 64 percent of the women were married, but only 18 percent of those in institutions. In Table 11.6, the comparison is limited to those of middle age to minimize the effect of variations introduced by differences in age distribution. The facts in succeeding paragraphs are very striking; the most modest observation this table suggests is that married men have only one-third, and married women two-fifths, the comparable rate of institutionalization for the general population.

The number of inmates of institutions per 10,000 population varied widely among the several categories of unmarried persons of middle age. It ranged from a "low" rate of 99 for widows, which is actually almost three times the rate of 37 for married women, to the extremely high rate of 935 for bachelors, which is nearly 21 times the rate for married men. Over 9 percent of all single men 45 to 64, and nearly 5 percent of all single women of the same age range, were residing in institutions.

Type of institution. As previously noted, middle-aged persons (here, 45 to 64 years old) are featured through much of this monograph. Among this group, mental patients in hospitals providing psychiatric care accounted for one-half of the men and two-thirds of the women in institutions. Inmates of correctional institutions accounted for one-fifth of the men but very few of the women in institutions. Residents in homes for the aged and dependent accounted for about one-sixth of the men and women in institutions. Far more men than women were in tuberculosis hospitals and in hospitals for the chronically ill. A substantial number of the men in chronic and tuberculosis hospitals were residing in facilities for military veterans because of disabling conditions incurred in or aggravated by war service.

Married persons. Residence in homes for the aged and dependent was most rare for the married. Only 4 out of every 10,000 middle-aged married men were in "domiciliary" and nursing homes for the aged, whereas the corresponding rates were about 25 to 35 times as high for separated, widowed, divorced, and single men. Divorced men in homes for the aged were more likely than other men to be residents of generally less desirable types of institutions, namely, places not known to provide nursing care. Extremely low rates of residence in hospitals for chronic conditions as well as in homes for the aged and dependent were recorded for persons with marriages intact. This fact is interpreted as evidence that persons who manage to live with their spouse "until death does them part" tend to provide mutual care and to reduce the physical and mental anguish of their spouse when the latter is stricken with a severe chronic ailment.

In general, married persons were spared much more than unmarried persons from being institutionalized for medical care, but they were the least spared with respect to residence in tuberculosis hospitals. Separated persons and divorced men, however, had especially high hospitalization rates for tuberculosis. These facts are closely related to the high incidence of tuberculosis among Negroes. Specifically, among all tuberculosis hospital patients in 1960, one-fourth of the men and one-third of the women were nonwhite (mostly Negro), whereas only one-tenth of the people 14 years old and over in the United States in 1960 were nonwhite.

Almost one-half of the 200,000 married persons in mental hospitals in 1960 were between the ages of 45 and 65 years. In this critical age range, from the viewpoint of the emphasis in the present study, married women were more than half again as likely to be in a state or local mental hospital under public control as were married men.

The far higher correctional-institution rate for married men than for married women stands in sharp contrast with the much lower mental-institution rate for married men than for married women. The forms which extremely deviant behavior usually takes among maladjusted men and the types of treatment usually prescribed by society for such behavior are quite differently distributed than they are for maladjusted women. Also, a husband who is on the borderline of mental illness may more likely be cared for by his wife at home than the reverse situation.

The far higher rates of federal hospital treatment of men than women of each marital status for mental illness probably are a consequence of the hospitalization of substantial numbers of ex-servicemen in facilities for veterans and the larger proportion of men who are being treated for drug addiction in a federal hospital.

Unmarried persons. Persons with marriages disrupted by separation or divorce had considerably higher rates of mental-hospital treatment than those whose marriages were intact or who were widowed. But the highest rates were for middle-aged single persons, with fully 5.5

percent of the bachelors and 3.0 percent of the spinsters 45 to 64 years old residing in a mental hospital.

Comparatively high rates of confinement for correctional treatment were found among separated and divorced persons. It is not known to what extent the divorce or separation is a consequence of the person's being so confined. Separated and divorced men, and separated women, likewise had distinctly high rates of hospital treatment for tuberculosis.

On the whole, nursing homes under private management[3] are likely to have much more satisfactory facilities than public homes for the aged without nursing care. This comment is relevant to the finding that widowed and single persons 45 to 64 years old were more likely than separated and divorced persons to use the better types of home for the aged.

Divorced men of middle age had very much higher rates of chronic hospitalization, incarceration in correctional institutions, and tuberculosis-hospital rates than did divorced women of similar age. This finding may actually be a function of a greater general propensity toward remarriage among divorced men than divorced women, so that a larger proportion of the competent divorced men (with regard to health, status, and the like) tend to remarry; hence the divorced men who remain unmarried would be more heavily weighted with the seriously ill or maladjusted. On the other hand, a higher proportion of quite competent divorced women evidently choose to remain unmarried.

Patients in mental hospitals. Mental-hospital rates in 1960 by marital status and sex, with and without standardization for age, are shown for persons 14 years old and over in the United States in Table 11.7. This table is of special interest because of the generally recognized close relationship between mental health and marital adjustment and also because mental patients account for such a large proportion of all inmates of institutions. Since the married population was used as the standard for age adjustment, the rates for this group are unchanged by the standardization process. The most pronounced effect of standardizing was to increase greatly the mental-hospital rates for single persons and to lower considerably the rate for widows.

As pointed out above, a very small proportion of married persons reside in mental hospitals. Moreover, among unmarried persons, the

Table 11.7. Mental-hospital residence rate per 10,000 population 14 years old and over, by marital status and sex, unstandardized and standardized for age: United States, 1960

Marital status	Unstandardized mental-hospital rate		Mental-hospital rate standardized for age				Women as percent of men
	Men	Women	Men		Women		
			Rate	Index	Rate	Index	
Total, 14 & over	54	45	61	339	42	183	69
Married[a]	18	23	18	100	23	100	128
Widowed	99	69	94	522	47	204	50
Divorced	200	120	188	1,044	105	457	56
Separated	168	126	169	939	132	574	78
Single	128	85	405	2,250	214	930	53

Source: U.S. Bureau of the Census, U.S. Census of Population: 1960, Subject Reports, Inmates of Institutions, Final Report PC(2)-8A, table 26; and Marital Status, Final Report PC(2)-4E, tables 1 and 4.

[a]Married, except separated.

mental-hospital rates for women were quite low by comparison with those for men. With the rates for persons currently married assigned an index number of 100, the rates for those in other marital categories ranged from 204 for widows to 2,250 for single men. The findings indicate that men and women who remain single into the middle years of life face by far the greatest risk of being residents of mental hospitals as of a given point in time.

Those receiving hospital care for mental illness in 1960 tended to have higher socioeconomic status than many other types of inmates. In fact, except for men in state and local hospitals, patients in each category of mental hospital had educational levels above the average of institutional inmates in general; among patients 45 to 54 years old in private mental hospitals the average educational level was actually above that of the general population.

Length of stay and recidivism. The residence rates for institutional inmates discussed here are affected by the differences in length of stay for those in the various types of institutions. Moreover, the length of stay in a hospital is likely to be shorter, and the hospital-residence rate correspondingly smaller, for adults with a spouse at home who can provide care to the patient after discharge. In addition, married persons, being of relatively higher economic status on the whole, are more likely to receive not only needed hospital care but also medical care before or at the onset of illness than are unmarried adults. The net effect of these and other factors in the situation is that married persons are evidently much less likely than the unmarried to require long-term hospitalization.

For a fuller understanding of the relationship between marital status and institutional residence, therefore, more information than that currently available is needed on average annual admission and discharge rates for patients in both short-stay and long-stay hospitals by type of hospital, marital status, age, and sex.[4] Meantime, the following data throw light on the combined effect of length of stay and recidivism. The findings are based on 1960 migration data for institutional inmates 5 years old and over and make no allowance for differences from one type of institution to another in the distributions of length of stay.[5] It was determined that mental-hospital patients included a larger proportion in the same institution in both 1955 and 1960 by the following factors:

Twice that for residents in homes for the aged and in chronic hospitals;
Three times that for tuberculosis-hospital patients and prisoners;
Seven times that for inmates of jails and workhouses.

The number of times a person is institutionalized for the same type of illness or conduct also affects the probability of eventual residence in an institution. The evidence available indicates a greater likelihood for persons to reside at some time in their life in a mental hospital than in any other type of institution.[6]

Mortality

Under almost all circumstances, married persons have lower death rates than comparable unmarried persons. Death rates range from a low level for white married women to high levels for nonwhite widowed and divorced men. The entire pattern of death rates by marital status reveals a negative correlation between these rates and the socioeconomic level of the marital status-color-sex subgroups in the population, wherein married women are assumed to derive their socioeconomic status largely from their husbands. The correlation is imperfect, however, because the selective factors which determine who

marries and who remains married include, besides socioeconomic
level, such partially independent factors as intelligence, temperament,
motivation, and pressures from the person's social group. Although
these factors are not measured in the present study, they undoubtedly
affect the person's way of life, including his chances of being married
and his chances of survival.

With the exception of Table 11.9, the data shown in the remaining
tables in this chapter are age-adjusted death rates for the range 15 to
64 years covering the period 1959 to 1961 or are ratios based on
such rates. Most marriages and divorces occur within this range of
ages.[7]

Death rates by color and sex. Among persons 15 to 64 years old
irrespective of marital status, men had death rates that were almost
twice as high as those for women (596 versus 313 per 100,000 population), according to Table 11.8; see also Figure 11.1. Moreover,
nonwhite persons had death rates that were roughly twice as high as
those for white persons, and widowed nonwhite persons had death
rates that were about twice as high as those for nonwhite married
persons. This pyramiding effect among the demographic differences
culminated in a remarkably large range between the very low death
rate of only 250 for white married women and the nearly eight-
times-as-high death rate of 1,936 for nonwhite widowed men 15 to
64 years old.

The amount by which the death rate for unmarried (single,
widowed, and divorced) persons exceeded that for married persons

Table 11.8. Average annual death rates per 100,000 persons 15 to 64 years old, by marital
status, color, and sex, standardized for age: United States, 1959 to 1961

Color and sex	Death rate by marital status					Percent of rate for married		
	Total	Single	Married	Widowed	Divorced	Single	Widowed	Divorced
Men, 15-64 years	596	888	510	1,282	1,422	174	252	279
White	559	826	485	1,080	1,385	170	222	285
Nonwhite	928	1,311	746	1,936	1,684	176	260	226
Rate for nonwhite as percent of rate for white	166	159	154	179	122	...	...	...
Women, 15-64 years	313	387	277	543	460	140	196	166
White	274	343	250	417	418	137	167	167
Nonwhite	666	776	537	1,059	749	144	197	139
Rate for nonwhite as percent of rate for white	243	226	215	254	179	...	...	...
Rate for men as percent of rate for women:								
Total	190	229	184	236	309	...	...	...
White	204	241	194	259	331	...	...	...
Nonwhite	139	169	139	183	225	...	...	...

Source: National Center for Health Statistics, unpublished data.

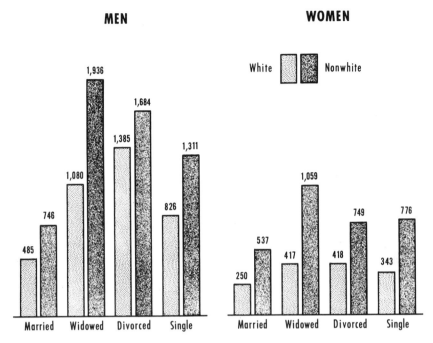

Fig. 11.1. Death rate per 100,000 persons 15 to 64 years old by marital status, standardized for age: United States, 1959 to 1961

Source: Table 11.8.

varied widely. The excess in the rate for single white women was only 37 percent and that for divorced nonwhite women was only 39 percent, as compared with corresponding married women; these two groups of unmarried women were the most highly educated groups among white and nonwhite women, respectively. By contrast, death rates for unmarried men exceeded those of married men by an upper limit of 185 percent for divorced white men and 160 percent for nonwhite widowers. Most of the deaths among persons 15 to 64 years old occur among those 45 to 64. Within this latter age range, single men had educational levels similar to those of widowers; nevertheless, the single had a smaller excess in their death rates as compared with married men than did widowed men. This is one of the situations in which variations in death rates cannot be explained entirely by differences in socioeconomic level as measured by educational attainment.

The advantages of life as a married person appear to be much more abundant for men than for women, insofar as such a life minimizes the death rate. In numerical terms, unmarried men had death rates which (on an unweighted basis) averaged 135 percent higher than those for married men, whereas unmarried women had death rates which averaged 67 percent higher than those for married women. According to this measure, therefore, being married was twice as advantageous to men as to women.

Reasons for this bonus for a man to be married remain speculative and deserve further study. Do married men, in fact, have such benefits as a more settled way of living, better food habits, more personalized care during illness, and more normal sex life than unmarried men? Are women — whether married or not — more likely than men to take care of those personal health needs which help to preserve their lives?

Recent changes in death rates by age. During the approximate generation between 1940 and 1963, several consistent changes occurred in death rates by marital status and age. For both men and women, the death rate of the married declined more than that of the unmarried in each age group from 25 to 64 years of age (see Table 11.9). Moreover, the proportional reductions in death rates for married persons were progressively larger toward the younger ages.

These changes occurred during a period when the proportion of the people who had ever married increased considerably, notably among women in the upper educational levels. Simultaneously removing these spinsters — with high probabilities of survival — from the ranks of the single and bolstering the ranks of married women with them apparently had the effect of slowing down the reduction in death rates during this period among single women and speeding that among married women.

The death rate was smaller in 1963 than in 1940 in almost every marital status-age-sex group. Among the single, widowed, and divorced there was a uniform tendency for the excess of the death rate over that for the married to diminish with age, both in 1940 and in 1963. Moreover, this pattern of differences became magnified over the approximately two decades.

The rising first-marriage and remarriage rates of the 1940's and 1950's may have progressively "skimmed the cream" from the ranks of the unmarried. Thus several questions arise, to which the expected answer is the affirmative: Did the "extra" persons who were marrying during this period — over and above the number required to keep up

Table 11.9. Death rates for 1963 as percent of those for 1940, and
death rates in 1963 and 1940 as percent of those for
married persons, by marital status, age, and sex:
United States

Year and marital status	Men by age (years)				Women by age (years)			
	25-34	35-44	45-54	55-64	25-34	35-44	45-54	55-64
1963/1940 death rate								
Single	81	84	92	91	71	98	83	68
Married	54	65	79	89	32	49	59	63
Widowed	94	79	92	93	55	65	72	71
Divorced	83	105	87	117	58	70	69	65
Percent of death rate for married								
1963: Single	271	248	190	147	275	235	159	121
Married	100	100	100	100	100	100	100	100
Widowed	764	361	260	181	463	255	196	155
Divorced	500	484	271	260	288	220	172	148
1940: Single	181	192	164	144	124	117	113	112
Married	100	100	100	100	100	100	100	100
Widowed	438	294	224	172	268	193	160	139
Divorced	323	298	248	197	160	154	147	144

Source: National Center for Health Statistics, Monthly Vital
Statistics Report, Vol. 12, No. 13, table 7; and Vital Statistics--Special
Reports, Vol. 23, No. 2, tables 1 and 2; and U.S. Bureau of the Census,
Current Population Reports, P-20, No. 135, table 1.

the pre-1940 level of the marriage rate — come largely from the
best of the unmarried from the standpoint of potential survival? Did
these persons include a high proportion of women but only a low proportion of men with good-to-moderate chances of survival? Would the
death rate of married men have fallen still more between 1940 and
1960 than it did if the high marriage rates during the period had not
transferred so many unmarried men with only moderate chances of
survival into the ranks of the married?

Cause of Death

Analysis of causes of death by marital status provides a unique insight into the relationship between mortality and marriage, just as
analysis of detailed occupation by marital status throws light on the
relationship between employment and marriage. The way people die

suggests much about the way they have lived. The ways that married men die are in many respects different from the ways that single or widowed or divorced men die. Data available for this study still leave open to question how much of the difference in death rates by marital status arises from factors which determine whether the person marries and how much from differences between the kinds of lives people lead after they are married compared with the kinds they would have lived if they had remained unmarried.

The process of selection in marriage tends, no doubt, to leave persons with ill health — in other words, poor mortality risks — among the unmarried.[8] Moreover, it may also leave among the unmarried those who are prone to take more chances that endanger their lives than married persons would ordinarily take in their jobs and in their recreation, because they have no spouse and probably no children to protect or because they are so inclined by temperament or long-standing habit. On the other hand, unmarried persons may be overly careful about their health or conduct to the point of withdrawal from the usual forms of sociable contacts where potential marital partners ordinarily meet. These considerations suggest a relevant question for further research: Are those who marry overrepresented by the kind who take rather good care of their health but who are not hypochondriacal?

Although this selection process generally occurs initially during the early years of adult life, the effects may continue to influence chances of death throughout the later years and to affect chances of remarriage among those who become widowed or divorced.[9]

Causes of death selected for analysis here include the dozen or so leading causes for which tabulated data for 1959 to 1961 were available and half a dozen or so other causes which have special relevance in the study of deaths by marital status.

The accompanying tables were designed to answer the questions: From what causes are married persons most likely to die? How different are their death rates from those of the single or the widowed or the divorced? Within each marital status, which causes of death tend to be especially high (or low) for men as compared with women, and nonwhite as compared with white persons? Related information from the same source was being prepared in 1969 for publication by the National Center for Health Statistics in a report, Series 20, no. 8, entitled "Mortality from Selected Causes by Marital Status: United States, 1959–61."

Table 11.10. Average annual death rates per 100,000 men 15 to 64 years old from selected causes, by marital status and color, standardized for age: United States, 1959 to 1961

Cause of death [a]	Death rate for white men				Death rate for nonwhite men			
	Single	Married	Widowed	Divorced	Single	Married	Widowed	Divorced
Coronary disease & other myocardial (heart) degeneration 420, 422	237	176	275	362	231	142	328	298
Motor-vehicle accidents E810-E835	54	35	142	128	62	43	103	81
Cancer of respiratory system 160-165	32	28	43	65	44	29	56	75
Cancer of digestive organs 150-159	38	27	39	48	62	42	90	88
Vascular lesions (stroke) 330-334	42	24	46	58	105	73	176	132
Suicide E970-E979	32	17	92	73	16	10	41	21
Cancer of lymph glands and of blood-making tissues 200-205	13	12	11	16	13	11	15	18
Cirrhosis of liver 581	31	11	48	79	40	12	39	53
Rheumatic fever (heart) 400-416	14	10	21	19	14	8	16	19
Hypertensive heart disease 440-443	16	8	16	20	68	49	106	90
Pneumonia 490-493	31	6	25	44	68	22	78	69
Diabetes mellitus 260	13	6	12	17	18	11	22	22
Homicide E964, E980-E984	7	4	16	30	79	51	152	129
Chronic nephritis (kidney) 592-594	7	4	7	7	18	11	26	21
Accidental falls E900-E904	12	4	11	23	19	7	23	19
Tuberculosis, all forms 001-019	17	3	18	30	50	15	62	54
Cancer of prostate gland 177	3	3	3	4	7	8	15	12
Accidental fire or explosion E916	6	2	18	16	15	5	24	16
Syphilis 020-029	2	1	2	4	10	6	14	15

Source: National Center for Health Statistics, unpublished data.

[a]Category numbers are from Seventh Revision of International Lists, 1955.

Death rates for married persons. Although death rates from nearly all causes are lower for married than unmarried persons, there is interest in knowing the most likely causes of death among married persons. Information on this subject is given for persons below old age on the first few lines of Tables 11.10 and 11.11.

White married men and women have in common four of the five

Table 11.11. Average annual death rates per 100,000 women 15 to 64 years old from selected causes, by marital status and color, standardized for age: United States, 1959 to 1961

Cause of death [a]	Death rate for white women				Death rate for nonwhite women			
	Single	Married	Widowed	Divorced	Single	Married	Widowed	Divorced
Coronary disease & other myocardial (heart) degeneration 420, 422	51	44	67	62	112	83	165	113
Cancer of breast 170	29	21	21	23	26	19	28	27
Cancer of digestive organs 150-159	24	20	24	23	33	25	41	35
Vascular lesions (stroke) 330-334	23	19	31	28	89	72	147	82
Motor-vehicle accidents E810-E835	11	11	47	35	13	10	25	20
Rheumatic fever (heart) 400-416	14	10	15	13	14	8	12	13
Cancer of lymph glands and of blood-making tissues 200-205	9	8	9	8	7	7	9	13
Hypertensive heart disease 440-443	8	7	10	9	63	50	97	56
Cancer of cervix 171	4	7	13	18	22	17	34	27
Diabetes mellitus 260	7	7	11	8	24	20	36	22
Cirrhosis of liver 581	6	7	15	20	20	9	23	20
Cancer of ovary 175.0	12	7	8	8	8	6	9	8
Suicide E970-E979	8	6	12	21	3	3	6	5
Cancer of respiratory system 160-165	5	5	6	7	6	5	9	10
Pneumonia 490-493	15	4	7	10	31	12	33	22
Chronic nephritis (kidney) 592-594	4	3	5	4	14	11	16	11
Homicide E964, E980-E984	1	2	7	9	17	14	33	25
Tuberculosis, all forms 001-019	5	2	4	5	24	8	19	16
Accidental fire or explosion E916	2	1	6	4	6	4	11	5

Source: National Center for Health Statistics, unpublished data.

[a]Category numbers are from Seventh Revision of International Lists, 1955.

leading causes of death: Coronary heart disease and other myocardial degeneration, motor-vehicle accidents, cancer of the digestive system, and vascular lesions or stroke. They accounted for 54 percent of all deaths among white married men and 37 percent of all deaths among white married women at ages 15 to 64 years in 1959–1961, according to data from the same source as Table 11.10. The other cause of death among the top five was cancer of the respiratory system among white husbands and cancer of the breast among white wives.

Diseases of the cardiovascular-renal system accounted for fully 49 percent of all deaths among white married men and 36 percent among white married women. The body systems which most often become fatally diseased by cancer are the digestive, the respiratory (among men),[10] and the reproductive (among women).

Nonwhite married men and women have in common three of four leading causes of death. These include two causes which ranked high for white persons, coronary disease and other myocardial degeneration, and vascular lesions; the third is hypertensive heart disease. Other causes of death for which the rates are conspicuously high for nonwhite as compared with white married persons are homicide (among men) and diabetes (among women). Comment about the magnitude of these differences by color and possible underlying factors is reserved for a later section.

Among nonwhite married persons, cardiovascular-renal diseases as a whole accounted for 44 percent of the deaths among men and 48 percent among women; thus the figure for nonwhite women is notably higher than that for white women (36 percent). Also noteworthy is the high incidence of deaths among nonwhite husbands by such violent means as homicide and accidental falls, fires, or explosions, which accounted for 8 percent of all deaths among these men as compared with only 2 percent among their white counterparts. Nonwhite wives had as their fifth highest cause of death diabetes mellitus; this cause ranked only tenth among white wives. On the other hand, motor-vehicle accidents ranked fifth among white married women but only eleventh among nonwhite married women.

Lung cancer is a leading cause of death among men but not among women, and tuberculosis, while no longer a leading cause of death, still claims the lives of four to five times as large a proportion of non-white (mostly Negro) as white married persons. For nonwhite wives, moreover, the death rate from tuberculosis is still half again as large as that from lung cancer.

Several causes of death are limited entirely to one sex, or nearly so. Cancer of the breast is a leading cause of death among both white and nonwhite wives but is very rare in men. Cancer of the cervix is an important cause of death among nonwhite women and claims twice as large a proportion of the lives of nonwhite as white wives.

Although suicide ranked sixth among causes of death among white husbands in 1959–1961, it ranked only fourteenth among nonwhite husbands; by contrast, homicide ranked third among nonwhite and thirteenth among white husbands. Suicide is one of the few causes of death for which rates were higher for white than nonwhite persons of every marital status.

Syphilis is at the bottom of the list of causes of death shown for white husbands and near the bottom also for nonwhite husbands. But the death rate from syphilis was six times as high for nonwhite as white husbands and (according to data not given in Table 11.11) seven times as high for nonwhite as white wives (2.2 versus 0.3 per 100,000).

Death rates for unmarried persons. The ratios of death rates shown in Table 11.12 are limited to *white* persons 15 to 64 years old in order to simplify the presentation. (Color differences are discussed in

Table 11.12. Death rate for unmarried as percent of death rate for married, for white persons 15 to 64 years old, by selected causes of death, marital status, and sex, standardized for age: United States, 1959 to 1961

One or more marital status-sex groups with--	Death rate for unmarried as percent of death rate for married							
	White men				White women			
	Single	Married	Widowed	Divorced	Single	Married	Widowed	Divorced
Large excess among rates for unmarried men								
Tuberculosis	485	100	529	876	313	100	247	300
Cirrhosis of liver	291	100	461	752	91	100	225	303
Accidental fire or explosion	246	100	733	658	146	100	454	331
Pneumonia	503	100	400	715	395	100	184	257
Homicide	166	100	359	673	61	100	394	494
Accidental falls	297	100	287	592	218	100	264	255
Suicide	184	100	538	426	146	100	214	393
Syphilis	211	100	233	467	167	100	167	267
Motor-vehicle accidents	155	100	411	371	103	100	442	328
Small excess among rates for unmarried men or women								
Coronary & other myocardial	134	100	156	206	117	100	154	142
Cancer of digestive organs	140	100	143	177	122	100	120	118
Cancer of respiratory system	117	100	155	234	102	100	129	164
Cancer of lymph glands & of blood-making tissues	106	100	92	128	115	100	114	96
Cancer of prostate gland	100	100	136	160	...	...	...	...
Cancer of cervix	...	...	...	...	60	100	179	244
Cancer of ovary	...	...	...	...	169	100	106	110
Cancer of breast	a	a	a	a	136	100	100	110

Source: Derived from Tables 11.10 and 11.11.

a Very small rates for men.

a later table.) The meaning behind the figures in this table can be more properly grasped by keeping in mind the differences in the general level of the death rates for men and women in Tables 11.10 and 11.11.

Nine causes of death are listed as having large excesses among the rates for unmarried men as compared with those for married men. The death rates from these causes were four to nearly nine times as high for at least one group of unmarried men (single, widowed, or divorced) as for married white men. This list also contains all causes of death which were three to five times as likely to occur among at least one group of unmarried white women as among married white women. Differences of such magnitude probably never would occur from errors in the basic data. For all these causes, the ratios were conspicuously high for divorced men and women and, for most of them, the ratios were also quite high for widowed men and women. For single persons, by contrast, several of these causes were associated with ratios which indicate death rates only moderately in excess of those for married persons, and for several the rates were actually below those for the married.

Speculation is offered as to why these nine causes of death are relatively so much more frequent among most of the categories of the unmarried. For instance, the unmarried who died of tuberculosis evidently had a distinct tendency not to marry at all after they had suffered from the disease, or not to remarry after becoming widowed or divorced if they had a history of illness from it. The once-tubercular unmarried person may feel that the potential advantages of marriage are outweighed by the danger that the responsibilities of marriage might bring on a recurrence or that the disease might be transmitted to a spouse. No doubt many widowed persons who died of tuberculosis had had a spouse from whom the disease was contracted. Also, many of the widowed and divorced persons who died of tuberculosis may have contracted the disease as a consequence of underlying neglect of personal health in the wake of the crisis surrounding the dissolution of the marriage, often aggravated by poverty, bad housing, and other circumstances which increase exposure to, and weaken resistance to, infection with the disease.

The ratio for deaths from pneumonia, in like manner, ranks high among all types of the unmarried. Interestingly, however, pneumonia struck down a much higher proportion of the divorced men and widowers than of the divorced women and widows. The lower remarriage rates of women than of men may leave a larger proportion of healthy women with the strength and resources to ward off conditions which tend to let persons drift into broken health and death by pneumonia before old age.

The ratio for deaths from cirrhosis of the liver, commonly but not exclusively associated with alcoholism, ranks second in Table 11.12 among the causes of death for divorced men and relatively high for all other types of the unmarried except single women. Evidently, spinsters tend to live in a "different way" from other unmarried persons.

The relatively high rates of accidental deaths involving motor vehicles, falls, and fires or explosions are noteworthy for widowed and divorced persons, especially in view of the concurrently high incidence of homicide and suicide in these groups as compared with the married. Widowed and divorced persons probably tend to be much more preoccupied with their adjustment problems — and have less help in solving them — than married persons and hence may tend to be more vulnerable to serious mishaps, self-inflicted wounds, or the taking of drugs which prove fatal. A longitudinal study of underlying tendencies toward instability of personal and social adjustment over the lifespan of a cross-section of the adult population might throw light on the extent to which such tendencies may have existed before marriage among persons who eventually become divorced.

Possibly to a small, but still unknown, extent the ratios for deaths from motor vehicle accidents among widowers and widows (as compared with married persons) are high because at least some husbands and wives die in the same accident but a few hours or days apart; the one who survives the longer is then recorded as having died while widowed rather than married. Likewise, an unknown amount of the concurrently very high ratios for death by homicide among divorced men and women as compared with married persons may reflect strong reactions to an impending remarriage or other conduct of the estranged spouse. Perhaps research can never establish even a rough estimate of the proportion of deaths involving motor-vehicle "accidents" that were really deliberate but classified as accidental in the absence of specific evidence otherwise.

Quite low ratios for deaths of single women by homicide, motor-vehicle accidents, and cirrhosis of the liver are shown in the upper portion of Table 11.12. This cluster of low ratios seems to provide further reason for inferring that spinsters usually live a more quiet and uninvolved life than married women. Although, as expected, white single males 15 to 24 years old have relatively high death rates from motor-vehicle accidents, the rates at older ages below 65 are very much lower.

The death rate from syphilis among white persons was nearly five times as high for divorced men as for married men and nearly three times as high for divorced women as for married women. Single and widowed persons had rates about twice as high as the married. These figures raise questions as to what extent the observed differences in death rates among those who have ever married reflect differences in the original source of the fatal infection (in marriage or outside).

Seven of the eight causes of death listed in the lower portion of Table 11.12 involve malignant neoplasms. Death rates from cancer of the digestive system and of the lymph glands and blood-making tissues (especially leukemia) differed by only about one-fifth or less for single, widowed, and divorced women from the corresponding level for married women — a level of difference low enough to conclude that selective factors in marriage and life events after marriage tend to have little to do with the chances that white women will become fatally ill with one of these types of cancer before old age. For all the other six causes of death in the lower list, the death rate for at least one of the three unmarried groups — single, widowed, or divorced — was likewise not to exceed one-fifth higher than that for married women of the same sex. Although, as Shurtleff says, "there is no disease that kills impartially, that kills the married and the unmarried alike," the causes of death listed in the lower portion of Table 11.12 come closest to doing so.[11]

The relatively low death rate from heart disease among single women as compared with married women may suggest to some readers that a key reason is the presence of Roman Catholic nuns among the spinsters and the relatively sheltered and secure life which they lead; this explanation is unlikely to be sound, however, because the nuns do not constitute a large enough proportion of all single women to affect the rates greatly. The low age-adjusted rate of lung cancer among single men and women — only slightly above that for married persons — contrasts sharply with the considerably higher rates for divorced persons; respiratory cancer and also heart disease are associated with heavy smoking. Moreover, lung-cancer deaths are also believed to be related to exposure to air pollution by downtown city living. City living and cigarette smoking are more characteristic of divorced persons than of the population in general; moreover, cigarette smoking is much less characteristic of single adults than of others.[12]

The last four causes listed in Table 11.12 relate to cancer of specific sites of the genitourinary system. Cancer of the prostate gland appears at an equal rate for single and married white men and cancer of the cervix at a rate only about six-tenths as high for single as for married white women. For the widowed and especially the divorced, the excess of the death rate from these causes over that of the married is substantial. It seems plausible to expect that these diseases tend to discourage the affected unmarried persons from remarrying. The virtual equality of death rates from cancer of the ovary and of the breast for married, widowed, and divorced women (the great majority of whom have been mothers) and the substantially higher death rates from these causes for single women have been observed in many studies. This fact provides quantification for the common observation that motherhood is a safer condition than childlessness from the standpoint of survival from diseases related to childbearing and childrearing.

Death rates for men and women. In this section death rates for men in the several marital-status groups are shown as percentages of those for women. As a caution in interpretation of the ratios, the fact is relevant that the ratios depend for their magnitude, in part, on whether the rate in the denominator is large or small. Thus a small absolute difference between the numerator and denominator will yield a ratio which differs greatly from 100 only if the denominator is small. One of the reasons for the groupings of the causes of death in Table 11.13 is to illustrate this point.

Coronary artery disease claimed the lives of more men and women in each marital status than any other cause of death; it also stood highest among the causes of death in the amount by which the death rate for white married men exceeded that for white married women. White married men were four times as likely as white married women to die of heart disease; this is true even though heart disease caused twice as many deaths among white married women as the next highest cause. The only other cause of death for which the rate among white married men exceeded that among white married women by a greater proportion was cancer of the respiratory system; this cause ranks third among married men but only fourteenth among married women.

Table 11.13. Death rate for men as percent of death rate for women, for persons 15 to 64 years old, by selected causes of death, marital status, and color, standardized for age: United States, 1959 to 1961

One or more marital status-color groups with--	Death rate for men as percent of death rate for women							
	White				Nonwhite			
	Single	Married	Widowed	Divorced	Single	Married	Widowed	Divorced
Rates for women high; rates for men still higher								
Coronary and other myocardial	465	400	410	584	206	171	191	264
Motor-vehicle accidents	491	318	302	366	477	430	412	405
Cirrhosis of liver	517	157	320	395	200	133	170	265
Cancer of digestive organs	158	135	163	209	188	168	220	251
Rates for women low; rates for men much higher								
Cancer of respiratory system	640	560	717	929	733	580	622	750
Syphilis	380	300	420	525	171	250	276	331
Suicide	400	283	767	348	533	333	683	420
Homicide	700	200	229	333	465	364	461	516
Tuberculosis	340	150	450	600	217	188	326	338
Pneumonia	207	150	357	440	219	183	236	314
Rates similar for men and women								
Chronic nephritis	175	133	140	175	129	100	163	191
Vascular lesions	183	126	148	207	118	101	120	161
Hypertensive heart disease	200	114	160	222	108	98	109	161
Rheumatic fever	100	100	140	146	100	100	133	146
Diabetes mellitus	186	86	109	213	75	55	61	100

Source: Derived from Tables 11.10 and 11.11.

Some of the highest sex ratios among death rates are for divorced and widowed persons. In the first section of Table 11.13, death rates from coronary artery disease for men divided by the corresponding rate for women yields an especially high ratio for white divorced persons (584). The ratios are even higher (in the second section) for cancer of the respiratory system among white (929) and nonwhite (750) divorced persons and for suicide among white widowed persons (767). Such results raise the question: To what extent does the selective process of remarriage tend to remove from the ranks of the widowed and divorced a larger proportion of men than women who are healthy and who have a strong sense of purpose in living?

A great excess of deaths by motor-vehicle accidents among men occurred in all marital-status groups. This finding is a likely reflection of the fact that men use motor vehicles much more in their daily round of duties, irrespective of marital status. Yet single men had five times as high a death rate (adjusted for age) as single women from this cause — the largest ratio for any category of marital status. This impressive difference, taken alone, does not prove that single men are more careless drivers than single women, but it is consistent with that hypothesis.

By contrast, cirrhosis of the liver caused death at widely different rates for men than women in the several marital-status groups. At one extreme are the married, for whom the rates among husbands were not especially far above those among wives. At the other extreme are white single persons 15 to 64 years old, among whom men were five times as likely to die of the cause as were comparable women; this observation has added meaning in the context that (1) cirrhosis of the liver is commonly associated with heavy drinking of alcoholic beverages, (2) this disease rarely causes deaths below the age of 25, and (3) there are substantially more unmarried women than unmarried men 25 to 54 years old (hence, evidently an adequate supply of women for bachelors to marry).

The death rate from cancer of the digestive organs for married men was low — in fact, nearly as low as that for married women. This finding may be the result, in part, of a tendency for husbands and wives to have diets that are optimal (as compared with those of unmarried adults) and essentially similar in regard to ingredients (spices, other irritants, starches, etc.) that tend to be related to cancer of the digestive system. Moreover, among women the death rate from this cause differed only slightly from one marital-status group to another.

The second group of causes of death in Table 11.13 displays the highest ratios, on the average. Behind these extreme differences is the fact that women had consistently moderate-to-low death rates from these causes, hence the bases for the ratios were quite small. Respiratory cancer easily tops the whole list in the table for uniformly high death rates among men and low death rates among women, regardless of marital status; but within this framework the unmarried had higher rates than the married. Exposure of men to irritating substances in the air while working and while going to and from work, as well as much higher rates of cigarette-smoking among men than among women, are believed to be closely related environmental factors.[13]

Divorced men ranked especially high as compared with divorced women in mortality from respiratory cancer and also from tuberculosis and pneumonia — all diseases of the respiratory system. This fact suggests that divorced men, far more than divorced women, neglect to protect themselves against exposure to the kinds of environmental conditions that affect respiration, and once they have contracted a respiratory disease, they are likely to neglect it for such a long time that it can no longer be arrested.

Syphilis is a relatively minor cause of death, but one for which men of each marital status, particularly the divorced, had much higher death rates than women in the period 1959 to 1961. The high death rate from syphilis for divorced men could have been related to their high remarriage rate, in the sense that a relatively large proportion of divorced men who remarry may comprise those without the disease.[14]

Suicide and homicide are significant as causes of death among men. They require overt aggressiveness in an extreme form. White widowers in 1959 to 1961 had an especially high suicide rate — the third-ranking cause of death among widowers — whereas white divorced men had an especially high rate of death by homicide, as compared with white men in the other marital-status groups and as compared with white women.

Several questions about these differences in suicide and homicide rates are suggested as possible areas for further study. Are widowers below old age more likely than widows of the same age to worry themselves to self-inflicted death over the loss of their spouse? Do social-security benefits to a surviving wife and the custom of leaving most of the insurance to the wife help significantly to minimize the shock at the death of the husband? Is the life of a widow more often eased by the demise of an ill and irritable spouse than is that of a widower? What proportion among those who commit homicide against divorced persons are former spouses of the divorced? (The far-higher suicide rates among white than nonwhite persons and the reverse for homicide rates are discussed in the next section.)

Certain other ailments take a relatively much higher toll of women than men. Although married men had death rates approximately twice the level of those for married women for all causes of death combined, the rates from causes in the final group in Table 11.13 averaged considerably less than that ratio. The first four causes in the list — chronic nephritis, vascular lesions (stroke), hypertensive heart disease, and rheumatic fever (and chronic rheumatic heart disease) — are among the cardiovascular-renal diseases. Some of these conditions are frequently associated with severe mental shocks which the person is not physically fit to absorb and which cause deterioration or inflammation of a vital body system. Nephritis is often related to the cramping of organs and resulting obstruction of the flow of body liquids during pregnancy.

Diabetes is one of the few causes of death for which the death rate is actually lower for married men than married women. It is more common among obese persons than among those of normal weight, and the untreated diabetic is susceptible to infection which is difficult to control. The development of obesity is often associated with overeating; in turn, overeating may be a consequence of frequent exposure to food during cooking or it may be a nervous reaction to frustration. It is hypothesized here that these conditions are relatively common among (underly active) housewives, and that they are less common among (overly active) husbands who are in the process of making a livelihood for the family.

Death rates for white and nonwhite persons. The differences in death rates according to color, shown in Table 11.14, range from one

Table 11.14. Nonwhite death rate as percent of white death rate, for persons 15 to 64 years old, by selected causes of death, marital status, and sex, standardized for age: United States, 1959 to 1961

One or more marital status-sex groups with--	Nonwhite death rate as percent of white death rate							
	Men				Women			
	Single	Married	Widowed	Divorced	Single	Married	Widowed	Divorced
Nonwhite rate very high as compared with rate for white								
Homicide	1085	1168	959	436	1536	783	470	285
Syphilis	532	611	657	355	1180	733	1000	563
Hypertensive heart disease	432	606	658	439	828	762	986	635
Tuberculosis	305	429	344	180	479	545	505	364
Cancer of cervix	...	...	...	...	507	238	257	154
Nonwhite rate relatively high								
Pneumonia	218	353	314	157	210	335	490	227
Vascular lesions	253	312	380	229	394	374	470	296
Cancer of prostate gland	268	300	447	290	...	...	...	...
Chronic nephritis	245	276	406	351	341	389	360	279
Nonwhite rate relatively low								
Accidental falls	160	187	207	82	192	209	128	121
Cancer of lymph glands & of blood-making tissue	98	88	139	113	80	89	100	166
Coronary & other myocardial	98	81	120	82	218	188	245	181
Cancer of breast	a	a	a	a	91	92	133	115
Nonwhite rate very low								
Motor-vehicle accidents	115	124	72	63	119	95	53	57
Cirrhosis of liver	130	110	80	68	331	138	155	101
Rheumatic fever	97	80	78	103	101	86	81	99
Cancer of ovary	...	...	...	...	68	80	121	108
Suicide	52	58	45	29	34	44	50	23

Source: Derived from Tables 11.10 and 11.11.
[a]Very small rates for men.

extreme, at which the death rate from homicide among nonwhite single women was 15 times as large as that for white single women, to the other extreme at which the death rate from suicide among nonwhite divorced persons was only one-fourth as large as that for white divorced persons. These facts reflect a tremendous range in the degree to which life seems frustrating to one group of persons as compared with their counterparts and the variation in destructive means used to express such extreme frustration.

As a cautionary note in the interpretation of white-nonwhite differences in death rates by cause of death, the fact deserves mention that white persons receive better medical care, on the average — a circumstance that may also be reflected in the quality of the medical information entered on the death certificate. Although probably most of the differences in death rates by color, aside from errors in the basic data, are the result of social and economic factors, there is a possibility that genetic influences may be present in some instances.[15] The following discussion, therefore, is more approximate than definitive.

Death rates among nonwhites tend to be quite high from the causes of death shown in the first group of Table 11.14. The contraction of syphilis (and inadequate treatment thereof) and the commitment of homicide are acts which are consonant with a depressed mental condition, or "anomie," a life of social or economic frustration, and a low degree of social control. Three types of communicable disease caused especially high death rates among married and widowed nonwhites — syphilis, tuberculosis, and pneumonia. Exposure to these diseases in the marriage relationship of husband and wife perhaps tends to increase their chances of being contracted and proving fatal.

Death from syphilis and from cancer of the cervix were quite frequent causes among nonwhite single women but rather rare among white single women. At the same time, the death rate from cancer of the ovary was more nearly alike for single and ever-married women among the nonwhites than the whites; this fact is very likely related directly to the far higher rate of illegitimate births to nonwhite women. The rate of death from hypertensive heart disease was exceptionally high among nonwhite as compared with white persons of all marital-status groups. This finding concurs with the results on chronic illness reported earlier in this chapter, and may be indicative of the heavier strain on the heart and nervous system which is typically experienced by nonwhite than by white persons in their daily activities.

Married and widowed nonwhite persons were especially likely to have death rates far in excess of those for married and widowed white persons from most of the causes in the second list as well as in the first list of Table 11.14. Besides the communication of certain diseases in the family setting, another factor may be the effect of dietary habits of the family members. Other experiences in the family, such as shock and mental strain arising out of deep disappointments about events affecting the spouse or children, may be significant contributing factors, both directly and as a condition which often increases food or liquid intake.

The full set of death rates from diseases of the reproductive organs by marital status throws light on the difference between mortality related to organs involved in the sex act, on the one hand, and in the bearing and nursing of children, on the other hand. Excess death rates for nonwhite persons as compared with the white were especially large from diseases associated with the former (cancer of the cervix and of the prostate gland), but death rates for single and married nonwhite women were even smaller than those for white women from diseases associated with the latter (cancer of the ovary and of the breast).

Some of the data in the foregoing tables suggest a relationship between the reputedly heavy responsibility which Negro women tend to assume in the management of family affairs (with corresponding mental strain) and the relatively high death rate from coronary disease among nonwhite married women (almost double that for white married women) in contrast to a lower rate for nonwhite than white married men. The differences are so great as to give support to the belief that they must be more than statistical artifacts. Still, the current situation may be only temporary. As more Negro men find opportunities to advance into less hazardous jobs and into positions that carry increased pressures due to responsibility, their illness and death rates may more nearly approach present health indexes for white men; moreover, at that time, a higher proportion of them may be living in stable family groups.

12 / LEGAL AND ADMINISTRATIVE
ASPECTS OF MARRIAGE
AND DIVORCE

Since the control of marriage lies with the states rather than with the federal government, each of the 50 states has enacted laws concerning marriage, divorce, and related matters. These laws are voluminous and varied in their provisions, and many court decisions interpret and apply them. In order to advise his clients wisely, the lawyer specializing in matrimonal law devotes considerable time to study of the statutes and decisions relating to them, especially those of his own state. The present discussion is concerned with a broad outline of legal provisions about marriage and divorce and with the major problems involved in their administration.

Marriage Laws

While an individual approaches divorce with trepidation, he approaches marriage with hope. There is a gay atmosphere at weddings as talk is heard of the beautiful bride and the handsome groom. Perhaps all this gaiety and hope are related to the regulation of marriage; there are few restrictions on getting married, and most of these are poorly enforced. The principal legal restrictions concern minimum age at marriage, delay between the application and the marriage, absence of certain communicable diseases, and degree of consanguinity.

Age at marriage. There are two provisions in state laws regarding age at marriage for men and women. One is the age at which young people may marry without the consent of their parents; the other concerns marriage with parental consent.[1] If there is no applicable state statute on the subject, age under the common law holds; this allows marriage at 14 years for males and 12 years for females.

Typically, however, state laws require that the groom be 21 years of age and the bride 18 in order to be married without parental consent. In about one-fourth of the states the bride must be older than 18, usually 21 years old. With parental consent, minimum ages are considerably lower — typically, 18 years for grooms and 16 for brides

— but a number of states provide lower minimum ages, frequently dropping two years lower for both sexes. Some states allow marriage at a very early age; in Massachusetts and Mississippi the minimums are 14 for males and 12 for females. Most states permit a judicial authority to lower age at marriage if the girl is pregnant. There appears to be a widespread opinion that if a girl is pregnant, regardless of her age, a marriage should take place. Thus the prevalent desire to prevent marriages at "too young" an age (however that term is defined) is thwarted in cases of premarital pregnancy.

The extent of premarital pregnancies in the United States and their probable effect on the possibility of future divorce of the couples involved have been the subject of careful research by Harold T. Christensen.[2] Using the method of record linkage, Christensen has provided convincing evidence that the likelihood of divorce is increased if the bride is premaritally pregnant. The certificate of the first birth, the marriage certificate, and the divorce certificate (if any) provided the evidence for his conclusions.

Evaluation of these objective data was complicated by the fact that some births are premature. In one study Christensen obtained data on birth weights, from which he could make an objective classification of probable premature births. He concluded from this study, based on Utah state records, that possibly 12 percent of the births were conceived before marriage. Using the same relationship between proportion of premature births and premarital conceptions in another study, based on Ohio records, he found that possibly some 20 percent of the Ohio marriages involved premarital pregnancies. Divorce followed 13 to 17 percent of the premarital pregnancies in the Christensen studies for various states of the United States. In Denmark, he found the percentage of such divorces to be higher.

Another study of premarital pregnancies was made by William F. Pratt.[3] This study was based on a probability sample for the Detroit metropolitan area and made use of birth and marriage records. Pratt concluded that between 20 and 26 percent of the brides in his study were premaritally pregnant. As age of bride decreased, the proportion who were premaritally pregnant increased.

It thus appears that attempts to enforce minimum age at marriage are often frustrated if pregnancy occurs and the laws permit waiving of age requirements.

"Age of consent" is a concept closely related to, but distinct from, the minimum age at marriage. No female may agree to marry if she is below the age of consent, which varies from 10 to 18 years under state laws. The age of consent is also the age below which a female is considered legally incompetent to agree to sexual intercourse.

Waiting period. A majority of the states have established a waiting period of several days between the application for a marriage license and the marriage.[4] In theory, this provides a check on "hasty" or "impulsive" marriages and an interval to investigate the character of any fascinating stranger who may not be eligible to marry. While 18 states do not require a waiting period, three of these provide legal restrictions of limited application. In North Carolina nonresidents in one county (Pamlico) must wait 2 days to obtain a marriage license. In Oklahoma there is a 3-day waiting period for minors. In Rhode Island there is a 5-day wait for nonresident females. In 32 states and the District of Columbia there are waiting periods of 1 to 7 days. Most of the laws provide either a 3-day waiting period (20 states) or a 5-day wait (9 states). Only Oregon specifies a 7-day wait, while South Carolina alone requires a 1-day wait.

The general concept of a waiting period before marriage seems reasonable on the face of it, although the effectiveness of present laws in preventing the hasty marriages that often end in divorce is unknown. The present waiting-period laws continue an old tradition of providing extensive publicity of intended marriages. Publication of the banns and announcement of an engagement to marry are inappropriate for most couples in the vast anonymity of modern urban society. Publication by many newspapers of the facts regarding local applications for marriage licenses and the requirement of a waiting period serve a similar purpose to a limited extent.

Physical examination. It is a general practice for the states to require some form of physical examination prior to obtaining a marriage license. It is generally held that individuals with certain conditions, particularly some contagious diseases, should not be permitted to marry.[5] Only four states do not require some form of premarital physical test. Nearly all of the tests are limited to venereal diseases. Usually a blood sample must be submitted to a licensed laboratory, where the test is performed and the results certified to the local marriage-licensing official. There has been some opposition to the tests among public-health officials because only a small proportion of the test results are positive. However, with numerous cases of syphilis prevalent in the population, there is widespread recognition of the educational and preventive value of such tests.

A few of the premarital tests go beyond venereal diseases and include tuberculosis, feeble-mindedness, insanity or mental illness, and uncontrolled epileptic attacks. In a few states chronic alcoholism is included. The intent of the state legislatures in passing these laws is clear: no one should be permitted to marry who might transmit a contagious disease to his spouse (or to his offspring) or who suffers from a condition, such as alcoholism, that would probably cause marriage failure. There is ample ground for disagreement with specific laws (for example, forbidding marriage of an epileptic or an alcoholic), but the general intent of safeguarding candidates for marriage from a known serious hazard doubtless has general support.

Clearly, many of the laws could be improved by providing for greater flexibility in enforcement, with special medical (including psychiatric) examinations of certain types of cases prior to issuance of marriage licenses. Doubtless many persons would feel that an epileptic should be permitted to marry a graduate nurse or some other person who could aid in treatment, or that a mature person who wished to marry an alcoholic undergoing suitable treatment should be permitted to do so. On the other hand, there seems to be no rational ground for permitting a person with syphilis in the communicable stage to marry, because the risk of infecting the spouse is great and because medical treatment can remove this risk.

Prohibited marriages. Certain types of marriages are forbidden by law; for example, within certain degrees of consanguinity — with considerable variation among states — marriage is unlawful.[6] In all of the states marriage is forbidden between the immediate members of a family. Because of the widely-held incest taboo, all states provide severe penalties for violations. The marriage of first cousins is generally forbidden; sometimes it is illegal for second cousins to marry. Prohibited marriages are not restricted to relatives by blood but also include a variety of relatives by marriage. In several states, a man may not marry his widowed or divorced mother-in-law or daughter-in-law. In Iowa a man may not marry his grandson's ex-wife. The latter restrictions indicate that state legislators are not exclusively concerned with prohibiting incestuous marriages as usually understood, but seek also to restrict marriages within a wider circle of affinal relationships.

Until recently, a complete discussion of prohibited marriages would have included forbidden interracial marriages. However, a 1967 United States Supreme Court decision in an interracial-marriage case declared a Virginia statute of this nature unconstitutional;[7] presumably similar laws of other states will also be held invalid if brought before the Supreme Court. In earlier years, many states had enacted laws prohibiting marriage between members of certain races. In 1963 there were 29 states with laws prohibiting marriage of a white person and a Negro; 15 states prohibited marriage of a white person and a Mongolian or an Oriental; and 7 states prohibited marriage of a white person and an American Indian.[8] Such marriages were, of course, entirely legal in the states that did not forbid them. However, as shown elsewhere in this monograph, the number of interracial marriages is small.

Marriage is usually forbidden to the feebleminded and the insane. The wording of state laws varies. Certain states forbid the marriage of idiots, imbeciles, feeble-minded persons, or persons of unsound mind. Regardless of the terms used, there doubtless is general agreement that persons seriously retarded or seriously mentally disturbed should not be permitted to marry. If a retarded person wishes to marry, however, elementary justice requires that he receive an objective test administered by a trained technician and that the minimum test result be specified. This service is rarely available. Also, if a person "of unsound mind" wishes to marry, he should be entitled to a psychiatric examination to determine whether he is sane, as that term is understood by psychiatrists.

Administrative mechanisms. State legislatures pass numerous laws concerning marriage, but implementing them is in the hands of an entirely different group of persons. A local official, frequently called a county clerk, has responsibility for issuing marriage licenses. The county clerk or, in many local areas, an employee in his office talks to each applicant for a marriage license, examines the entries on the application forms, and issues the license. If an applicant fails to qualify under any provision of the state laws, this is the point at which he is stopped.

What can be said of the qualifications of the persons filling these important positions? While conditions vary widely, it is not unusual for the county clerk to be elected to his post. Frequently, he is paid on a fee basis; often he is an important local politician. The employees in his office are likely to have little or no civil-service job tenure but hold their posts at the pleasure of the county clerk. Moreover, the issuing of marriage licenses is not usually considered a responsible and skilled duty but is frequently combined with various routine tasks, such as the issuing of fishing licenses. If in doubt about the eligibility of the person for a marriage license, the county clerk is likely to give full consideration to the political implications of his decision.

Control of the provisions concerning age at marriage would seem to be a simple, straightforward task. Provisions of the state laws on age are clear and proof of age, if by birth certificate, is simple. How well are these age provisions enforced? The author of this chapter must conclude, after talking to a large number of local officials, that enforcement is most uneven. In some places it appears to be good; after several hours of observing the operation in the Manhattan office of the City Clerk, New York City, he concluded that that office is reasonably efficient in its enforcement of the age provisions.

On the other hand, the author has had numerous experiences that point in the opposite direction. In a state where the girl *must* be at least 16 to marry, one local clerk was asked what he did when an underage couple, the girl pregnant, presented themselves for a marriage license. With evident satisfaction, he told of aiding a couple to evade the provisions of the law. His method was simple. He told the couple that many a person did not know his true age; the clerk suggested that the young couple consult their parents to determine their correct ages. Later the couple returned, reported qualifying ages (obviously false), and was issued a marriage license.

Another county clerk was asked about cases in which the ages of the couple would require parental consent but such consent was not given. The clerk stated that over the years he had had a considerable number of mothers come to his office to advise him that he should not issue a marriage license to their underage son or daughter. The county clerk stated that in such cases he informed the parent that marriage licenses were issued on the basis of the stated age of the applicants; however, the parent could bring an action in court to establish the facts regarding age. In this county the marriage license was routinely issued without proof of age by birth certificate or otherwise. As a result, the parental-consent provision of the law was inoperative for couples misstating their ages.

A recent study was made by D. L. Womble of the accuracy of reporting of age at marriage in Ohio.[9] Concentrating upon stated ages of 16 to 21 for females and 18 to 24 for males, Womble disregarded minor variations of less than one month and analyzed only the cases where there was strong reason to believe that the falsification was deliberate. In 13 southeastern Ohio counties he found that between 1954 and 1963 there was an increase in the percentage of marriage applications with reported falsification of age as indicated by the birth certificates. Among females the proportion with false ages increased from 7.4 to 11.5 percent; among males the percent with false ages increased from 8.3 to 14.7 percent. Although Womble's sample was small, his findings are consistent with other information on this subject.[10] Womble stated that the Ohio probate judges accepted the sworn statement of age without requiring proof.

It is quixotic to assume that reasonable controls regarding minimum age at marriage will be enforced by the present organization of county officials. Standards of operation vary widely among the more than 3,000 counties (or equivalent local units) in the United States. A large number of the rural counties have been losing population and experiencing difficulty in raising through taxation the minimum sums needed to meet modest county budgets. These budgets are often designed on the assumption that county officials will receive a substantial part of their income from license fees. Undoubtedly the administration of controls would be improved if marriage licenses were issued by state officials; in any event, there would be greater uniformity of enforcement within a state. Setting educational and other standards for marriage-license clerks would also be possible if the clerks had reasonable job security and were otherwise in a better position to resist local pressures in issuing licenses than are the local officials.

The most adequately enforced premarital laws appear to be those concerning the detection of syphilis in the communicable stage — the so-called "blood tests." Commercial laboratories meeting specified standards are licensed by the state, perform most of the tests for a modest fee, and certify the results to the marriage-licensing official. Frequently, the state public-health department also performs this testing service, without charge or for a nominal fee.

Perhaps a similar approach could be used in enforcement of other marriage laws. The retarded individual, for instance, could be tested by a clinic or other agency licensed by the state to determine whether he met the minimum specified standards set forth in state law. These tests would differ from the "blood tests" in that they generally would be unnecessary. Some simple screening test could be utilized, such as certification by a school official that the individual has completed a specified grade in school (perhaps the fifth). However, any approach of this type to the testing of applicants for marriage would not eliminate the urgent need to upgrade the caliber and status of the officials who issue marriage licenses. Until this is done, enforcement of marriage laws will continue to be inadequate.

Divorce Laws

Every individual classifiable as "divorced" has reached this status through elaborate legal proceedings. In a court action, or trial, he has appeared as a plaintiff — usually through an attorney — or as a defendant, perhaps remaining away from the court on advice of his lawyer and allowing the action to go uncontested. In any event, various documents have been examined and signed, fees and costs have been paid, long conferences have been held with an attorney, and, after delays and probably after unexpected complications, he has been informed that he is divorced. He is now free to marry again, unless there are restrictions in the decree requiring him to wait a specified time.

Divorce actions, within the jurisdiction of the states, include many variations in administrative process. Sometimes almost all legal hearings are conducted before court-appointed referees; in other jurisdictions the evidence normally comes directly before a presiding judge. Increasingly, in cities, the case comes before a family court. The legal grounds, or "causes," for divorce vary widely among the states. Since a divorce is difficult to obtain in certain states, many persons migrate temporarily to another state for the specific purpose of obtaining a divorce. At the time it is granted, a determination must be made regarding the custody of children, support payments by the husband, and division of jointly owned property. If such questions are not adjudicated wisely, they may arise later to embitter relations between the former husband and wife.

Today a growing body of opinion emphasizes a different approach to divorce. Preventive measures are stressed; greater precautions to prevent the marriage of persons where a high probability of divorce exists and help to couples whose marriages are in serious trouble are urged. Further, when it seems clear to trained and disinterested observers that a marriage is disrupted beyond hope of repair, they would recommend a different legal approach in divorce actions from that of accuser versus accused.

Legal grounds for divorce. Each of the states has a body of laws relating to divorce, and the United States Congress has enacted laws for the District of Columbia. The following list of principal legal grounds for divorce is of interest; the number shown after each indicates how many of the 51 jurisdictions had such grounds in their code in 1965: adultery (51); desertion (47) (to be effective, the period of desertion varied from 6 months to 5 years, with 1 year the most frequent); felony conviction or imprisonment (44) (with imprisonment for varying periods of time); cruelty, mental or physical, or both (43); alcoholism, or drunkenness, variously defined (41); impotency (33); nonsupport (30); insanity (30) (for varying periods of time, with various definitions); separation or absence (25) (for 1 to 10 years, with a majority specifying 3 years or less); pregnancy at marriage by another man (14); drug addiction (12); bigamy (10); infamous crime (10); prior decree of limited divorce (9); fraud, force, or duress (8); blood relationship to spouse within prohibited degree (4). This list could be greatly extended by indicating grounds included in only one or two states.[11]

Two types of legal actions closely related to absolute divorce are not included in this list of legal grounds for divorce. First, there are the so-called limited divorces, which are sometimes cited as divorce from bed and board, but which are more properly referred to as legal separations because the possessor of a limited divorce is not entitled to remarry. (An essential element of divorce, as the term is generally used, is the right to remarry.) Second, there are the legal grounds for annulment. An annulment is a judicial finding that a valid marriage has not occurred; the marriage is void or voidable. If, for example, a prior marriage existed when a second marriage took place, the latter is void. Or, if "force or duress" was involved, then the marriage is void as soon as facts to this effect are established to the satisfaction of the court. In most states annulments are few in number; in the statistical reports of some states annulments are combined with divorces.

To a lawyer considering a matrimonial action for a client, legal grounds for divorce are in the nature of gates through which his client may pass to be released from the bonds of matrimony. Perhaps the client qualifies to pass through more than one gate, in which case the lawyer, as a technician, advises the client on the preferred course under the circumstances. He also points out the differences in personal distress that will be caused the defendant spouse by using one or another of the legal grounds. On occasion, a plaintiff is so angry that he (or she) is ready to bring forward the most serious charges — to "throw the book" at the offending spouse. In such an event the lawyer probably points out that the proposed action may provoke the defendant to file a cross-complaint charging various offenses, with resultant delay, uncertainty, and added expense. Consequently, it is not surprising that the vast majority of divorce actions are uncontested and that they are brought under some of the legal grounds, such as cruelty, that are minimally offensive to the defendant.

Legal grounds most frequently used. The legal grounds for divorce most used in the states of the Divorce Registration Area are shown in Table 12.1. By far the most frequent of these was cruelty, with more than one-half of the cases falling under this heading. It was followed by desertion, covering nearly one-fourth of the cases, and nonsupport, covering one case in 25. Such grounds as adultery, bigamy, conviction of crime, drunkenness, fraud and insanity appear in only a trivial proportion of the cases. Obviously, there are marked differences among the states shown.

The following legal grounds are especially important in the states indicated: adultery (Virginia), desertion (Virginia, Alabama, Pennsylvania, Georgia, Tennessee), drunkenness (Nebraska), and nonsupport (Tennessee, Kansas). Also, the following legal grounds listed in the table under "other," as indicated, are overwhelmingly important: incompatibilty (Alaska), indignities (Pennsylvania), and intolerable indignities (Wyoming). State laws and judicial practices regarding the nature of the evidence required lead attorneys to bring actions under one cause rather than another wherever alternatives are relevant to the case.

Underlying causes of divorce. If a representative sample of people were asked the causes of divorce, the views expressed would reflect each individual's background. An experienced marriage counselor would doubtless respond in terms of his own clinical experience and that of his colleagues, and he might point out that he did not know whether these "causes" were truly representative. Other respondents

Table 12.1. Divorces by legal grounds: 16 states of Divorce Registration Area, 1959

| Area | Total divorces | | Legal grounds | | | | | | | | | | | |
	Number	Percent	Adultery	Bigamy	Conviction of crime	Cruelty	Desertion	Drunkenness	Fraud	Insanity	Non-support	Under age	Other[a]	Not stated
Divorce Registration Area	84,927[b]	100.0	1.2	0.5	0.6	51.6	23.2	1.2	0.3	0.1	4.1	0.1	13.1	4.1
Alabama	14,975	100.0	2.7	0.2	0.0	51.6	41.4	2.2	-	0.1	0.2	0.0	0.7	0.9
Alaska	679	100.0	0.1	-	0.1	7.8	4.0	0.1	-	0.1	1.2	-	86.3	0.1
Georgia	8,609	100.0	0.6	0.1	0.5	60.1	15.4	2.3	0.3	0.1	0.3	0.0	0.8	19.6
Idaho	2,652	100.0	0.3	-	0.6	83.0	4.4	0.6	0.8	0.1	1.0	0.2	2.9	6.0
Iowa	4,594	100.0	0.7	0.4	1.4	90.6	4.9	1.0	0.0	0.1	0.1	0.1	0.4	0.3
Kansas	4,963	100.0	0.3	0.6	0.5	70.3	6.8	0.2	0.6	0.1	20.2	-	0.4	0.0
Montana	2,062	100.0	0.5	0.4	1.3	80.8	8.1	0.2	4.8	0.2	2.6	0.5	0.4	-
Nebraska	2,201	100.0	0.8	1.5	0.4	67.9	6.6	13.3	0.8	0.3	7.6	0.7	0.1	-
Oregon	6,009	100.0	0.2	-	0.9	86.2	7.8	0.3	-	-	-	-	0.3	4.2
Pennsylvania	13,891	100.0	0.3	0.5	0.5	7.3	20.4	-	0.1	-	-	-	63.7	7.4
South Dakota	763	100.0	0.3	0.4	0.8	82.7	9.6	0.4	0.8	0.1	4.6	0.3	0.1	-
Tennessee	9,205	100.0	1.3	0.4	0.9	63.3	10.4	0.6	-	-	22.5	-	0.4	0.1
Utah	1,336	100.0	0.8	0.5	0.6	79.9	2.6	-	1.1	0.1	1.9	0.2	2.6	9.6
Virginia	7,111	100.0	3.6	1.3	1.7	-	92.3	-	0.2	0.0	-	0.1	0.5	0.2
Wisconsin	4,657	100.0	0.5	1.5	0.3	87.9	4.0	0.2	0.4	0.0	0.8	0.2	3.8	0.4
Wyoming	1,220	100.0	-	0.2	0.7	5.3	3.9	0.1	-	0.4	1.9	0.3	87.0	-

Source: National Center for Health Statistics, Vital Statistics of the United States, 1959, Section 2, Marriage and Divorce Statistics, table 2-X; Section 10, table 20.

[a] Percents where the number of divorces and annulments granted on specified grounds included in this group formed 10 percent or more of the total number in a state are as follows: Alaska--incompatibility, 85.6; Pennsylvania-- indignities, 63.6; Wyoming--intolerable indignities, 87.0.

might stress factors that had come under their own observation; one person might stress the role of alcohol, another might emphasize inadequate moral training, and so on. One fact seems clear to students of the family: the real causes of divorce are numerous and complex. But under the prevailing applicable laws it is necessary to be specific.

When a state legislative committee is drafting a law under which an individual may obtain a divorce, it must provide specific guidance to the courts in order that a determination can be made concerning an individual's eligibility. This is based upon proof that one spouse has been grievously wronged by the other spouse. There is thus established the pattern of the innocent and the guilty parties; the innocent, as a redress for grievance, seeks release from the bonds of matrimony. The "causes" for divorce, in legislative terms, become a series of wrongs any one of which, if proven, entitles the innocent spouse to freedom from the guilty spouse. As previously indicated, these legal grounds for divorce are of general interest as indicating the wrongs which are widely held to be so serious as to entitle a wife (or a husband) to a divorce, but they are not to be confused with the underlying causes of marital disruption. Some of the more recent thinking on this subject is reviewed in later paragraphs.

Migratory divorce. One result of extremely restrictive divorce laws in some states and less restrictive laws in others has been the Alice-in-Wonderland phenomenon of individuals going to a state where the laws are less restrictive than in their own, establishing residence there (temporarily), obtaining a divorce, and returning to their permanent home in their own state. This practice seems to have prevailed since the early days of the republic. Statistics on migratory divorce are not readily available; all divorces granted in Reno are to residents of Nevada, according to law. The legal fiction is widely recognized, but for statistical data one must use an indirect approach. Three bits of evidence on migratory divorce are presented: (1) data on place of marriage and place of divorce; (2) data on residence of the defendant in the state where the decree was granted or elsewhere; (3) an estimate of migratory divorces in 1960, based on county divorce rates in several states.

(1) The most likely place for a divorce to be granted is in the state where the marriage was performed; however, in the Divorce Registration Area in 1961 more than one-third of the decrees were not granted in the state where marriage occurred (see Table 12.2).

Table 12.2. Divorces and annulments by state of occurrence, distributed by place where marriage was performed: Divorce Registration Area and each registration state, 1961

| State | All divorces and annulments | Place where marriage was performed | | | |
		In same state	Percent	In other area	Percent
Total	95,235[a]	55,703	58.5	39,532	41.5
Alaska	909	405	44.6	504	55.4
Hawaii	1,554	1,106	71.2	448	28.8
Idaho	2,512	1,288	51.3	1,224	48.7
Iowa	4,740	2,810	59.3	1,930	40.7
Kansas	5,110	2,820	55.2	2,290	44.8
Maryland	4,360	3,020	69.3	1,340	30.7
Michigan	16,000	10,700	66.9	5,300	33.1
Missouri	11,340	6,640	58.6	4,700	41.4
Montana	2,024	1,364	67.4	660	32.6
Nebraska	2,340	1,406	60.1	934	39.9
Oregon	5,890	2,190	37.2	3,700	62.8
Pennsylvania	13,500	8,800	65.2	4,700	34.8
South Dakota	840	488	58.1	352	41.9
Tennessee	9,220	4,320	46.9	4,900	53.1
Utah	1,770	870	49.2	900	50.8
Virginia	7,570	4,190	55.4	3,380	44.6
Wisconsin	4,270	2,680	62.8	1,590	37.2
Wyoming	1,286	606	47.1	680	52.9

Source: National Center for Health Statistics, Vital Statistics of the United States, 1961, Vol. 3, table 4-1.

[a]Excludes 2,653 divorces with no report on place of marriage.

Here is evidence bearing on migratory divorces, but it is difficult to evaluate because of the unrelated migration that constantly occurs between states. The American population is highly mobile, especially young adults — the age group in which most first marriages occur. Accordingly, many persons who applied for divorce in a state other than the one in which marriage occurred were bona fide residents of the second state. However, the table indicates marked differences between states; at one extreme are those in which more than one-half of the dissolved marriages had taken place outside the state's boundaries (Alaska, Oregon, Tennessee, Utah, and Wyoming) and at the other extreme are states in which about one-third or fewer of the marriages had taken place elsewhere (Hawaii, Maryland, Michigan, Montana, and Pennsylvania). Such wide variations, and others indicated in the table, cannot be explained entirely in terms of normal migration; part of the difference is evidently due to migratory divorces.

(2) Another indirect approach to migratory divorce considers whether the defendant was a resident of the state where the decree was granted (see Table 12.3). If a husband and wife "agree to disagree," they frequently agree that the wife will file the suit. If they reside in a state where it is difficult to obtain a divorce, say New York, and if they can afford all the expenses involved, the wife takes up residence temporarily in another state, say Nevada, until the final decree is granted. In such instances the defendant husband maintains his usual residence. In the great majority of the divorces tabulated the defendant was the husband, and in 85 percent of these divorces

Table 12.3. Divorces and annulments by resident status of defendant husband or wife in state where decree was granted: 13 states, 1961

Resident status of defendant	Defendant	
	Husband	Wife
Total divorces & annulments	48,998	17,316
Percent	100.0	100.0
State where decree granted	85.0	73.6
Other state in same region	7.2	12.8
Different region	7.8	13.6

Source: National Center for Health Statistics, Vital Statistics of the United States, 1961. The states included in this table are: Georgia, Hawaii, Idaho, Iowa, Missouri, Montana, Nebraska, Oregon, Pennsylvania, South Dakota, Tennessee, Virginia, and Wisconsin.

he resided in the same state as his wife. In the remaining 15 percent his residence was in another state, often in a different region.

The present tabulation is limited to the 13 states with data available. None of these falls in the extreme groups of states with either the most rigid or the most lenient divorce laws. Such data are not readily available, for example, from New York or Nevada. Again, however, many of these marriage terminations are not migratory divorces. There is usually a considerable interval of time between the final separation of husband and wife and formal application for divorce, and the normal migratory tendencies of individuals would lead to changes of residence. The wife, in particular, may be seeking employment, or she may be returning to live with her parents, and this frequently involves moving to a different state. Table 12.3 shows that more than one-fourth of the wives who were defendants were nonresidents. These bits of evidence indicate that probably a substantial proportion of these nonresident defendants represent migratory divorces, but they provide no estimate of the number.

(3) Migratory divorces for the year 1960 were estimated by Alexander Plateris to total slightly over 19,000 cases, or about one in every 21 divorces.[12] His estimate is based on county divorce rates and was concentrated among those counties having rates at least one and one-half times the state rate, excluding the counties with unusually high rates. In Florida he found seven counties with high rates of divorce and, using these county figures minus the rate for the remainder of the state, estimated a total of 1,600 migratory cases for Florida in 1960.

Plateris' is an interesting, although conservative, estimate of the volume of migratory divorce. It includes figures from five states. Excluded are the other 45 states and all divorces obtained in Mexico and other countries outside the United States. One excluded type of migratory divorce involves residence in an adjoining state. It is evident that a couple or an individual seeking a divorce will do so in an area that involves a minimum of expense and inconvenience, and where the divorce can be obtained quickly. A few years ago there was a strong movement in Washington, D.C., to modify the divorce laws in order to make a divorce easier to obtain there. Lawyers were prominent in this legislative push. In private conversations attorneys stated that persons were moving to Maryland to obtain divorces and pointed out that such persons could continue to be employed in the District while residing in Maryland. In the same manner, persons residing near other state lines may move across, temporarily, to facilitate obtaining a divorce. Local courts may have a considerable backlog of cases leading to undue delay, or local judges may have a reputation for being unusually strict in the application of divorce laws. These and other factors often lead to temporary migration.

Putting together these bits and pieces of evidence suggests that possibly one divorce in ten is migratory. However, the situation is constantly changing. The new law in New York, discussed elsewhere, will doubtless reduce migration from that state in order to obtain a divorce. Plateris estimated that Alabama granted 8,400 migratory divorces in 1960 but that the number had declined substantially by 1963 because of stricter enforcement of residence requirements by Alabama courts. This illustrates the situation that has prevailed since the earliest days of the republic; the states have different and changing divorce laws, and divorce-seekers go to the areas where it is easiest to be released from the bonds of matrimony.

Although one year is the usual residence requirement in a divorce action, eight states require longer residence and in several states the round trip may be completed in a shorter time. Some states, judging by residence requirements, desire to attract persons seeking divorces. Six months normally establishes residence in six states (Florida, Georgia, Maine, North Carolina, Oklahoma, and Vermont); a period of two months is ample in Arkansas and Wyoming, and six weeks is adequate in Idaho and Nevada.[13]

Throughout our history the favorite state in which to obtain a divorce has shifted many times. One of the earliest was Pennsylvania; later it was successively Ohio, Indiana, and Illinois, where Chicago held a prominent place. For a time lawyers advertised the advantages of certain locations and offered their services. For a short time in the 1890's Sioux Falls, South Dakota, was considered the divorce capital of the country, and later it was Fargo, North Dakota. Among other states, Oklahoma, Wyoming, Arkansas, and Florida have been prominent. Today Nevada is the best-known state to those seeking divorce.[14] Frequently, a state attracted divorce-seekers because of an unplanned loophole in the law, which was later corrected. For example, many far-western states enacted into law a very brief period of required residence to enable migrants from the East to qualify to vote. The early miners were a highly migratory group, and the western territories, striving to register enough population to qualify for statehood, were anxious to accommodate them with voting rights. In doing so, they opened the door to those desiring speedy divorce.

Administration of divorce laws. The winds of social change are blowing vigorously through the field of matrimonial law. An illustration of this is the new legislation adopted in New York State in the spring of 1966. Prior to adopting the new grounds for divorce, New York had long been the most restrictive of the 50 states in its legal provisions. In 1966 five grounds for divorce (in addition to the long-established grounds of adultery, unexplained absence for 5 years, and presumed death of spouse) were set up: (1) cruel and inhuman treatment, (2) abandonment for a minimum of 2 years, (3) imprisonment for 3 years, (4) separation for 2 years under a court decree, and (5) separation for 2 years under a written agreement of separation filed with a county clerk. This last ground deserves special notice, for it is removed entirely from the innocent-guilty dichotomy of the traditional adversary divorce proceedings. Under this provision it is not necessary for one spouse to pose as an innocent victim; however, it is necessary to wait at least 2 years to obtain a divorce. Since the person seeking divorce is characteristically in a hurry, this provision will probably be less frequently used than if the required waiting period were less than 2 years. Consequently, it seems probable that in New York, as in so many other states, cruelty will become the most frequently used legal ground for divorce.

Under the same 1966 legislation, provision was made for a comprehensive conciliation service in New York State. Under the new law, before there is further action on a divorce petition the parties to the dispute are required to appear, on pain of contempt of court, for a conciliation conference. Any relevant records or documents may be subpoenaed. Unless it appears unwise to the presiding official, a counselor is appointed who attempts to bring about a reconciliation. The counselor may, with the consent of the parties, make use of clergymen, psychiatrists, and others who might be of assistance. Time limits are fixed by law for this conciliation effort, and if it has not succeeded within the specified time the court proceeds to take evidence and act upon the divorce petition.

When two people are granted a divorce, a great deal more is involved than simply freeing them from the bonds of matrimony. In a large proportion of divorces the custody of minor children must be determined and visitation and other rights established for the spouse who does not obtain custody. If there is jointly owned property, a determination must be made regarding its disposition. If the husband has been the principal financial support of the family, there must be a determination as to a reasonable level of regular payments to be made by him for the support of his children and his former wife. Suitable arrangement of these matters cannot be made without a full examination of all the relevant facts. Unfortunately, the courts in most divorce cases do not examine all important information before making a decision. And there are compelling reasons why this is so.

Normally, the state courts having jurisdiction in divorce cases also hear a great variety of other cases and are not staffed with persons specially trained to deal with matrimonial questions. The large backlog of cases frequently found in such courts creates pressure to act quickly to clear the docket. Under such circumstances it is not surprising that settlements worked out by the opposing attorneys and agreed to by husband and wife are accepted by the court with only a passing glance or, if questions are in dispute, they are settled without comprehensive review of the facts. In a small but growing number of courts, divorce questions — along with other questions concerning family relations — are handled by specialized family courts. These courts will be discussed in later paragraphs.

Part of the difficulty in administering divorce laws results from their very slow rate of change since colonial days. Attitudes toward divorce among the American people have undergone significant modification in the years since 1890, but during this period changes in the divorce laws, while important, have been far less comprehensive.[15] At the end of the nineteenth century several of the major Christian churches, both Protestant and Roman Catholic, took a strong line against divorce. Prominent church leaders expressed opposition to church-sanctioned weddings for divorced persons, except to the "innocent party" where divorce had been granted for adultery.[16]

With the passage of time many Protestant groups softened their stand, whereas the Catholic church continued to oppose divorce. At the end of the Victorian era and in the early years of this century, many popular writers attacked the traditional marriage institution and the inferior position of women in society. Not only did "votes for women" become a burning issue with feminists, but the restrictions placed upon women in business, industry, and the professions were attacked as unjust. Wider educational opportunities for women were urged and easier divorce was supported. True emancipation of women, it was held, required the ability to terminate an intolerable marriage.

At about this time, sociologists who specialized in the study of the family added their voices to those who had been urging that divorce under certain circumstances was desirable and inevitable. George E. Howard, whose monumental *History of Matrimonial Institutions* made this point, was joined by others. James P. Lichtenberger in 1909 published *Divorce, a Study in Social Causation,* and in 1915 appeared Willystine Goodsell's *History of the Family.* These writers and others took the widely accepted current view of marriage and divorce. However, the laws under which divorces are granted have changed far more slowly than popular attitudes. Persons seeking divorce have been compelled to do so under laws that frequently do not reflect prevailing views on the subject.

This lag in divorce legislation strikes lawyers especially hard, and they constitute the key professional group that must administer divorce laws. A person seeking a divorce retains a lawyer, and the ranks of lawyers are the source for recruiting judges to preside over divorce actions. Consequently, the attitudes of lawyers toward, and their adjustment to, the administration of divorce laws are relevant. A recent study by Herbert J. O'Gorman[17] gives the results of comprehensive interviews with a sample of New York City lawyers who had handled a divorce case in that city a few weeks previously. The interviews were conducted in 1958, before the recent (1966) changes in the New York divorce law; thus the study is not representative of conditions in the country generally, but illustrates the situation when there is extreme cleavage between the law and public opinion about divorce. For this reason the study merits detailed review.

When O'Gorman asked his panel of lawyers what they thought of the existing New York divorce law, there was overwhelming disapproval of it; only four of the 92 attorneys gave it their approval. The great majority indicated that the law was unrealistic; couples who wanted divorces would get them. It discriminated against the poor (who could not afford to go to Reno), and it tended to produce deviant behavior (for which much of the evidence frequently had been manufactured). The author of the study also cited legal literature indicating widespread dissatisfaction with matrimonial laws in general and with divorce laws in particular.

Among his 92 lawyers O'Gorman found some who rarely — and reluctantly — handled divorce cases. As a favor to a regular client, often for a reduced fee, they would accept a divorce case. Such lawyers at times advised an out-of-state divorce. At the opposite extreme were the lawyers who specialized in matrimonial actions, accepted many divorce cases on referral from other attorneys, and regarded such cases as "all in the day's work." There were many lawyers in an intermediate position, frequently in general practice, who took the cases (sometimes reluctantly) that chanced to come their way because they needed the money.

The lawyers' attitudes can be partly understood in terms of their experience with divorce clients. One often-mentioned characteristic of such clients was their emotionalism and another was their marked ignorance of the law; both of these characteristics were especially marked among women clients. Not surprisingly, some of the lawyers mentioned the strain of handling divorce cases. Moreover, they indicated that one of the standard procedures of the courts increased emotionalism at the outset of a case. Before a presiding judge could approve an order for the husband to pay his wife temporary alimony (and a fee to her attorney) it was necessary to convince the court that the wife would probably win her case. This led her attorney to encourage preparation of a strongly worded statement to be filed with the court indicating the wrongs she had suffered from her husband. The effect of such statements upon a husband is easy to surmise.

All of this emotionalism led, at times, to extreme actions by the divorce clients. One husband proposed to support his children on 50 cents a day, and one wife slashed all the tires on her husband's car. Some of the clients frequently changed their minds; others made outrageous demands. The lawyer was sometimes at a loss to know what was best for his client, or even to know what his client actually wanted. Some of the lawyers contrasted this situation with their cases which did not involve matrimonial disputes. In a commercial case, for example, the client is out to make money, and the attorney is there to help him.

The lawyers recognized the desirability of a possible reconciliation between the estranged husband and wife, but they did not feel themselves professionally equipped to bring this about. O'Gorman found that New York City lawyers were confronted with clients wishing to be divorced and a general climate of public opinion that usually supported these clients, but with an ancient body of laws that made divorce difficult to obtain; consequently, they resorted (often unhappily) to various stratagems. Sometimes they advised clients to consider an out-of-state divorce, and sometimes they advised an annulment rather than a divorce because on occasion it was easier to bring about. But when a New York divorce was the only feasible method of terminating a marriage, they had to advise clients as to exactly the type of evidence (adultery) that would be acceptable to the courts. O'Gorman does not indicate what the next steps were in the lawyer-client relationship; however, many of the attorneys evidently were not happy with the situation, and a number of them indicated that some New York lawyers of their acquaintance refused to accept divorce cases. The lawyers felt themselves caught in the middle of an unfortunate situation. The law was clearly out of tune with current social realities.

The difficulties and complexities of unraveling a marriage by divorce, as well as the exasperating and perplexing questions that frequently arise between the ex-spouses after the decree has been granted, have led students of the family to indicate that conventional court procedures should be replaced by new ones, as exemplified in the idea of the family court. A commission appointed by the Governor of California advised in a report filed in 1966 that all actions for divorce should be heard by family courts. Although there are variations in the family-court idea, the California proposals deserve examination; they relate to the state with far more divorces than any other.[18] The commission would establish in every county of California a family court, as a part of the regular state court system, to be given jurisdiction over all matters relating to the family, including marriage, legal separation, declaration of nullity, dissolution of marriage, child custody and support, alimony and division of community property, paternity and legitimation of children, adoptions, emancipation of children, guardianship of minors and incompetent persons, approval of contracts for minors, juvenile-court matters, and all other legal relationships within the family. An adequate staff trained in the social sciences would be a part of each court or, in rural areas, each group of local courts.

The commission proposed the following divorce procedures:

(1) A "petition of inquiry regarding the marriage of A and B" would be filed. This first move toward divorce would make no charges of cruelty or other wrongdoing to inflame emotions. The petition could be filed either by the husband or the wife.

(2) An evaluation interview would permit sounding out both parties, noting areas of agreement and disagreement, gaining insight

regarding the underlying causes of the marriage failure, and determining whether marriage counseling would be beneficial.

(3) The first report to the court would indicate whether counseling was advisable. If so, the couple could use private community resources or the personnel of the court.

(4) The second report to the court would be made not later than 120 days after the first hearing, and after consulting the attorneys for both parties the court would be advised of points of agreement and whether the marriage was viable. If advisable, a further delay of not to exceed 90 days would be allowed for further counseling. If not, an order for dissolution of the marriage would be issued. Neither the first delay of 120 nor the second of 90 days would be mandatory; the court could issue the dissolution order when convinced that the marriage was not viable.

This California commission made other recommendations:

(1) The California law (as of 1966) requiring one year of delay prior to remarriage under an interlocutory decree should be repealed. (It may be noted that if this occurred, the migratory divorce business of neighboring Nevada would be substantially reduced.)

(2) Children in divorce cases should have their interests protected by a court-appointed attorney as guardian *ad litem* to speak for them.

(3) Alimony and support orders should be issued solely on the basis of needs and ability to pay. Questions of guilt should not be considered. The court should be allowed to order wages and the like paid directly to the court.

Although a long delay usually occurs between the issuing of a report containing a commission's recommendations and the final enactment — if ever — of its proposals, nevertheless this report is an important indication of the direction of public opinion regarding the legal dissolution of marriages. At the same time, it must be emphasized that the family court is not a magic formula and that there are practical difficulties in implementing it.

First of all, only with an adequate staff is it possible for a family court to function effectively. Certain special skills are required. Moreover, a great deal more money is needed to operate the family court, and taxpayers must be convinced of the desirability of the added expense. The family court must have available a marriage counselor to work with couples who request such assistance and to advise the court whether counseling is desirable. Sometimes individuals do not seek the legal dissolution of marriage bonds until after the emotional bonds have been severed. Although this is doubtless true of many marriages, it is not true for all of them. For example, a considerable number of couples are divorced and then remarry each other. Evidently individuals differ regarding the point in a deteriorating marital relationship at which they seek divorce. A considerable amount of emotional ambivalence may exist in the husband-wife relationship even after the decision is made to obtain a divorce. Consequently, after a formal application for divorce is made, the skills of a marriage counselor may be useful to determine whether therapy is indicated.

Another skill needed by the family court is that of a down-to-earth economist; someone is required who is familiar with family budgets, wage rates, and standards of living to advise the court on all the money matters involved. This is an important function and requires a high degree of skill. One of the bleak facts about many, if not most, divorces is that insufficient financial resources are in sight to maintain the accustomed standard of living. After the divorce two households usually replace the original one, and most of the persons who obtain divorces are in modest or poor circumstances. Thus the court's decision on the level of payments is of crucial importance. If payments seem exorbitantly high to the husband and if he is left without hope of meeting them, he may refuse to pay and be sent to jail for contempt of court; or he may disappear and become a fugitive from the law. Under either alternative, the wife and children as well as the husband suffer. On the other hand, if payments are unduly low, the wife and children obviously suffer. A wise decision must be based upon all relevant facts.

Another essential function of a family court is to evaluate its own work. For this purpose it needs the services of a research sociologist or other social scientist to establish the necessary record-keeping and reporting procedures and to prepare evaluative studies on various phases of the court's work. Such studies may be valuable in building public support if the court is doing a satisfactory job, or in indicating remedial action if it is failing in certain respects. Such staff members could also serve as a link with academic and other research persons interested in preparing analytical studies on various aspects of the court's work.

Whether one thinks of a family court, a traditional court, or some other administrative mechanism for granting divorces, clearly the whole procedure could profit from revision. Consideration might be given to directing the procedure toward carrying out a healing process rather than one that further inflames the already aroused emotions of the husband and wife who seek divorce. For this reason, the question can be raised as to whether any good purpose is served by the airing of sensational charges. The court might review the kinds of statements that go to the press after an application for divorce has been filed and continue to do so until after the decree has been granted. Consideration could be given to hearing divorce cases in private, unless there are unusual and compelling reasons for conducting open hearings.

Also, the court might take steps to anticipate the probable points of friction that will arise after the decree has been granted and take preventive action. One potential source of friction is the irregular or tardy payment for alimony and child support. If this situation is anticipated, the payments might be made to the court. Another frequent source of friction concerns the children. The husband who has been given visitation rights on Saturday afternoons may repeatedly find on arrival at his former home that the children are not there; accordingly, he may feel so frustrated that he consults his lawyer. The lawyer may advise him to withhold alimony payments. This may lead the wife to consult *her* lawyer, and the case may find its way back into court through a contempt citation, or the husband may suddenly find himself in jail without a hearing.

No easy method can prevent this melancholy sequence of events if a high level of emotion prevails, but certain actions can make it less likely. If the court makes a determined effort to have husband and wife appear at the time the final decision is announced, the terms of the decision can be explained; a firm statement can be made of the nature of compliance expected, with a warning as to the consequences of noncompliance. Moreover, compliance can be facilitated if husband and wife have informal access to a minor official of the court to whom they can raise questions without the bother and expense of requesting formal action by a lawyer. This can be done more easily with a family court which is staffed for such services than with a traditional court which is not staffed in this way.

Aid to Marriages in Trouble

The help that comes through a family court to a marriage in trouble is given rather late in the day. The marital relationship may have deteriorated to a point where one or both partners have concluded that a divorce is desirable. Married couples wishing professional help when serious trouble first appears may look in one of several directions for such help. Traditionally, they turn to a clergyman or a physician without psychiatric specialization. Some evidence shows that these two groups are consulted more frequently by persons concerned about their marriages than by all other professional groups combined.[19] The devout naturally consult their ministers about personal problems, and physicians also are asked about family matters. No doubt the advice given by clergymen and physicians is often excellent, but neither is a specialist in marriage counseling.

Welfare clients, especially the clients of private welfare agencies, frequently receive expert assistance with marital troubles. Special training in the treatment of such problems is given to graduate students in schools of social work.

A few persons with marital problems turn to psychiatrists or to clinical psychologists, and a small number turn to professional marriage counselors. This last group represents a new profession. The American Association of Marriage Counselors was founded in 1942, and in 1962 had only about 450 members.[20] To qualify for membership, an individual must complete extensive graduate-school training and undergo a long period of supervised marriage counseling. Unfortunately, the number of qualified persons is much too small to meet the need.

The effectiveness of a professional marriage counselor cannot be properly measured by his success in "keeping the marriage from breaking up," but rather in guiding the couple to the best available solution to their unique problem. This may mean divorce, or it may involve continuing the marriage by resolving or compromising the role conflicts that have caused the trouble. The professional marriage counselor is in a position analogous to that of a physician; the patient with abdominal pain may require surgery or a change of diet.

The individual who has moved so far down the road of marital difficulties as to apply for a divorce clearly deserves a careful and unhurried examination such as that provided by a trained marriage counselor in an adequately staffed family court. If the marriage, even at this late date, is viable after therapy it can begin to function again; if it is not, it can be terminated. Even if the marriage ends, the counseling will still have served a useful purpose, for it will have aided the former husband and wife to see their problems more clearly and will have furthered the process of adjustment to their changed situation.

13 / RECENT CHANGES
IN MARRIAGE AND DIVORCE

Development of New Statistics

Vital records on marriage and divorce. In recent years some advances have been made in marriage and divorce statistics based on reports of those vital events that are recorded by the various states. There are now state files of marriage and divorce records in nearly all states. Three states — Arizona, New Mexico, and Oklahoma — still lack state files of both marriages and divorces, and one state — Indiana — lacks state files of divorce records. Unfortunately, many states with such files fail to meet the moderate standards of completeness and accuracy of reporting to qualify for the established registration areas. However, the number of states qualifying has increased gradually. Two states — Minnesota and South Carolina — were recently added to the Marriage Registration Area (MRA), bringing the total to 41 states plus the District of Columbia. Three states — Kentucky, New York, and South Carolina — have been added to the Divorce Registration Area (DRA), bringing the total to 29 states. A glance at the map on page 10 indicates that while the MRA is reasonably complete except in the southwestern states, the DRA is incomplete in all sections of the United States. In fact, neither the MRA nor the DRA satisfactorily represents the entire United States; neither area constitutes a properly drawn sample for the whole country.

Moreover, reporting from the established registration areas leaves much to be desired. Before a state is admitted to a registration area, a test of completeness and accuracy is conducted by federal and state officials. If the completeness is less than 90 percent, the state is not admitted. However, after a state has been admitted to the MRA or DRA, federal officials have not participated in retesting the state to determine whether the reporting still meets minimum standards. This is in contrast to the action taken 50 years ago when the birth and death registration areas were being developed. At that time retests were conducted and states were dropped from a registration area for incomplete reporting.

New report forms (see page 12) were adopted by all states for use in recording each marriage and divorce beginning with the year 1968.

States were urged to provide additional socioeconomic information regarding persons at the time of marriage or divorce. Among the new items was education, which was recommended for both the marriage and divorce forms. However, the new items were not adopted by very many of the states. In April 1975, less than one-half of the MRA states had added the education item to their state forms; in the much smaller DRA slightly over half the states had added this item. For 1972, the latest available year, the reporting of education was decidedly better on the marriage form than on the divorce form; for 12 reporting states in the MRA the completeness was more than 95 percent, but for the remaining states it was less than 75 percent. By contrast, for the DRA the completeness in only 6 of the reporting states was over 90 percent; in the other states it was lower, being less than 50 percent in 3 of them.

Social scientists, especially sociologists and demographers, have made major efforts to improve the registration and reporting of marriages and divorces.[1] A committee on marriage and divorce statistics of the American Sociological Association has informed state and local officials of the interest of sociologists in having better data made available. In each state where reporting was inadequate, a sociologist residing in that state has urged the local officials to stimulate better reporting.

Census data on marital status. Between the mid-1960's and the mid-1970's, several new types of marital statistics became available by the introduction of a new question in the 1970 census and several in the Census Bureau's Current Population Survey. In 1970, the census included the two marital questions that were asked in 1960 (marital status and whether married more than once) plus a new question for remarried persons on how their first marriage ended. This innovation permitted a determination of the number of adults who were "known to have been divorced" (or widowed) after their first and/or most recent marriage. Since about three of every four divorced women and five of every six divorced men eventually remarry, the proportion of adults who are known to have been divorced is generally several times as large as the proportion currently divorced, as can be seen by the data for 1971 in Table 13.1.

A whole battery of marital questions was included in surveys conducted by the Bureau of the Census in 1967, 1971, and 1975. These questions provided information on the number of times married (up

Table 13.1. Marital history measures for women born between 1910 and 1934: United States, June 1971

| Measure | Born in 1930–1934 | | | Born in— | |
	All races	White	Black	1920–1924	1910–1914
Percent by number of times married	100.0	100.0	100.0	100.0	100.0
Never married	4.3	3.8	8.4	4.2	4.9
Married once	82.0	82.7	74.5	78.7	77.8
Married twice	12.0	11.8	15.0	14.2	14.8
Married 3+ times	1.7	1.7	1.9	2.8	2.5
Percent ever married by survey date	95.8	96.2	91.6	95.7	95.1
Percent currently divorced at survey date	5.4	4.8	11.2	5.5	4.4
Percent with first marriage ended in divorce	16.0	15.3	24.1	16.7	13.8
Percent known to have been divorced	16.7	15.4	24.3	17.9	14.8
Median age at first marriage	20.3	20.2	20.4	21.2	22.0
Median age at divorce after first marriage	27.8	27.6	28.3	29.6	33.3
Median age at remarriage after first marriage ended in divorce[a]	29.8	29.8	30.1	32.1	36.6
Median age at redivorce after second marriage[a,b]	38.1	38.3	37.5	c	c

Source: U.S. Bureau of the Census, Current Population Reports, Series P-20, No. 239, "Marriage, Divorce, and Remarriage by Year of Birth: June 1971," tables A, C, D, E, F, G, and 1.

[a] Based on women married twice.

[b] Based on women born in 1900 to 1954 for adequate number of cases.

[c] Median not shown where base is less than 75,000.

to three or more), on when the first and most recent marriages occurred, and on when and how they ended (if they had ended) for persons who survived to the survey date. The information in Table 13.1 from the 1971 survey illustrates the magnitude of the differences in results by race and by birth cohort. The new measures greatly broaden our perspective with regard to experience with marriage, divorce, and widowhood. However, the results by birth cohort should be interpreted with caution; they do not provide strictly comparable information on change over time, because the younger cohorts have had less time to become married, divorced, and remarried than the oldest cohort.

Another innovation is the availability of more data for Negroes (here reported as blacks) in place of data for "nonwhites."

In 1970 and 1960, efforts were made to evaluate the reporting on marital status by comparing reports for identical adults most of whom were enumerated in April or May for the decennial census and during the third week of March of the corresponding year for the Current Population Survey (CPS). For both years, the results showed that the reporting on the two largest categories (married, excluding separated, and single) was between 97 and 99 percent in agreement. However, reporting on other categories (separated and divorced) was moderately inconsistent, partly as a consequence of changes in marital status that had actually occurred between the dates of the census and the CPS. The degree of inconsistency was similar in 1970 and 1960, but was slightly less in 1970. About 16 percent of both men and women in 1970 who were classified as divorced in the CPS were tabulated in a different marital category in the census; for separated persons, the corresponding difference was about 30 to 40 percent.

Although this study revealed no clear pattern of bias, there was an apparent tendency in 1970 for some persons who were reported (through direct interviews) in the CPS as separated to be reported (largely through self-enumeration) in the census as divorced.

The limitations in the coverage of the vital statistics on marriage and divorce, as well as the weaknesses in the reporting of both the vital and census statistics, tend to reduce the precision of the data from both types of sources. However, attempts are being made to improve the data and to make them more timely. In the meantime, the findings from these sources may be used with a reasonable degree of confidence that the patterns they reveal are essentially correct.

Comparative International Trends in Marriage and Divorce

Changes in marriage rates. Although 16 of the 22 countries shown in Table 13.2 had a higher marriage rate in the early 1970's than was recorded for them in 1965, a substantial majority of the marriage rates showed a decline after 1965 or after the early 1970's. Five of the countries shown in the table experienced only lower rates after 1965 — Austria, Denmark, Germany (Federal Republic), Sweden, and Switzerland. Among the latter the one with the most marked decline was Sweden, where the marriage rate fell from 7.8 to 4.7 per 1,000 population, then rose slightly to 5.5. An official publication of the Swedish government attributes this decline in the number of marriages to an increase in the number of couples living together without being legally married.[2]

Table 13.2. Marriage rates per 1,000 population: Selected countries, 1965 to 1974

Country	1974	1973	1972	1971	1970	1965
Australia[a]	8.3[b]	8.6	8.8	9.2	9.3	8.3
Austria	6.5	6.6	7.7	6.5	7.1	7.8
Canada		9.0	9.2	8.9	8.8	7.4
Chile[a]				8.6	7.3	7.6
Denmark		6.1	6.2	6.6	7.4	8.8
Egypt		9.4	10.4	10.2	9.8	9.8
Finland	7.5	7.5	7.7	8.2	8.8	7.9
France	7.6	7.7	8.1	7.9	7.8	7.1
Germany (Fed. Rep.)	6.1	6.4	6.7	7.1	7.3	8.3
Ireland[a]	7.3	7.5	7.3	7.3	7.1	5.9
Israel	9.5	9.1	9.5	9.4	9.1	7.9
Italy	7.3	7.6	7.7	7.5	7.4	7.7
Japan[a]	9.2[b]	10.0	10.4	10.5	10.1	9.7
Mexico[a]		8.3	8.1	7.5	7.3	6.9
Netherlands	8.1	8.0	8.8	9.3	9.5	8.8
Norway	6.8	7.0	7.3	7.6	7.6	6.5
Spain	7.6	7.7	7.6	7.5	7.4	7.2
Sweden	5.5	4.7	4.9	4.9	5.4	7.8
Switzerland	6.0	6.2	7.0	7.1	7.5	7.6
United Kingdom[a] (England and Wales)			8.6	8.3	8.5	7.8
United States[c]	10.5[b]	10.9	11.0	10.6	10.6	9.3
U.S.S.R.		10.1	9.4	10.0	9.7	8.7

Source: United Nations, Demographic Yearbook, 1973, table 19; and 1969, table 47. Also, unpublished data from the United Nations.

[a]Data by year of registration rather than year of occurrence.

[b]Provisional.

[c]Official publications of the U.S. National Center for Health Statistics.

Note: Rates are number of legal (recognized) marriages performed and registered per 1,000 population, excluding unions established by mutual consent or by tribal or native customs. For population and territorial inclusions and exclusions, see source.

The United States continued to have the highest marriage rate of any country included in Table 13.2. The rate hit a peak of 11.0 per 1,000 population in 1972 and subsequently declined to 10.5 in 1974 and to 10.1 during the 12 months ending September 1975, according to official publications for the U.S. National Center for Health Statistics. An important reason for this high rate is the fact that this country has the highest divorce rate, and a large majority of divorced persons remarry. Other countries shown in the table with marriage rates of 9.0 or higher for at least one year include Australia, Canada, Egypt, Israel, Japan, Netherlands, and the U.S.S.R. When vital rates for the next year or two become available in the United Nations reports, more are expected to show a downward movement of marriage rates because of the currently widespread downturn in business conditions.

Changes in age at marriage. Although earlier marriage for women than for men must be nearly universal, Table 13.3 features the wide range of differences among countries in the proportion of marriages that occur at a relatively young age, here defined as under 25 years old. The table also shows that early marriage tended to increase be-

Table 13.3. Percent of marriages occurring to persons under 25 years old: Selected countries, 1972 and 1965

Country	Men			Women		
	1972[a]	1965[b]	Change	1972[a]	1965[b]	Change
Japan	32.6	24.1	8.5	69.0	65.3	3.7
Sweden	36.1	49.5	−13.4	57.6	71.7	−14.1
Switzerland	40.3	39.1	1.2	63.7	63.0	0.7
Austria	48.1	45.7	2.4	70.4	67.0	3.4
Germany (Fed. Rep.)	49.0	42.8	6.2	71.3	66.0	5.3
Netherlands	58.9	47.6	11.3	78.6	72.8	5.8
United States	59.0	58.9	0.1	71.5	72.2	−0.7
Canada	59.7	56.5	3.2	75.5	77.2	−1.7
U.S.S.R.	60.8	31.8	29.0	73.4	51.6	21.8
Australia	62.5	55.7	6.8	79.2	77.5	1.7

Source: United Nations, Demographic Yearbook, 1966 to 1973, various tables, and official publications of the U.S. National Center for Health Statistics.

[a]1971 for Germany (Federal Republic), Switzerland, and Australia.

[b]1966 for U.S.S.R.

tween 1965 and the early 1970's. The range of early marriage was much wider for men than for women, with the proportion of men marrying before age 25 in the early 1970's being nearly twice as high in Australia (63 percent) as in Japan (33 percent), and with the corresponding proportion for women being one-third larger in Australia (79 percent) than in Sweden (58 percent).

Since the data refer to all marriages, regardless of whether first or subsequent marriages, countries with high divorce rates and therefore with relatively large proportions of marriages that are remarriages might be expected to have fewer of their total marriages occurring at an early age. However, the United States and the U.S.S.R. have high divorce rates and yet they have two of the highest proportions of early marriages. Perhaps the very fact that these countries have so much early marriage helps to account for their high divorce rates, inasmuch as the two variables tend to be closely correlated.

The shift toward more early marriage is apparent for most of the countries shown in the accompanying table. However, Sweden shows a sharp decline in early marriage for both men and women, and the United States and Canada show small decreases in early marriage for women. Whether or not these shifts are the forerunners of a general reversal of the recent tendency toward more early marriage remains to be seen.

The rate of increase in relatively young marriage was generally greater among men than among women, and this change brought the ages of husbands and their wives closer together. Illustrative marriage rates for Norway that appear in Table 13.4 show that an increasing proportion of marriages has been taking place among persons in their

Table 13.4. Marriages per 1,000 unmarried persons 15 to 24 years old, by age and sex: Norway, 1969–70 and 1949–52

Age	Men		Women	
	1969–70	1949–52	1969–70	1949–52
15–19 years	10.1	2.7	47.5	23.0
20–24 years	132.4	57.0	226.3	146.6

Source: Norway, Central Bureau of Statistics, Socialt Ulsyn, Oslo, 1974, table 1.26.

teens and early twenties (both men and women), but the percent of increase in the rates has been especially large for men.

The more rapid increase in early marriage among men is particularly evident in countries where the proportion of youthful marriages has been historically small. For example, according to findings cited in a report on social trends in England and Wales,[3] the proportion of persons born in 1930 who had joined the ranks of the "ever-married" group by the time of their twentieth birthday was only 3 percent for men and 18 percent for women. This is in sharp contrast to persons born in 1950; by their twentieth birthday, 8 percent of the men and 27 percent of the women had married. Although the average age at marriage in England and Wales had been in the neighborhood of 27 or 28 years for men from early in the century until World War II, it fell to just over 24 years in the early 1970's; meantime, the average age for women to marry, which had been about 25 to 26 years, fell to just over 22 years.

Changes in divorce rates. Between 1965 and the early 1970's, all but 2 of the 17 countries listed in Table 13.5 experienced a rising divorce rate; the two exceptions were Egypt and Israel. The amount of the increase in the rate varied: in Austria, France, and Japan it was a nominal rise of 0.1 or 0.2 point, but for most countries the increase was substantial, in a few instances doubling or tripling during the period.

In some countries — United States, U.S.S.R., and Canada — both the marriage rate and the divorce rate were higher than the average, and in others — Austria, Germany (Federal Republic), and Switzerland — both rates were lower than the average. But for many of the other countries both rates were about average or were of mixed levels.

The United States has continued to have the highest divorce rate, according to available data from the United Nations. After reaching a low point of 2.1 per 1,000 population in 1958, the U.S. divorce rate climbed to 2.5 in 1965 and to 3.5 in 1970. Moreover, according to official publications of the U.S. National Center for Health Statistics, the divorce rate continued to rise through 1974, when it reached 4.6. It stood at 4.7 for the 12 months ending in September 1975. Thus the tendency for the rate to rise was continuing as this book went to press.

One factor in the rising divorce rate has been a change in the divorce laws. An official Canadian publication states: "Due to the significant easing of divorce laws in 1969, divorce rates prior to 1969

Table 13.5.   Divorce rates per 1,000 population: Selected countries, 1965 to 1973

Country	1973	1972	1971	1970	1965
Australia	1.2	1.2	1.0	1.0	0.8
Austria	1.3	1.3	1.3	1.4	1.2
Canada	1.7		1.4	1.4	0.5
Denmark	2.5	2.6	2.7	1.9	1.4
Egypt[a]	2.1	2.2	2.1	2.1	2.2
Finland	1.8	1.8	1.6	1.3	1.0
France		0.9	0.9	0.8	0.7
Germany (Fed. Rep.)		1.4	1.3	1.2	0.9
Israel	0.8	0.9	0.8	0.8	0.9
Japan[a]	1.0	1.0	1.0	0.9	0.8
Netherlands	1.3	1.1	0.9	0.8	0.5
Norway	1.2	1.0	1.0	0.9	0.7
Sweden	2.0	1.9	1.7	1.6	1.2
Switzerland	1.3	1.2	1.1	1.0	0.8
United Kingdom (England and Wales)	2.1	2.4	1.5	1.2	0.8
United States[b]	4.4	4.0	3.7	3.5	2.5
U.S.S.R.	2.7	2.6	2.6	2.6	1.6

Source: United Nations, _Demographic Yearbook_, 1973, table 21; and 1969, table 49.

[a]Data by year of registration rather than year of occurrence.

[b]Official publications of the U.S. National Center for Health Statistics. Data include annulments.

Note: Rates are number of final decrees granted under civil law per 1,000 population. Annulments and legal separations are excluded unless otherwise specified.

are not comparable and therefore are not shown." [4] Also, in Great Britain the Divorce Reform Act of 1969, which came into effect at the beginning of 1971, had important effects including a shortening of the time between the actual end of the marriage and its legal termination.

The relation between early marriage and a high divorce rate is illustrated by the following information concerning marriages that took place in England and Wales in 1966: if the wife was less than 20 years old at marriage, 33 of every 1,000 marriages had ended in divorce within five years; if she was 20 to 24 years old at marriage, 18 of every 1,000 marriages had ended in divorce within five years; and if she was 25 to 29 years old at marriage, only 14 of every 1,000 marriages had ended in divorce within five years.[5]

A list of nine countries that did not grant full divorce is presented on page 27 of the British report, *Social Trends*. Little has happened recently in these countries regarding legal granting of divorce. Brazil, the largest of these countries, still does not allow divorce, although a prolonged internal struggle has been under way. In the spring of 1975 a scant majority of the national legislature voted to amend the constitution to allow divorce. The measure failed to become law, however, since the majority fell short of the required two-thirds, according to an article in the Washington *Post*, May 10, 1975.

An inquiry in 1975 regarding possible changes in the laws was sent by one of the authors to the embassies of these nine countries. In only one had a significant change occurred. The Divorce and Matrimonial Causes Act became Law 898 in Italy on December 1, 1970. It was submitted to and approved by national referendum, thereby approving the right to divorce. The struggle in the Italian Parliament had been a prolonged one. In none of the other seven countries — Argentina, Chile, Colombia, Ireland, Paraguay, the Philippines, and Spain — was there a reported change in the law to allow divorce with the right to remarry.

Changes in age at divorce. Various measures may be used to analyze the typical or average age at which divorce usually occurs. During the late 1950's and early 1960's the modal age groups of men and women at divorce varied widely (Table 2.7). For many countries women were usually in their twenties (20 to 29) and men in their late twenties or early thirties (25 to 34). Later information given in the *Demographic Yearbook* for 1968 shows a slight trend toward earlier ages at divorce. More countries show 20 to 24 years as the typical ages of women at divorce, and 25 to 29 years for men. For the United States, the modal ages at divorce did not change and in 1970 stood at 20 to 24 for women and 25 to 29 for men. The earlier the typical ages at divorce, the greater the probability that the persons who divorce will remarry.

Changes in Marriages, Divorces, and Marital Status

Changes in marriage and divorce rates. During most of the decade and a half since 1960, marriage and divorce rates in the United States have been rising substantially (Table 13.6). However, the marriage rate per 1,000 population hit a peak of 11.0 in 1972 and was still declining at the time of this writing. Since about three of every four persons at the time of marriage have not been previously married, and since an avalanche of young people born after World War II were reaching the age to enter marriage during and after the mid-1960's, the changing age composition of the population strongly favored an upturn in the marriage rate. But the increase of 25 percent in the marriage rate during the 1960's was less than half the increase in the population 18 to 24 years old (57 percent).

Meantime, the divorce rate in the United States more than doubled between 1960 and the mid-1970's. Even in 1975, when economic recession and widespread unemployment prevailed, the upward climb

Table 13.6. Number of marriages, number of divorces, crude marriage rate, and crude divorce rate: United States, 1960 to 1975

Year	Marriages			Divorces		
		Per 1,000 population			Per 1,000 population	
	Number (000's)	Rate	As percent of 1960	Number (000's)	Rate	As percent of 1960
1975[a]	2,149	10.1	119	1,002	4.7	214
1974	2,223	10.5	124	970	4.6	209
1973	2,284	10.9	128	915	4.4	200
1972	2,282	11.0	129	845	4.1	186
1971	2,190	10.6	125	773	3.7	168
1970	2,159	10.6	125	708	3.5	159
1969	2,145	10.6	125	639	3.2	145
1968	2,069	10.4	122	584	2.9	132
1967	1,927	9.7	114	523	2.6	118
1966	1,857	9.5	112	499	2.5	114
1965	1,800	9.3	109	479	2.5	114
1964	1,725	9.0	106	450	2.4	109
1963	1,654	8.8	104	428	2.3	105
1962	1,577	8.5	100	413	2.2	100
1961	1,548	8.5	100	414	2.3	105
1960	1,523	8.5	100	393	2.2	100

Source: U.S. National Center for Health Statistics, Monthly Vital Statistics Report, Vol. 24, No. 9, "Births, Marriages, Divorces, and Deaths for September 1975," p. 1; Vol. 24, No. 5 Supplement, "Summary Report, Final Marriage Statistics, 1973," table 2; Vol. 24, No. 4 Supplement, "Summary Report, Final Divorce Statistics, 1973," table 2; Vol. 23, No. 13, "Annual Summary for the United States, 1974," tables J and K.

[a]Based on the 12 months ending September 1975.

of the divorce rate continued. In that year the number of divorces reached 1.0 million for the first time, whereas the number of marriages declined to 2.1 million. The annual number of divorces was approximately 600,000 higher than in 1960, whereas the number of mar-

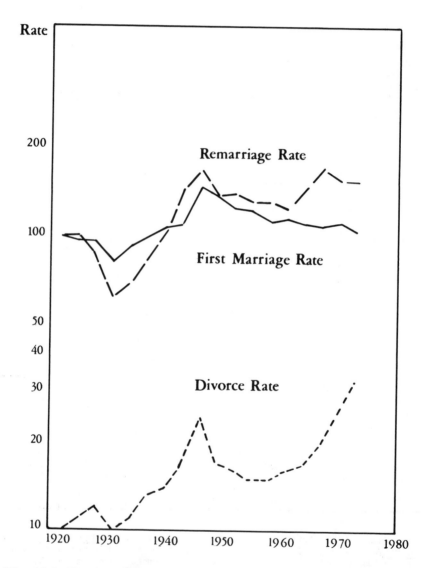

Fig. 13.1. First-marriage, remarriage, and divorce rates per 1,000: United States, 1920 to 1974

Source: Table 13.7.

riages was only 700,000 higher. Accordingly, much of the credit for the 25-percent increase in the marriage rate during this period was a consequence of a sharp increase in the number of persons who were remarrying.

Dramatic contrasts among the trends of first marriage, divorce, and remarriage rates over the last half-century are evident in the accompanying Figure 13.1 and Table 13.7. These rates are more refined than those in Table 13.6, not only because the two types of marriage are identified, but also because the bases are limited to the most eligible population in each case.

The first-marriage rate per 1,000 single women 14 to 44 years old has been declining almost continuously since it reached a peak soon after World War II ended. The divorce rate per 1,000 married women 14 to 44 years old likewise hit a peak in 1945 to 1947 and then de-

Table 13.7. Number and rate of first marriages, divorces, and remarriages: United States, 3-year averages, 1921 to 1974

Period	First marriages		Divorces		Remarriages	
	Thousands	Rate[a]	Thousands	Rate[b]	Thousands	Rate[c]
1921–23	990	99	158	10	186	98
1924–26	992	95	177	11	200	99
1927–29	1,025	94	201	12	181	84
1930–32	919	81	183	10	138	61
1933–35	1,081	92	196	11	162	69
1936–38	1,183	98	243	13	201	83
1939–41	1,312	106	269	14	254	103
1942–44	1,247	108	360	17	354	139
1945–47	1,540	143	526	24	425	163
1948–50	1,326	134	397	17	360	135
1951–53	1,190	122	388	16	370	136
1954–56	1,182	120	379	15	353	129
1957–59	1,128	112	381	15	359	129
1960–62	1,205	112	407	16	345	119
1963–65	1,311	109	452	17	415	143
1966–68	1,440	107	535	20	511	166
1969–71	1,649	109	702	26	515	152
1972–74	1,662	103	907	32	601	151

Source: Arthur J. Norton and Paul C. Glick, "Marital Instability: Past, Present, and Future," Journal of Social Issues, Vol. 32, No. 1, 1976 (in press).

[a]First marriages per 1,000 single women 14 to 44 years old.

[b]Divorces per 1,000 married women 14 to 44 years old.

[c]Remarriages per 1,000 widowed and divorced women 14 to 54 years old.

clined, but after more than a decade with little change, the divorce rate resumed its historical upward trend, and during the early 1970's it climbed well above the post–World War II level. The remarriage rate per 1,000 widowed and divorced women 14 to 54 years old also reached a peak in the mid-1940's and declined to a level where it remained for more than a decade; then, like the divorce rate, it resumed its historical upward trend. However, the level that it reached in the late 1960's was very little above that of the mid-1940's, whereas the recent divorce rate was far greater. In fact, the latest estimates, shown in Table 13.7, indicate that the remarriage rate had started to decline well before 1975 even though the divorce rate continued to rise.

These findings add up to a general slackening of entrance into marriage, a continued high rate of divorce, and an apparent beginning of a tendency for a smaller proportion of divorced persons to "make another try at it" by remarrying.

The probable future trend of the divorce rate is of great interest and a subject about which there is much speculation. In this setting, an attempt was made by Glick and Norton[6] to use the actual divorce experience of women about 30 to 70 years old in 1971 in order to project the eventual proportion of young women who would ever end their first marriage in divorce. This was done by starting with the proportion of women born in 1940 to 1944 whose first marriages had already ended in divorce and assuming that the increments of divorce during the 1960's for those of successively older ages in 1971 would likewise apply to the future divorce experience of the women born in 1940 to 1944 when they would be in these older age groups. Using data based on experience of the 1960's, these authors reached the conclusion that eventually 25 to 29 percent of young women in their late twenties and early thirties were likely to end their first marriage in divorce. Comparable projections for older women included 19 percent for those 20 years older and 12 percent for those 40 years older.

But between 1971, when the data for this projection were collected, and 1975 the divorce rate had increased by about one-fourth. It is not surprising, therefore, that a similar study made in 1975 yielded a likelihood that at least one-third of the first marriages of couples about 30 years of age would eventually end in divorce. Moreover, the 1975 study showed that redivorce after remarriage was, as expected, somewhat more likely to occur than divorce after first marriage. These and other related facts imply that somewhere between 35 and 40 percent of all married couples under middle age in 1975 are likely to have their marriages end in divorce. However, the proportion likely to become divorced varies inversely with socioeconomic level. Therefore the proportion of marriages that eventually end in divorce is probably much smaller than 35 percent for couples at the upper range of the income distribution.

Marital status by age and sex. Marital patterns of men differ widely from those of women in early adulthood and old age, but are much more nearly the same during the intermediate phase of the adult life cycle (Table 13.8). Moreover, differences between the marital status distribution for men and that for women are largest at the extremes of adult life because of earlier marriage, lower remarriage rates, and longer survival among women than men. Within this context, additional changes occur over time (Table 13.9).

Table 13.8.   Percent distribution by marital status for persons 14 years old and over, by age and sex: United States, 1974

(Numbers in thousands)

Marital status and sex	Total, 14 years and over	Age (years)					
		14-24	25-34	35-44	45-54	55-64	65 and over
Men, 1974	75,040	20,873	14,222	11,007	11,360	9,051	8,528
Percent	100.0	100.0	100.0	100.0	100.0	100.0	100.0
Single	29.0	80.4	17.2	8.3	5.9	6.1	4.6
Married, wife present	63.1	17.7	75.7	82.6	85.6	82.9	76.8
Married, wife absent	2.4	1.1	2.6	3.9	2.6	2.9	2.1
Separated	1.5	0.6	1.8	2.4	1.9	1.8	1.3
Other	0.9	0.6	0.8	1.5	0.7	1.1	0.8
Widowed	2.5	...	0.2	0.5	1.5	4.1	14.4
Divorced	3.1	0.7	4.3	4.7	4.4	4.0	2.2
Women, 1974	82,244	21,406	14,750	11,608	12,242	10,164	12,074
Percent	100.0	100.0	100.0	100.0	100.0	100.0	100.0
Single	22.5	68.1	10.2	4.9	4.2	5.5	6.3
Married, husband present	57.5	27.6	77.1	80.1	77.5	66.4	37.3
Married, husband absent	3.6	2.7	5.6	5.5	3.9	3.0	1.4
Separated	2.7	1.5	4.5	4.5	2.9	2.2	0.8
Other	0.9	1.2	1.1	1.0	0.9	0.8	0.6
Widowed	11.9	0.1	0.8	2.6	7.8	20.5	52.4
Divorced	4.4	1.4	6.3	6.9	6.6	4.7	2.6

Source: U.S. Bureau of the Census, Current Population Reports, Series P-20, No. 271, "Marital Status and Living Arrangements: March 1974," table 1.

All but 4 percent of the women about 50 years old in 1974 had married, as compared with 7 percent in 1960 and 10 percent in 1920. However, because of the recent tendency for more women to delay marriage well into their twenties (a fact that is documented further in the section on single men and women), a reasonable prospect is developing for the proportion of women who never marry to reach at least 5 percent again by the time those currently in their twenties reach 50 years of age. By way of comparison, all but 6 percent of the men 50 years old in 1974, 7 percent in 1960, and 12 percent in 1920 had ever married.

The decline in singlehood among those about 40 to 50 years old, however, has not resulted in an increase in the currently married population, as might have been expected. Instead, women about 40 years old in 1960 had the highest proportion married with husband present (83 percent), but after the mid-1960's this figure declined until it reached 80 percent by 1974. A comparison of the data in Tables 13.8 and 13.9 facilitates analysis of the components of change between

Table 13.9. Percent distribution by marital status for women by age: United States, 1960 and comparison with 1974

(Numbers in thousands)

Marital status and sex	Total, 14 years and over	Age (years)					
		14-24	25-34	35-44	45-54	55-64	65 and over
Women, 1960	64,913	13,445	11,637	12,336	10,487	8,145	8,882
Percent	100.0	100.0	100.0	100.0	100.0	100.0	100.0
Single	19.0	62.7	8.6	6.1	7.0	8.0	8.5
Married, husband present	62.1	32.6	82.5	82.7	75.8	62.5	34.7
Married, husband absent	3.9	3.5	5.0	4.4	4.2	3.5	2.7
Separated	2.0	1.2	2.8	2.7	2.4	1.8	1.0
Other	1.9	2.3	2.2	1.7	1.8	1.7	1.7
Widowed	12.1	0.2	0.9	3.0	8.8	22.3	52.1
Divorced	2.9	0.9	2.9	3.8	4.3	3.7	2.0
Women, 1974 ──────── Women, 1960	1.27	1.59	1.27	0.94	1.17	1.25	1.36
Single	1.18	1.09	1.19	0.80	0.60	0.69	0.74
Married, husband present	0.93	0.85	0.93	0.97	1.02	1.06	1.07
Married, husband absent	0.92	0.77	1.12	1.25	0.93	0.86	0.52
Separated	1.35	1.25	1.61	1.67	1.21	1.22	0.80
Other	0.47	0.52	0.50	0.59	0.50	0.47	0.35
Widowed	0.98	0.50	0.89	0.87	0.89	0.92	1.01
Divorced	1.52	1.56	2.17	1.82	1.53	1.27	1.30

Source: U.S. Bureau of the Census, 1960 Census of Population, Vol. II-4E, Marital Status, table 4; and 1974 data for women in preceding table.

1960 and 1974 for women; data are not shown for men in Table 13.9, partly to keep the presentation brief and partly to avoid giving data that are affected by the changing size of the Armed Forces, many members of which are not covered by the available figures for 1974.

Besides declines in the proportions of women who were single or married with husband present, a decline was also recorded in the proportion widowed. Altogether these three categories of women about 40 years old constituted 4.2 percent less of the total in 1974 than in 1960. The corresponding increase of 4.2 percent was distributed between married women with husband absent (1.1 percentage points) and divorced women (3.1 percent). Thus, more women about 40 years old had ever married, but fewer were still married with husband present in 1974 than in 1960.

The *rate* of change since 1960 in the proportion of women in the several marital categories is shown in the lower tier of Table 13.9. Especially large rates of change occurred among divorced women, who constituted half again as large a proportion of all women in 1974 as in 1960 (4.4 percent versus 2.9 percent, or 1.52 times as large a proportion at the more recent date); and among married women whose husbands were reported as absent for reasons other than separation, who constituted only about one-half as large a proportion of all women in 1974 as in 1960.

Rates of increase in the percent divorced were largest among women under 45 years old, but were also substantial among older women. In other words, all age groups were sharing in the trend toward more divorce. Moreover, all but the elderly women showed considerable increases in the percent separated, perhaps as an indication that a growing proportion of women below old age were moving toward divorce. Significantly, however, the increase in the percent divorced was consistently larger than the increase in the percent separated. This finding is interpreted as evidence that more and more couples with marriages that have failed beyond a reasonable chance of regeneration are completely ending their marriages by divorce, rather than lingering in a state of separation. In these circumstances, one or both spouses are concluding that they prefer to make a transition to another marriage they believe would be more satisfactory than the one they are ending — or to nonmarriage.[7]

One of the reasons why the proportion classified as "other married with husband absent" has shrunk so consistently among all age groups is that a smaller proportion of married persons in the 1970's than in

1960 were living apart from their spouse in an institution. Another probable reason is that more unmarried mothers were frank in reporting their marital status as single.

Being married and living with a husband has become somewhat less characteristic of younger women and more so of older women since 1960. Delayed marriage and more marital disruption probably explain most of the change for younger women, and higher marriage rates two or three decades ago plus longer joint survival of husbands and wives through late middle age probably explain most of the change for older women.

Changes in marital status among white, black, and Mexican American women. The two largest minorities among ethnic groups in the United States today are blacks (11 percent) and persons of Spanish origin (5 percent). Three-fifths of the Spanish-origin population are of Mexican descent and nearly all (97 percent) are white. The best means for showing changes since 1960 in characteristics of the Mexican Americans is to compare information from the 1960 and 1970 censuses on persons of Spanish surname in the five southwestern states where this group is most concentrated. Moreover, the best age-sex group to feature in showing these changes is women 35 to 44 years old. Because of the relatively high fertility among Mexican American women (who are more likely than the general population or blacks to be Roman Catholic), and because of the large amount of immigration from Mexico among young adult persons, the adult population of Mexican origin in the United States has a much younger age profile than that of either blacks or whites as a whole. Within these constraints, the following discussion relates to the data for women 35 to 44 in Table 13.10.

In both 1970 and 1960, the marital status distribution for Mexican American women was consistently intermediate between that for white women as a whole and that for black women, but in 1970 it was consistently closer to that for white women. (Incidentally, the same observation is relevant whether the comparison is made for women of all adult ages or for those 35 to 44 years old.) White women 35 to 44 were the most likely of the three groups to be married and living with their husband and least likely to be in any of the other categories. Black women deviated most from either the white or the Mexican American women with regard to their very high proportion reported as married but living apart from their husband — mostly separated.

Table 13.10. Percent distribution by marital status, for women 35 to 44 years old by race for the United States, and by Spanish surname for five southwestern states: 1970 and 1960

Race, Spanish surname,[a] and year	Women, 35-44 years	Single	Married, husband present	Married, husband absent	Widowed	Divorced
White:						
1970	100.0	5.3	83.6	3.5	2.5	5.1
1960	100.0	6.0	84.8	3.0	2.5	3.6
1970/1960	...	0.88	0.99	1.17	1.00	1.42
Black:						
1970	100.0	8.8	58.8	17.6	6.6	8.3
1960	100.0	7.0	63.3	16.6	7.2	5.9
1970/1960	...	1.26	0.91	1.11	0.96	1.46
1970 Black/White	...	1.66	0.70	5.03	2.64	1.63
Spanish surname:						
1970	100.0	6.6	77.9	6.5	3.1	6.0
1960	100.0	6.5	79.0	6.0	3.6	4.8
1970/1960	...	1.02	0.99	1.08	0.86	1.25
1970 Spanish/White	...	1.25	0.93	1.86	1.24	1.18

Source: U.S. Bureau of the Census, 1970 Census of Population, Vol. II-1D, Persons of Spanish Surname, table 8; Vol. II-4C, Marital Status, table 4; 1960 Census of Population, Vol. II-1B, Persons of Spanish Surname, table 7; Vol. II-1C, Nonwhite Population by Race, table 19; and Vol. II-4E, Marital Status, table 4.

[a]For five states: Arizona, California, Colorado, New Mexico, and Texas.

All three groups had a larger rate of increase in the proportion divorced than in the proportion married with husband absent, thereby suggesting an increasing tendency to resolve marital problems by divorce rather than to leave them unresolved. Puerto Rican women in the United States are like Mexican American women in that they are mostly of Spanish origin; but the Puerto Rican women 35 to 44 years old have a relatively high proportion divorced (7.3 percent). In this respect, the Puerto Rican women are nearer to black women than to Mexican American women; this fact is demonstrable by comparing Table 13.10 with Table 5 of a 1970 census report, *Puerto Ricans in the United States.*

As a result of the changes during the 1960's the distribution for Mexican American women moved a little nearer to that of white women as a whole and farther from that of black women. By contrast, the gap between black and white women 35 to 44 widened somewhat with respect to the proportions who had entered marriage and who had remained married; the already high percent single among blacks increased whereas that for whites decreased, and the already low percent married with husband present among black women declined even more than that for white women. These changes during the 1960's for black women and white women amounted to a continuation of directions of change that occurred in the 1950's.[8]

Changes in marital status by educational level. Some social and economic groups have experienced a considerably greater rate of change than others in their marital status distribution during recent years. One of the most appropriate variables to use in documenting this assertion is educational level; as pointed out in an earlier chapter, this variable applies to all adults, whereas occupation and income do not apply to a substantial proportion of women. The results in Table 13.11 show where the rates of change have differed most from that for the average of persons in all educational levels combined. These results are for persons 35 to 44 years old. This is a good age group to study for the present purpose, because persons of this age range are old enough to have had considerable opportunity to marry, to become divorced, and to remarry, yet they are young enough to reflect relatively recent practices with respect to marriage. The fact remains, however, that persons in this age group were more likely to marry and less likely to become divorced by the age of 25 to 34 in 1960 than those who were 25 to 34 in 1970.

The third tier of Table 13.11 is most relevant in the present context. It shows clearly that the largest rate of change in marital status at each educational level has been that for the proportion separated or divorced. Persons in all educational levels have contributed to the sharp increase in these types of marital disruption. Two findings in the table are especially noteworthy:

(*a*) Upper-group men have experienced the highest *rate* of increase in the proportion separated or divorced, but these men have the lowest *proportion* separated or divorced for men; and

(*b*) Women college graduates with no further education have experienced the lowest *rate* of increase in the proportion "separated or divorced," and these women also have the lowest *proportion* separated or divorced for women.[9]

Thus, the proportion of upper-group men 35 to 44 with marriages disrupted by separation or divorce has been *converging* most toward

Table 13.11. Percent in selected marital categories, for persons 35 to 44 years old, by years of school completed and sex: United States, 1970 and 1960

Census date and years of school completed	Percent of men 35 to 44 who were--			Percent of women 35 to 44 who were--		
	Never married	Married once with wife present	Sepa-rated or divorced	Never married	Married once with husband present	Sepa-rated or divorced
1970, total	7.9	72.9	5.5	5.7	69.3	8.8
0-11 years	9.2	67.4	6.8	5.8	61.7	11.2
12 years	6.6	74.9	5.1	4.5	74.3	7.2
13-15 years	6.7	73.7	5.3	5.1	72.8	8.2
16 years	6.7	81.5	3.4	7.6	78.4	5.2
17 years or more	8.4	80.4	3.4	18.8	62.0	8.7
Median years	12.1	12.4	12.0	12.3	12.4	12.1
1960, total	8.1	74.7	4.3	6.1	70.9	6.5
0-11 years	9.1	70.6	5.4	5.4	66.4	8.0
12 years	6.9	77.7	3.5	5.5	75.6	5.1
13-15 years	6.2	77.1	3.8	6.5	74.0	5.7
16 years	7.0	83.3	2.2	9.9	77.5	3.9
17 years or more	9.0	81.3	2.0	24.0	59.5	6.1
Median years	10.9	12.1	10.5	12.3	12.2	11.1
1970/1960	0.98	0.98	1.28	0.93	0.98	1.35
0-11 years	1.01	0.95	1.26	1.07	0.93	1.40
12 years	0.96	0.96	1.46	0.82	0.98	1.41
13-15 years	1.08	0.96	1.39	0.78	0.98	1.44
16 years	0.96	0.98	1.55	0.77	1.01	1.33
17 years or more	0.93	0.99	1.70	0.78	1.04	1.43

Source: U.S. Bureau of the Census, 1970 Census of Population, Vol. II-4C, Marital Status, table 14; and 1960 Census of Population, Vol. II-4E, Marital Status, table 11.

the average proportion for all men in the age group, whereas the corresponding proportion for women with exactly four years of college has been *diverging* from the average for all women in the age group. These contrasting changes, as one consequence, have brought the proportion divorced or separated for upper-group men closer to that for the women college graduates.

The highest proportion separated or divorced in both 1970 and 1960 was that for men and women who had not completed a high school education. Moreover, persons who started college training but did not complete a full four years continued to have a higher percent separated or divorced than either those with 12 or 16 years of school.

Evidently these persons have more difficulty than the average in maintaining amicable marital adjustment.[10]

Women with graduate school training also continue to have a high proportion separated or divorced. In addition, they still have by far the highest proportion never married and one of the lowest proportions still married to their first husband. In each of these respects, however, women in this top educational level have converged toward the average since 1960, with a much smaller (but yet large) proportion remaining never married and with a somewhat larger (but yet relatively small) proportion still married to their first husband. These changes in marital status appear to reflect an increasing degree of compatibility between marriage and a career for these highly educated women. According to 1970 and 1960 census reports entitled *Employment Status and Work Experience,* about three-fourths of all women 35 to 44 years of age in this educational level were in the labor force in 1970, as compared with two-thirds in 1960; only one-half of the other women in 1970 and a little over four-tenths of them in 1960 were in the labor force. The highly educated women no doubt have more options with regard to the life styles and roles they may adopt than women with less education. Moreover, a larger proportion of the most highly educated women obviously tend to place a higher priority on satisfaction through work outside the home than other women.

Marital status of men by socioeconomic level. Table 13.12 was designed to illustrate the extremes to which marital status distributions vary when classified by socioeconomic status (SES). The data are for 1970 and feature men age 45 to 54, who were near the period of life when their earnings were the highest. The distribution in the upper tier of the table for men of high SES indicates that those who "had everything going for them" in regard to education, occupation, and earnings were nearly all currently married — among both the white men (95 percent) and the black men (92 percent). Far more of the white than black men of high SES were still living with their first wife, whereas far more of the black than white men were known to have been divorced or widowed and to have remarried. Only a few (2 percent) of the upper SES white men of middle age had never married; for black men, the proportion was also small (5 percent). An even smaller proportion of the high-level men had been widowed but were not currently remarried (under 1 percent).

Table 13.12. Percent distribution by marital status, and mean earnings in 1969 by marital status, for white and black men 45 to 54 years old of high and low socioeconomic level: United States, 1970

Marital status	White men			Black men		
	High SES[a]	Low SES[b]	High⁄Low	High SES	Low SES	High⁄Low
Total, 45-54 years old	584,054	107,799	5.42	6,353	70,388	0.09
Percent	100.0	100.0	...	100.0	100.0	...
Single	2.2	13.4	0.16	4.5	10.6	0.42
Married	95.4	76.8	1.24	91.6	79.5	1.15
Widowed	0.6	2.6	0.23	0.9	5.3	0.17
Divorced	1.8	7.1	0.25	3.0	4.6	0.65
Married once, wife present	84.2	57.7	1.46	68.5	49.8	1.38
Known to have been divorced	10.0	18.9	0.53	22.0	18.6	1.18
Mean earnings for all men 45-54 years old	$19,350	$5,660	3.42	$12,437	$4,501	2.76
As percent of that for all men	100	100	...	100	100	...
Single	59	76	...	85	79	...
Married	103	105	...	102	104	...
Widowed	87	86	...	81	88	...
Divorced	83	75	...	86	89	...
Married once, wife present	103	108	...	103	106	...
Known to have been divorced	99	93	...	101	102	...

Source: U.S. Bureau of the Census, 1970 Census of Population, Vol. II, 4-C, Marital Status, table 9.

[a]In the upper tier, professional and managerial workers with 4 or more years of college and with earnings of $15,000 or more in 1969; in the lower tier, the earnings criterion is omitted.

[b]In the upper tier, nonfarm laborers with no high school education and with earnings of $1 to $5,999; in the lower tier, the earnings criterion is omitted.

By contrast, the low SES men who "had very little going for them" were far more likely to have remained single (over 10 percent) or to have become widowed or divorced and not remarried (another 10 percent); consequently, only a little over three-fourths of them were currently married. Both black and white men of low SES included high proportions known to have been divorced after their first or most recent marriage (19 percent).

Surprisingly, *upper*-level black men included an even higher proportion known to have been divorced than *lower*-level black men (22 percent versus 19 percent). Among white men, the situation was the reverse, with nearly twice as large a proportion of lower-level men known to have been divorced (19 percent versus 10 percent). The reasons for the atypical pattern for black men are not apparent, but the pattern is nonetheless noteworthy.

In the lower tier of Table 13.12, socioeconomic level is defined in terms of only two characteristics, education and occupation. Within this framework, comparisons are made between the mean annual earnings of men of middle age in the several marital status categories.

The married men had consistently higher earnings, on the average, than men in any other marital status. This significant finding was the same for men of high and low SES, for both white and black men, and for not only men still in their first marriage but also currently married men as a whole including those who had remarried. The fact that the earnings of all men known to have been divorced were higher, on the average, than those of currently divorced men implies that those who remarry also tend to have greater earnings than those who remain divorced (at least for a longer time).

Men who have low earnings are the ones who most often remain single, either voluntarily or because they are passed over in the process of marital selection. A small proportion of these men are well-educated, single clergymen who choose not to marry. The relatively low earnings of widowed men of middle age suggests that many of these men had not been able to afford very healthful conditions for their wives. Moreover, their low earnings were often complicated by the presence of dependent children; these conditions placed many widowers at a disadvantage in competing for a partner in remarriage.

Age at Marriage

Changes in age at first marriage. After a historic decline, the median age at first marriage reached a low level in the mid-1950's; since that time it has been rising gradually. In 1956, the median dipped to 22.5 years for men and 20.1 years for women, according to data from the Bureau of the Census. By 1965 it had risen by 0.3 year for men and 0.5 year for women, and by 1974 it had risen again by the same amounts. The overall result was that the median age at first marriage has been rising more slowly for men than for women — the latter having risen by a full year during the two-decade period. This means that the historic trend toward a narrower gap between the ages of men and women at first marriage has continued until now the difference is only 2 years. Thus, by 1974 the median age at first marriage for men was 23.1 years and for women was 21.1 years (Table 13.13).

A useful means of describing the changing distribution of ages at marriage is the interquartile range. This measure shows the age bracket within which the central one-half of the marriages fall — with one-fourth occurring at younger ages and one-fourth occurring at older ages. In other words, it is the difference between the first quartile of ages and the third quartile; the second quartile is the median age. The last column of Table 13.13 shows that the interquartile range of age at first marriage has been increasing during the last decade, with the increase being twice as large for women as for men. A comparison of the changes in the other columns shows that the main source of the rising age at marriage has been a substantial upward movement of the third quartile, meaning that only a few more persons are marrying at a very young age but that many more are marrying at a relatively high age through longer postponement of marriage.

Differences in age at marriage by marital status. Age at marriage varies widely according to the marital status of both partners to the union. This can be effectively demonstrated by comparing ages at marriage for couples whose marital status before marriage is the

Table 13.13. Quartiles of age at marriage: United States, 1974, 1970, and 1965

Sex and year	First quartile	Median	Third quartile	Interquartile range
Men				
1974	20.1	23.1	26.6	6.5
1970	20.1	23.2	26.2	6.1
1965	20.0	22.8	25.9	5.9
Women				
1974	18.9	21.1	24.3	5.4
1970	18.9	20.8	23.3	4.4
1965	18.7	20.6	22.7	4.0

Source: U.S. Bureau of the Census, Current Population Reports, Series P-20, No. 271, "Marital Status and Living Arrangements: March 1974," table B.

same. By far the youngest age at marriage is that for brides and grooms who are both single (never married). One-half of the brides in this category are just over 20 years old, and one-half of the grooms are about 2 years older, just over 22, according to vital statistics for 1973 from the National Center for Health Statistics (Table 13.14). The interquartile range for these single-single couples is surprisingly narrow, rounding off to only 4 years for both brides and grooms. Thus, half of these brides fell between the ages of 18.6 and 22.5 years, and half of the grooms between 20.3 and 24.7 years.

Table 13.14. Quartiles of age at marriage for brides and grooms with the same marital status: Marriage Registration Area, 1973

Marital status	First quartile	Median	Third quartile	Interquartile range
Age of bride				
Total	19.3	21.9	26.9	7.6
Bride and groom:				
Single	18.6	20.3	22.5	3.9
Divorced	26.5	31.9	40.1	13.6
Widowed	52.5	59.5	66.2	13.7
Age of groom				
Total	21.2	24.1	30.2	9.0
Bride and groom:				
Single	20.3	22.2	24.7	4.4
Divorced	29.8	36.3	44.8	15.0
Widowed	57.3	64.7	71.4	14.1

Source: Unpublished tabulation from U.S. National Center for Health Statistics.

Age at marriage for persons who have been divorced is somewhat older, and for those who have been widowed it is, of course, much older. The median ages at marriage for brides and grooms who had both been divorced were in the thirties, and those for brides and grooms who had both been widowed were another 25 years older. Most of these persons were marrying for the second time, but some were entering their third or subsequent marriage. Despite the wide differences in median ages at marriage for the divorced-divorced and the widowed-widowed, the interquartile range is about the same (14 or 15 years). Moreover, the difference between the median ages of brides and grooms is also very similar for both-divorced and both-widowed couples (4 or 5 years). This is evidence of the strong tendency for marriage partners not to be very far apart in age regardless of their marital status at the time of marriage. The fact remains, however, that the age gap is much wider for those who are remarrying than for those who are marrying for the first time.

Since more than two-thirds of all unions involve single-single marriages, it is not surprising that the ages at marriage for all brides combined, and for all grooms combined, are closest to those for persons who are entering their first marriage.

Relation between age at marriage and marital stability. One of the best ways to show the close relation between age at first marriage and the probability that the marriage will remain intact for a period of at least 5 to 10 years is found in Table 13.15. This table makes it clear that men are least likely to dissolve their first marriage within a few years if they enter it between their middle twenties and their early thirties. The same applies to both white and black men in both 1970 and 1960. The corresponding optimum period for women to enter their first marriage to ensure stability is during their twenties. An important reason for low dissolution rates for persons who marry for the first time in their mid-twenties is that college graduates are most likely to marry during that period of life, and their marriages are generally among the most stable.

The table also shows that white persons whose first marriages do *not* occur during the optimum age range for stability are more likely to have their marriages dissolved within 5 to 10 years if they marry when they are quite young than when they are a few years older than the optimum range. Within this optimum range, the proportion of black persons with dissolved first marriages has been consistently higher than for their white counterparts. Moreover, among white persons the dissolution rates were higher in 1970 than in 1960 for persons in each group by age at first marriage.

Additional information about age at first marriage and at remarriage by race and period of birth is given in Table 13.1. In addition, a discussion of factors related to the recent increase in the postponement of marriage in the United States is presented below in the section on single men and women.

Table 13.15. Percent of persons whose first marriage was dissolved through death or divorce by the census date, by year of first marriage, age at first marriage, race, and sex: United States, 1970 and 1960

| Sex and age at first marriage | Percent of first marriages dissolved by census date[a] | | | |
| | White persons who first married in-- | | Black persons[b] who first married in-- | |
	1960-64	1950-54	1960-64	1950-54
Men	12.9	9.2	13.0	12.3
14-19 years	20.0	14.7	14.0	15.2
20-24 years	11.9	8.5	12.9	16.6
25-29 years	8.8	6.7	11.2	10.7
30-34 years	9.8	8.0	11.2	10.4
35 years and over	14.4	10.8	16.3	14.6
Women	15.5	11.0	17.3	15.5
14-17 years	25.2	18.6	19.1	16.4
18 and 19 years	17.3	11.1	17.6	14.6
20-24 years	10.1	7.4	15.1	13.4
25-29 years	10.0	8.7	14.6	16.2
30 years and over	18.8	14.2	22.1	20.3

Source: U.S. Bureau of the Census, 1970 Census of Population, Vol. II-4D, Age at First Marriage, table 4; and 1960 Census of Population, Vol. II-4D, Age at First Marriage, table 4. (See Tables 8.11 and 8.12.)

[a]1960-64 marriages dissolved by 1970 and 1950-54 marriages dissolved by 1960.

[b]Persons of races other than white in 1960.

Education and Race of Husband and Wife

Education of husband and wife. Since 1960, the educational distribution of husbands and their wives has moved sharply upward. Attrition through death reduced the proportion of marital partners who were elderly persons with relatively low levels of education; and increments through marriage augmented the proportion of partners who were young adults with relatively high levels of education. Only three-fifths (58 percent) as many relatively young couples who entered their first marriage in the 1960's as in the 1950's consisted in husbands and wives who had not graduated from high school (lower tier of Table 13.16). By contrast, more than twice as large a proportion of couples first married in the 1960's as in the 1950's consisted in husbands and wives who had completed 17 or more years of school, the vast majority of whom had completed at least one year of graduate school.

Table 13.16. Percent distribution of husband's years of school completed by
wife's years of school completed, for married couples with both
the husband and wife in first marriage at census date, married
in decade before the census: United States, 1970 and 1960

Census year and years of school completed by husband	Total	Years of school completed by wife					
		0-11	12	13-15	16	17 or more	Median
1970, total	100.00	23.44	48.22	15.82	9.60	2.92	12.6
0-11 years	25.15	13.96	9.74	1.09	0.27	0.08	11.4
12 years	38.06	7.63	25.33	3.90	0.99	0.20	12.5
13-15 years	16.84	1.40	8.37	5.20	1.56	0.32	12.8
16 years	10.38	0.27	3.05	3.19	3.38	0.50	14.8
17 years or more	9.57	0.18	1.73	2.45	3.40	1.82	16.1
Median years	12.7	10.8	12.6	14.7	16.6	17.2	...
1960, total	100.00	35.11	45.38	11.78	6.24	1.48	12.3
0-11 years	39.72	24.20	13.73	1.44	0.29	0.06	10.7
12 years	33.00	8.58	20.80	2.79	0.70	0.13	12.4
13-15 years	12.29	1.68	6.22	3.19	1.02	0.18	12.7
16 years	8.65	0.44	3.09	2.55	2.28	0.29	13.9
17 years or more	6.34	0.22	1.54	1.81	1.96	0.82	15.3
Median years	12.3	10.5	12.4	14.6	16.5	17+	...
1970/1960	1.00	0.67	1.06	1.34	1.54	1.97	...
0-11 years	0.65	0.58	0.71	0.75	0.96	1.34	...
12 years	1.15	0.89	1.22	1.40	1.41	1.57	...
13-15 years	1.37	0.83	1.35	1.63	1.53	1.80	...
16 years	1.20	0.63	0.99	1.25	1.48	1.71	...
17 years or more	1.51	0.79	1.12	1.36	1.74	2.21	...

Source: U.S. Bureau of the Census, 1970 Census of Population, Vol. II-4C,
Marital Status, table 14; and 1960 Census of Population, Vol. II-4E, Marital
Status, table 11.

Recently married husbands tend to have more education than their
wives, with the exception of those who have not graduated from high
school (that is, who have completed fewer than 12 years of school).
Recently married (and relatively young) wives are still more likely
than their husbands to have completed exactly 12 years of regular
school, and recently married husbands are still much more likely than
their wives to have completed a given number of years of college
training. In 1970, young husbands who were college graduates were
"only" 1.6 times as numerous as young wives who were college
graduates; this ratio was down from 1.9 times as numerous in 1960.

As one consequence of these developments, more and more college-
educated persons now can — and in fact do — marry persons with a

similar amount of education. That this tendency has continued into the 1970's is suggested by the larger rate of increase between 1970 and 1974 in the number of college graduates among women (up 30 percent) than among men (up 25 percent). The narrowing of the gap between the numbers of young men and women college graduates means, among other things, that fewer men must now "marry down" with regard to education (or remain unmarried); likewise, competition must now be increasing among college-educated women for marriage to available college-educated men.

The general rise in the educational level among young adults since 1960 has increased the pool of skilled persons who are seeking acceptable jobs and marriage partners. Moreover, the higher educational level among young adults today than a decade or two ago has presumably increased the store of information and skills that is brought to bear in making decisions about selecting jobs, marriage partners, recreational activities, and so on. As personal competence has presumably increased through advancement of educational levels, more choices in regard to entering marriage and remaining married are presumably depending less on traditional parental control and more on individual decisions.

Race of husband and wife. More than 99 percent of all married couples living together at the time of the 1970 and 1960 censuses comprised husbands and wives of the same "race," as the term is used in census statistics — 99.26 percent in 1970 and 99.60 percent in 1960. But, as these percentages imply, the number of couples involving partners who were reported as being of unlike race was actually twice as large in 1970 (330,000) as in 1960 (164,000). The increase during the decade undoubtedly was at least partially a result of more interracial marriages after the Supreme Court invalidated the ban against such marriages in 1967. Another factor that probably contributed to this result, but that cannot be documented, is more frankness in 1970 than in 1960 in the reporting of race for persons in racially mixed marriages. To reduce the disturbing effect of some of these factors, and to focus on recent experience, the remaining discussion in this section is limited to first marriages in the 1960's that were still intact at the time of the 1970 census.

In 1970, married couples with the husband and wife of different race constituted 1.17 percent of all intact first marriages of the 1960's (Table 13.17). This was half again as large a proportion as that for all married couples in 1970, regardless of when or how often each partner had married (0.74 percent). A majority of the interracial couples involved a white person married to a black, Indian, or Japanese person. In 1970, as in 1960 (see page 129), the number of black men married recently to white women far exceeded the number of white men married recently to black women.

Table 13.17. Race of husband by race of wife, for couples married in 1960 to 1970, both married once and living together: United States, 1970

Race of husband and wife	Couples married in 1960 to 1970		Race of husband and wife	Couples married in 1960 to 1970	
	Number	Percent		Number	Percent
All couples			Husband black	920,461	100.00
married once	10,272,498	100.00	Wife black	901,073	97.89
Both same race	10,152,766	98.83	Wife white	16,419	1.78
White	9,142,816	89.00	Wife other	2,969	0.32
Black	901,073	8.77			
Indian	22,037	0.21	Husband Indian	34,994	100.00
Japanese	26,003	0.25	Wife Indian	22,037	62.97
Other	60,837	0.59	Wife white	11,940	34.12
Different race	119,732	1.17	Wife other	1,017	2.91
Husband white	9,200,496	100.00	Husband Japanese	31,998	100.00
Wife white	9,142,816	99.37	Wife Japanese	26,003	81.26
Wife black	7,352	0.08	Wife white	4,213	13.17
Wife Indian	11,952	0.13	Wife other	1,782	5.57
Wife Japanese	13,462	0.15			
Wife other	24,914	0.27	Husband other	84,549	100.00

Source: U.S. Bureau of the Census, 1970 Census of Population, Vol. II-4C, Marital Status, table 12.

The pattern was reversed among white-Japanese couples in both 1970 and 1960, with far more white men married to Japanese women than Japanese men married to white women. A large proportion of the 16,000 white (husband)-Japanese (wife) marriages of the 1950's recorded in the 1960 census no doubt involved Japanese war brides. The number of white-Japanese marriages of the 1960's recorded in the 1970 census (13,000) was nearly as large, but probably for other reasons; one of these could be a change in the racial classification in Hawaii, where the category "part-Hawaiian" was used in 1960 but not in 1970, and many Japanese-Hawaiian mixtures may have therefore been classified as Japanese in 1970.

The pattern for mixed couples involving an American Indian partner differed from that involving either blacks or Japanese. Virtually
identical numbers (12,000) of white-Indian and Indian-white first
marriages of the 1960's were tabulated in the 1970 census. In 1960,
the census showed only 6,000 white-Indian and 4,000 Indian-white
first marriages of the 1950's that were still intact at the 1960 census
date. A part of the sharp increase over the 10-year period in these
types of mixed marriages may reflect the fact that more Indians have
moved to urban areas, where they have mingled closely with white
persons. Another factor may have been a growing tendency for Indians
(or part-Indians) to assert their racial identity because of heightened
attention to problems of minorities during this period. Still another
factor may have been the request in 1970 but not in 1960 for American Indians to report their tribe in the decennial census.

Intermarriage by socioeconomic status. Two measures of the socioeconomic level of husbands and wives in the most frequent type of
mixed marriage — black-white — are presented in Table 13.18. These
measures, education and income, show the proportion of black men
who had entered their first marriage with a single white woman during
the 1960's and whose marriages were still intact in 1970. Overall,
nearly 2 percent of the black men had married a white woman. However, about two to four times as large a proportion of black men in
the top level as in the lowest level shown had married a white woman.
Likewise, more than twice as large a proportion of the upper-level as
of the lower-level wives were involved in these marriages. Although
the cross-classification of levels for husbands and wives in these mixed
marriages does not show a completely consistent pattern, one general
conclusion nonetheless seems warranted: black-white intermarriage
has a greater probability of occurrence among persons of high education or income than among other persons.

Stability of interracial marriages. Although there are some indications that interracial marriages are not as likely as other marriages to
end in divorce,[11] the preponderance of evidence is to the contrary.
According to statistics for the United States as a whole, the proportion
of interracial marriages involving couples who married for the first
time in the 1950's and whose marriages were still intact in 1970 was
considerably smaller than the corresponding proportion of couples
who were of the same race. Thus, data from the 1960 and 1970

Table 13.18. Percent of black men married to white women, both married once, married 1960 to 1970, by years of school completed and income in 1969 of husband and wife: United States, 1970

Years of school completed by--		Percent of black men married to white wives	Income in 1969 of--		Percent of black men married to white wives
Husband	Wife		Husband	Wife	
Total	Total	1.8	Total	Total	1.8
	0-8 years	1.4		Under $3,000	1.6
	9-12 years	1.5		$3,000-$6,999	2.0
	13 or more	3.2		$7,000-$9,999	2.3
				$10,000 or more	3.7
0-8 years	Total	1.1	Under $3,000	Total	1.6
	0-8 years	1.1		Under $3,000	1.3
	9-12 years	1.1		$3,000 or more	2.7
	13 or more	1.6	$3,000-$6,999	Total	1.7
9-12 years	Total	1.6		Under $3,000	1.5
	0-8 years	1.6		$3,000 or more	2.0
	9-12 years	1.5	$7,000-$9,999	Total	1.9
	13 or more	2.0		Under $3,000	2.0
13 or more	Total	3.5		$3,000 or more	1.8
	0-12 years	2.7	$10,000 or more	Total	2.9
	13 or more	4.2		Under $3,000	2.9
				$3,000 or more	2.8

Source: U.S. Bureau of the Census, 1970 Census of Population, Vol. II-4C, Marital Status, tables 15 and 16.

censuses show that 90 percent of the white-white and 78 percent of the black-black first marriages of the 1950's were still intact in 1970, as compared with 63 percent of those involving a black husband and a white wife and only 47 percent of those with a white husband and a black wife.[12] Results of the 1980 census will be watched for evidence of either an increase or a decrease in the relative stability of these four types of marriage.

Children and parents of different race. An interesting sidelight on racial intermarriage is the reported race of the child when the parents are of unlike races. According to a tabulation on which a forthcoming census report is to be based, 1 percent of the 78 million children living with one or both parents in 1970 had a race reported for them that was different from that of one or both parents in the household. This proportion varied widely from one-half of 1 percent for white children to 1 percent for black children, 11 percent for Chinese, 13 percent for Japanese, and 24 percent for Indian children. Among children living with two parents of unlike race, five were classified according to the race of the father for every two who were classified according to the race of the mother. Within this framework, Indian and Japanese children were assigned the race of the mother nearly as often as that of the father; by contrast, white and black children were classified as having the same race as the mother less than half as often as that of the father; and only one-sixth of the Chinese children with parents of unlike race were classified as having a Chinese mother. These contrasting findings evidently have grown out of substantial differences among the racial groups in the degree of equality with which the children's fathers and mothers regard each other.

A very small but sociologically significant group of 85,000 children in 1970 were identified as living with two parents but were classified as of a different race from that of either parent. Presumably most of these were adopted children. About 70,000 of the children lived with two parents of the same race; two-thirds had white parents. About half as many of the children were white with two black parents as were black with two white parents (8 percent versus 18 percent of the 85,000); 13 percent were American Indians with two white parents, 7 percent Korean with white parents, and 4 percent Japanese with white parents. Of the 15,000 children living with a lone parent of a race different from the child's race, nine of every ten lived with a white parent. These results are consistent with a tendency for white couples to adopt children of other races on a selective basis; but, of course, the level of the numbers and some of the differences among the results may reflect difficulties in obtaining accurate reporting on race in households with members of different races.

Living Arrangements of Children and Adults

Living arrangements of children. In the usual situation, young children live in a home with both of their parents. Although this is still the predominant living arrangement, it is much less typical now than a decade or two ago, and it is also much less characteristic of some social groups than others. Thus, the proportion of children under 18 years of age who were living with two parents declined from 89 percent in 1960 to 81 percent in 1974, and the proportion living with two parents in 1974 varied widely from 87 percent for white children to only 51 percent for black children under 18 (Tables 9.12 and 13.19).

Table 13.19. Living arrangements of children under 18 years of age, by race and age of child and marital status of parents: United States, 1974 and 1970

(Numbers in thousands)

Year and marital status of parents	Children under 18			Children under 6		
	Total	White	Black	Total	White	Black
Total, 1974	67,047	56,431	9,526	19,852	16,586	2,914
Percent	100.0	100.0	100.0	100.0	100.0	100.0
Living with two parents	81.4	86.7	50.7	83.2	89.2	49.3
Living with one parent	15.6	11.6	39.6	13.8	9.6	38.5
Mother only	14.4	10.4	37.8	13.2	9.0	37.3
Father only	1.3	1.2	1.8	0.6	0.6	1.1
Parent never married	1.5	0.4	7.9	2.8	0.9	14.0
Parent separated	4.9	2.9	16.7	4.8	3.1	14.7
Parent divorced	5.4	5.1	7.0	3.9	3.8	4.6
Other	3.9	3.2	8.0	2.3	1.7	5.3
Living with neither parent	3.0	1.7	9.7	2.9	1.2	12.2
Total, 1970	69,523	59,125	9,463	20,931	17,671	2,949
Percent	100.0	100.0	100.0	100.0	100.0	100.0
Living with two parents	83.1	87.2	57.5	84.7	89.2	57.9
Both in first marriage	68.7	72.6	44.7	71.9	79.5	48.1
Both previously divorced	3.7	3.9	2.5	3.0	3.2	1.7
One previously divorced	9.0	9.2	8.2	8.8	9.2	6.9
Other	1.6	1.5	2.0	1.0	0.9	2.2
Living with one parent	13.4	10.3	33.1	12.3	8.9	32.8
Mother only	11.5	8.5	30.2	10.8	7.6	30.4
Father only	1.9	1.8	2.9	1.5	1.3	2.4
Parent never married	1.3	0.5	6.6	2.4	0.9	11.3
Parent separated	3.6	2.1	13.2	3.6	2.2	11.8
Parent divorced	3.8	3.6	5.3	2.8	2.7	3.7
Other	4.7	4.1	8.1	3.5	3.1	6.0
Living with neither parent	3.5	2.5	9.4	3.0	1.9	9.3

Source: U.S. Bureau of the Census, Current Population Reports, Series P-20, No. 271, "Marital Status and Living Arrangements: March 1974," tables 4 and 5; 1970 Census of Population, Vol. II-4B, Persons by Family Characteristics, tables 1 and 8.

Further refinement of the data reveals a major finding in Table 13.19, namely, that only a little over two-thirds (69 percent) of the children under 18 in 1970 were living in families with both natural parents present and in their first marriage. Even more revealing is the fact that this proportion was well below one-half (45 percent) for black children under 18, although it was still quite low (73 percent) for white children. Corresponding figures limited to children of school age were lower, 43 percent and 71 percent, respectively.[13]

These findings imply that in 1970 more than one-half of the black school children and more than one-fourth of the white school children were living in an atypical home in the sense that they were living with one or both parents who were stepparents; or were living with a separated, divorced, widowed, or never-married parent; or were living apart from either parent.[14] Moreover, the proportion of children living thus has undoubtedly been increasing since 1970, in view of the fact that by the mid-1970's the separation and divorce rates were higher and the proportion of births that were illegitimate had risen still higher. For those who are greatly concerned about this situation, one relevant thought is that children from these homes at least have more company now than before; that is, they have less reason to feel unique and different from other children than those in similar circumstances a few years ago. In addition, certainly a minority — perhaps a majority — of the children whose parents have been divorced become better adjusted in their new living arrangements than they were formerly.[15]

Preschool children are more likely than older children to be living with a never-married mother, as can be seen by the information in Table 13.19. Most of the mothers of these children eventually marry, but some unpublished research[16] suggests that a majority of them probably do not marry the father of their illegitimate child(ren). On the other hand, school-age children are more likely than younger children to be living with a divorced or widowed mother, perhaps in part because the presence of children in this age range may tend to make couples with marital problems postpone divorce longer than the average interval (7 years) between marriage and divorce.

A frequently occurring arrangement for black children is that they live in the home of their grandparents. According to data in the 1970 source cited in Table 13.19, 9 percent of the black children under 18 years of age in 1970 were grandchildren of the head of the household where they lived. Over half these children had neither parent present. By contrast, only 2 percent of the white children under 18 lived with their grandparents, and close to two-thirds of them had at least one parent present also.

Young children have better-educated but less affluent parents than older children who still live at home. Again, data from the 1970 source cited in Table 13.19 show that 16 percent of the children under 6 years of age have a college graduate as the head of their family, as compared with 9 percent of those 18 to 24 years old. On the other hand, the younger children live in families with only two-thirds as much income ($9,000 in 1969) as the older children ($13,000). These findings reflect not only the younger parents of the preschool children, but also the older average age at which upper-group sons and daughters marry or leave their parental homes for other reasons.

The quality of life among children living with two parents contrasts sharply with that among children living with only one parent, on the average, at least in the sense that median family incomes for the two groups are quite different ($11,000 versus $4,500 in 1969). When the contrast involves additional factors, including race and age of child, the range of the difference in family income is much greater. The median family income in 1969 for black children under 6 years of age living with their mother but not their father was a meager $2,600; whereas the comparable income for families of white children 18 to 24 years old living with two parents was $14,500, according to data in the 1970 report cited in Table 13.19. Of course, the majority of the very young children in single-parent families will eventually have two parents, but their available resources for a healthful livelihood generally will be more limited in the meantime.[17]

Living arrangements of adults. Although the foregoing discussion of the living arrangements of children and the earlier discussion of changes in marital status have a close relation to the living arrangements of adults, nearly three of every five households contain no young sons or daughters of the head, and nearly 4 percent of the adults live in "nonhouseholds," that is, in institutions or other group quarters (rooming houses, college dormitories, military barracks, and the like). In this context, the 70 million households maintained by adults in 1974 had an average size of 3.0 persons, including 2.0 persons 18 years old and over and 1.0 child under 18. These averages are down from 3.3 persons per household in 1960 (comprising 2.1 persons 18 and over and 1.2 under 18) when there were 53 million households. The decline in adult household members is largely a consequence of an increasing amount of voluntary and involuntary exclusion of both young adult and elderly relatives of the household head, so that households with middle-aged heads are becoming increasingly "nuclear."[18] The decline in child members is, of course, a result of falling fertility rates during the last decade or so. The practice of married couples living in with relatives ("doubling up") is now limited to only 1 percent of all couples, as compared with 2 percent in 1960.

Between 1960 and 1974 the rate of growth in the number of households differed widely by type of household. With the delay in marriage and the increase in separation and divorce, the number of husband-wife households increased by only 18 percent; meantime, the number of households with a female head and no husband present increased much faster, by 67 percent or nearly four times as rapidly, and the much smaller number with a male head and no wife present increased even faster, by 79 percent. A primary reason for the faster increase in the number of households with no spouse of the head present was the nearly doubling during the 14-year period in the number of persons living entirely alone in a house or apartment. Interestingly, the number of men living alone grew by 107 percent in this period, while their female counterparts grew by 88 percent. Table 13.20 confirms that these differential rates of increase were still in full force during the early 1970's, as well as during the 14-year period considered as a whole.

The largest *numerical increase* in households in the period from 1970 to 1974 was that for households with a woman as the head and no husband present, namely, 2.7 million. This increase was evenly divided between those living alone (mostly elderly widowed and divorced women) and those with young children present (mostly separated, divorced, and never-married mothers). Although husband-wife households involved a far larger proportion of the households, their number went up only 2.4 million during the four years.

The largest *rate of increase* in households during the early 1970's was for households with a man as the head and no wife present, namely, 37 percent. Two-thirds of the 1.9 million increase in this type of household occurred among men living alone; also, two-thirds of the increase occurred among men who were under 35 years old. Again, the largest rate of increase occurred among households with a man as the head who had no relatives present but who was sharing his living quarters with one or more partners or other nonrelatives (78 percent increase). Among such men who were under 35 years old, the number more than doubled between 1970 and 1974.

Unrelated adults living together. For 1960 and 1970, census figures show how many heads of households with no relatives present were

Table 13.20. Living arrangements of household members 14 years old and over, by sex: United States, 1974 and 1970

(Numbers in thousands)

Living arrangements of persons in households	Male, 14 years old and over			Female, 14 years old and over		
	1974	1970	1974/1970	1974	1970	1974/1970
Total in households	74,740	68,730	1.09	81,957	75,955	1.08
Head or spouse of head	53,862	49,588	1.09	62,784	57,696	1.09
Husband or wife	46,787	44,408	1.05	46,787	44,408	1.05
No children under 18	20,930	18,397	1.14	20,930	18,397	1.14
Some under 18	25,857	26,011	0.99	25,857	26,011	0.99
Head, no spouse present	7,075	5,180	1.37	15,997	13,288	1.20
No relatives present	5,654	3,970	1.42	9,288	7,795	1.19
Living alone	4,742	3,458	1.37	8,626	7,234	1.19
With nonrelatives	912	512	1.78	662	561	1.18
With relatives present	1,421	1,210	1.17	6,709	5,493	1.22
No children under 18	916	782	1.17	2,204	2,195	1.00
Some under 18	505	428	1.18	4,505	3,298	1.37
Not head or spouse of head	20,879	19,142	1.09	19,173	18,259	1.05
Living with relatives	19,291	17,968	1.07	18,029	17,365	1.04
Child 14 to 17 of head	7,979	7,443	1.07	7,532	7,093	1.06
Other relative of head	11,312	10,525	1.07	10,497	10,272	1.02
Living with nonrelatives	1,587	1,174	1.35	1,144	894	1.28

Source: U.S. Bureau of the Census, Current Population Reports, Series P-20, No. 276, "Household and Family Characteristics: March 1974," table 17; No. 271, "Marital Status and Living Arrangements: March 1974," tables 2 and 6; No. 218, "Household and Family Characteristics: March 1970," table 17; and No. 212, "Marital Status and Family Status: 1970," tables 2 and 6.

sharing their living quarters with nonrelatives who were recorded as "partners" or "resident employees" of the opposite sex; such data are not available for 1974. Summary data for this "quasi-family" type of living arrangement at the two census dates are presented in Table 13.21.

The most striking feature of this table is the manifold increase in the number of men and women reported as partners living in the same house or apartment without being married. The number recorded in 1970 was over eight times as large as that in 1960. Even though the absolute number in 1970 was still small, it nonetheless involved the lives of at least 143,000 men and 143,000 women, or a total of nearly 300,000 adults. Moreover, Current Population Survey data in press at the time of this writing (December 1975) show that the number

Table 13.21. Household heads sharing their living quarters with an un-related partner or resident employee of opposite sex and no related persons, by sex, age, and race: United States, 1970 and 1960

Sex, age, and race of head of household	Sharing quarters with unrelated partner of opposite sex			Sharing quarters with resident employee of opposite sex		
	1970	1960	1970/1960	1970	1960	1970/1960
Total	142,848	17,320	8.2	49,981	53,729	0.9
Male head	104,516	9,359	11.1	46,571	48,864	1.0
Under 25 years	22,183	444	50.0	1,536	101	15.2
25-44 years	36,661	3,252	11.3	5,698	4,496	1.3
45-64 years	28,773	3,320	8.7	17,348	19,028	0.9
65 and over	16,899	2,379	7.1	21,989	25,239	0.9
White	83,837	5,903	14.2	41,830	43,955	1.0
Other race	20,679	3,456	6.0	4,741	4,909	1.0
Female head	38,332	7,925	4.8	3,410	4,865	0.7
Under 25 years	7,733	469	16.5	46	...	...
25-44 years	8,792	1,316	6.7	268	289	0.9
45-64 years	12,795	3,828	3.3	1,084	1,860	0.6
65 and over	9,012	2,312	3.9	2,012	2,716	0.7
White	28,698	6,394	4.5	2,557	3,453	0.7
Other race	9,634	1,531	6.3	853	1,412	0.6

Source: U.S. Bureau of the Census, 1970 Census of Population, Vol. II-4B, Persons by Family Characteristics, table 11; and 1960 Census of Population, Vol. II-4B, Persons by Family Characteristics, table 15.

of household heads with nonrelatives but no relatives present increased by 94 percent between 1970 and 1975. Therefore, it seems reasonable to assume that the number of heads together with their partners of opposite sex had climbed far above the 300,000 level by the mid-1970's. Of course, some of the recorded increase may result from a growing tendency to report such living arrangements more frankly, but even that is a symptom of social change. Many couples who live in this way regard doing so as an extension of the courting process.[19]

The increase in "partnering" during the 1960's was twice as large among men sharing their home with a female partner as among women sharing their home with a male partner. As of 1970, about three white men to every one white woman shared their home in this manner, but among household heads of other races (mostly black persons) men thus sharing their homes exceeded women sharers by only two to one.[20] For both males and females, partnering increased most among the young (those under 25) but also at a rate above average for those in the next older age bracket for which data are available (25 to 44). Among those under 25 years of age involved in partnerships, about one-fifth of the men and one-third of the women were students enrolled in college. The age distribution of partners shifted from only 32 percent under 45 in 1960 to 53 percent of this age range in 1970. The practice of maintaining such informal living arrangements has been going on for some time at a more extensive level among older people, often in the form of common-law marriages. The thirteen states that recognize common-law marriages are listed below in the section on legal and administrative aspects of marriage and divorce.

Another living arrangement, which may be identified as "companioning," involves a household head and a resident employee of opposite sex but no relatives of the head present. Examples include a man who has a woman living with him as a housekeeper, nurse, or hired companion, and a woman with a handyman living in. Persons maintaining a home in this manner are generally older than those living as partners: more than 90 percent of the companioning household heads were over age 45 in 1960 and 85 percent were in this age range in 1970. More than 90 percent at both dates were maintained by a man with a female companion sharing the house or apartment. About 100,000 adults lived in this manner in 1970, a decline of nearly 10 percent from 1960. White persons were more heavily represented than in the general population.

Both head-partner and head-companion couples in many instances seem to operate in many exterior ways like conventional husband-wife families. In fact, the Bureau of the Census has been asked by some of its data-users to consider providing more data for these quasi-families and for communes, which in a sense constitute family economic units, so that the results can be compared with, or combined with, those for conventional families. The population in these types of "variant family forms" numbered close to one-half million in 1970 and seems likely to be much more numerous by 1980.

Another 1.2 million adults in 1970 were sharing the living quarters of another person of the *same* sex as "partners," with no relatives of the household head present. The 600,000 households involved in 1970 were three times as numerous as in 1960, according to the sources cited in Table 13.21. The number in 1970 constituted 3 percent of adults who were not married. Most of the same-sex partners were young and white; they were about evenly divided between men and women. This type of living arrangement probably less often involved dependence of one partner on the other for economic sustenance than either the opposite-sex partners or the head-companion couples.

This discussion of the living arrangements of adults has not covered the marital status of the persons involved, except for those in husband-wife families and quasi-families. In later sections the living arrangements of separated, divorced, widowed, and single adults will be analyzed in some detail.

Employment and Income of Wives and Mothers

Trends and variations in employment. The more rapid increase in the labor-force participation of women than men since 1960 has been one of the most significant economic changes of that period. Between 1960 and 1974, the number of female workers rose by 12.6 million, from 23.3 million to 35.9 million or by 50 percent, while that for male workers rose by only 8.4 million from 48.9 million to 57.3 million or by only 17 percent. Thus, the number of working women was less than one-half the number of working men in 1960 but was nearly two-thirds as great by 1974. These dissimilar overall changes reflect not only a sharp increase in the employment rates for women of nearly all age groups but also declining employment rates for both young men of college age and elderly men of retirement age. A still longer time perspective shows that the number of women in the labor force has more than doubled since the end of World War II, while the corresponding number of men has increased by only 30 percent. However, women are much less likely than men to work full time. The 1970 census showed that only 43 percent of women who worked in 1969 had worked 50 to 52 weeks; the comparable figure for men was 67 percent.

Almost all of the increase in the employment of women during the last decade or two has occurred among married women, the group that is featured in this section. In 1960, 31 percent of the married women with husband present were in the labor force (Table 7.3), whereas 43 percent were in the labor force in 1974 (Table 13.22). Several developments during the period may have contributed to this substantial rate of change. The high level of business activity, partly on account of the Vietnam conflict, attracted more women into the labor market as more men were being drawn into military service; with a diminished supply of men of marriageable age, more women remained in school longer and thus built up their skills for the performance of paid work; marriages were delayed, and the birth rate fell, as an increasing number of women used more of their energy for work outside the home than for rearing children; and as more married women gained work experience — usually in locations quite apart from those of their husbands — they were inclined more often to develop a sense of economic and personal independence that may have contributed to the increase in separation and then divorce for a while before remarriage.[21] At the same time, millions of couples would no longer have their marriage healthily intact if it were not for the contribution of the wife's employment, which raises the family income into the middle range.

The worker rates for married women varied widely according to their age, education, and number of children, and by the income of their husbands. The range among subgroups of women, shown in Table 13.22, is from a little over 20 percent to nearly 80 percent in the labor force. Especially high rates occurred in 1974 among young

Table 13. 22. Percent of wives in the labor force, by presence and age of own children, age and years of school completed by wife, and income of husband in 1973: United States, 1974

Characteristics	All wives	With no children under 18	Some 6 to 17 only	Some under 6
All wives	43.0	43.1	51.2	34.4
Age:				
16-24 years	52.3	72.3	60.5	35.9
25-34 years	46.1	77.7	56.6	34.5
35-44 years	50.1	60.0	53.4	32.2
45-54 years	49.6	53.5	45.5	24.1
55 years and over	23.6	22.9	38.8	...
Education of wife:				
0-11 years	32.2	27.5	43.9	30.5
12 years	46.0	49.5	53.1	33.5
13-15 years	48.1	53.2	52.7	37.0
16 years and over	58.8	67.3	62.0	43.0
Income of husband:				
Under $3,000	35.5	32.0	54.6	36.8
$3,000-$4,999	35.8	31.2	53.6	38.8
$5,000-$6,999	43.3	40.4	54.4	40.6
$7,000-$9,999	49.3	51.7	56.9	39.8
$10,000 and over	43.4	48.1	48.9	30.1

Source: U.S. Bureau of Labor Statistics, Special Labor Force Report 173, "Marital and Family Characteristics of the Labor Force, March 1974," tables F and P.

childless wives; the rates were only moderately lower for wives whose children were all of school age, but were much lower for those with children of preschool age. Nonetheless, the worker rate for mothers of preschoolers went up abruptly between 1963 (Table 7.9) and 1974 from 23 percent to 34 percent — a faster rate of change than that for either childless women or mothers of school-age children only.

Worker rates were higher for wives with successively larger amounts of education, within each category according to presence of children. Thus the level of educational attainment tends to determine the degree of employability of wives and/or the degree of interest wives have in being employed. The especially low worker rates for childless women of low education — as well as for childless older women and for childless women with low-income husbands — should be recognized as being heavily weighted by elderly wives who are generally too old to work outside the home.

The highest worker rates for wives were reached among women whose husbands' incomes were one or two intervals below the top, as shown by Table 13.22. This finding is interpreted as evidence that the employability and/or work interest of wives tends to increase as the income level of the husband increases, but that an upper point is reached where counteracting factors tend to reduce worker rates for wives. Among these factors may be a decreasing sense of need for the wife to work and/or a feeling that the prestige of an upper-group family tends to be negatively affected by even partial dependence on the employment of the wife to supplement the husband's income.

The discussion of employment deserves to include mention of the sharp upturn in unemployment during the 1970's. As recently as 1966 to 1969, the unemployment rate was at the low level of 3 percent for men and 5 percent for women. But by 1974, the average unemployment rate for the year was 5 percent for men and 7 percent for women, and during the first half of 1975 the rate for men zoomed to 8 percent and for women to 10 percent, according to data from the Bureau of Labor Statistics. A continuing high unemployment rate would probably tend to reduce both marriage and divorce rates.

Contribution of wives to family income. Table 13.23 shows that black children in 1974 were about one-fourth more likely than white children to have a working mother. It also shows that the average income of black families with the mother in the labor force was about $2,300 higher if the mother worked than if she did not work; the comparable figure was only about $1,000 for families of white children. Even so, the median family income of white children with working mothers remained about half again as high as that of black children with working mothers ($14,500 versus $9,700). Children with a mother but no father present were more likely to have a working mother (53 percent) than those with both parents present (41 percent); the median family income of the fatherless children was only about one-third as high as that of the children with both parents present.

An indication of how much working wives strengthen the family's economic situation is summarized in the fact that wives with earnings contributed about one-fourth (26 percent) of their family income during the preceding year, on the average, according to 1974 statistics from Table U of the report cited in Table 13.23. The wife's contribution to family income was especially large, on the average, if she worked full time for the entire year (38 percent) or if the family income was quite low (35 percent for families with less than $2,000 income). However, only one-half of the wives had earnings in 1973.

Table 13.23. Number of own children under 18 years old and their median family income in 1973, by type of family, labor force status of parents, and race: United States, March 1974

(Number of children in thousands)

Type of family, race, and employment status of father	Number of own children under 18			Median family income	
	Total	With mother in labor force		Total	With mother in labor force
		Number	Percent of total		
All own children under 18	63,542	26,768	42.1	$12,795	$13,762
White	54,504	22,292	40.9	13,485	14,470
Black	8,068	4,028	49.9	7,365	9,673
In husband–wife families	54,154	22,165	40.9	13,909	15,000+
Father employed	50,624	20,820	41.1	14,226	15,000+
Father unemployed	1,482	588	39.7	10,285	11,818
Father not in labor force	2,048	757	37.0	7,327	9,148
In families with female head, no husband present	8,648	4,603	53.2	4,729	6,193
In other families	740	...	...	11,867	...

Source: U.S. Bureau of Labor Statistics, Special Labor Force Report 174, "Children of Working Mothers, March 1974," tables 1, A, A-1, and B.

In at least one segment of the population the gap between the income of blacks and whites has been closed, thanks to the contribution of black wives. In the North and West, black husband-wife families with the husband under 35 years old, in which both the husband and wife were earners, had as much income in the early 1970's as their white counterparts. However, this impressive achievement applied to only 6 percent of the black families in the United States. Details of this development are presented in a Census Bureau report entitled *The Social and Economic Status of the Black Population in the United States, 1974.*

Wives with more income than their husbands. Another noteworthy development in family economics has been a rapid rate of increase in the minority of wives who have more income than their husbands. Several different approaches can be used to throw light on the extent of the change and on how the wives with more income are distributed. One of the most direct measures of the increase during the 1960's in this group of wives consists in a comparison of data on the "chief income recipient" in the family; this type of information is shown in reports from the 1960 and 1970 censuses entitled *Persons by Family Characteristics* (Table 26 for 1960 and Table 14 for 1970).

According to these sources, 5.7 percent of the wives in husband-wife families in 1960 had more income from all sources than their husbands, and in 1970 the comparable figure was 7.4 percent. Although these proportions are small, the rate of change was substantial, three-tenths within one decade. During the same period of time, the corresponding increase for white wives was from 4.9 percent to 7.0 percent; for wives of other races the figure was 7.6 percent in 1960, and for black wives in 1970 it was 11.1 percent. Thus, as might have been expected, a considerably larger proportion of black than white wives have more income than their husbands. Moreover, above-average proportions of wives with more income than their husbands were found in 1970 among families with the husband under 25 years old (16 percent) and with the husband 55 to 64 years old (10 percent). These age groups include relatively large proportions of wives who have not yet had any children or whose children have already left home.

A great deal can be observed about wives' versus their husbands' incomes by studying Table 13.24. Here the line is not drawn between those with a dollar more or less than the other, but between those in

the same or a higher or lower *income interval* than the other, as
defined by the categories shown in the table. According to this approach, 6.3 percent of the 44 million wives in husband-wife families
in 1970 had more income than their husbands, 5.6 percent had about
the same income as their husbands, and 7.0 percent had incomes in
the next higher interval than their husbands. For the entire 19 percent
of wives in these three categories, the great majority of husbands had
quite low median incomes, below $4,000. For the other 81 percent of
wives, the husbands had incomes that were "very perceptibly higher"
than theirs, that is, the husbands had incomes that were two or more
intervals higher than that of their wives; in these families the husbands'
median income was more than twice as high, $8,800. These findings
show that families in which the husband has less income or not much
more income than his wife tend to have small total incomes.

Another approach throws additional light on the relatively low
income of families in which the wife has some income but not a very
large one. Data from the same source as Table 13.24 show that the

Table 13.24. Income of husband in 1969 by income of wife in 1969:
United States, 1970

(Numbers in thousands)

Income of husband	All husband-wife families		Husband's income interval—				
			Lower than wife's	Same as wife's	Higher than wife's		
					Total	By one interval	By 2+ intervals
	Number	Percent					
Total	44,002	100.0	6.3	5.6	88.1	7.0	81.1
Without income	447	100.0	57.3	42.7	...	...	...
With income	43,555	100.0	5.8	5.2	89.0	7.1	81.9
$1-$999 or loss	1,155	100.0	34.2	33.7	32.1	32.1	...
$1,000-$1,999	2,322	100.0	24.1	15.9	60.0	29.7	30.2
$2,000-$2,999	2,239	100.0	18.6	9.1	72.3	14.5	57.8
$3,000-$3,999	2,512	100.0	13.1	9.0	77.8	9.2	68.6
$4,000-$4,999	2,616	100.0	9.0	7.5	83.6	9.8	73.8
$5,000-$5,999	3,233	100.0	6.0	5.6	88.3	8.0	80.4
$6,000-$6,999	3,625	100.0	3.9	4.1	92.0	6.0	86.0
$7,000-$7,999	4,109	100.0	2.4	2.7	94.9	4.2	90.6
$8,000-$9,999	7,320	100.0	1.0	2.4	96.5	2.6	93.9
$10,000 and over	14,425	100.0	0.5	1.7	97.8	2.7	95.2
Median income	$7,992	...	$2,723	$3,734	$8,504	$3,705	$8,802

Source: U.S. Bureau of the Census, 1970 Census of Population, Vol. II-8A,
Sources and Structure of Family Income, table 9.

18.8 million wives with no income at all were married to husbands with more income than the average (median of $8,800 versus the overall median of $8,000). The medians for husbands of the relatively few (1.5 million) wives with incomes above $8,000 were the highest ($9,500 for husbands whose wives had incomes of $8,000 to $9,999 and $11,700 for husbands whose wives had $10,000 and over). Thus, wives with both no income and the highest incomes tend to be married to men with above-average incomes.

Separated and Divorced Persons

Separation prior to divorce. Generally the divorcing couple separate before the final decree of divorce is issued, and different places of residence are established for the husband and the wife. The duration of marriage prior to the final separation as well as the time interval between separation and divorce is of interest to students of the family. While national statistics are not available, information on these subjects for 1973 from ten states is presented in Table 13.25, along with statistics on duration of marriage prior to divorce for the Divorce Registration Area.

Before final separation prior to divorce, more than one in four of the marriages had lasted for 10 years or longer and half of them had lasted for at least 5 years. However, there is a strong concentration of cases in which the final separation came within a short interval after marriage: one-third of the separations came in 2 years or less.

The time interval between separation and divorce is usually a short one. In more than two-thirds of the cases it was 1 year or less, and in nine cases out of ten it was 4 years or less.

Marriages that end in divorce now last, on the average, for slightly less than 7 years. In 1973 the median stood at 6.6 years, as compared with 6.9 years in 1969 and 7.2 years in 1965, according to published and unpublished data from the U.S. National Center for Health Statistics (see Table 13.25). Many of these marriages are of long duration; more than one in three of them lasted for 10 years or longer. One in five ended within 2 years, and one in three ended in 4 years or less.

Age and living arrangements. During the 1950's, the number of divorced persons in the United States who had not remarried increased by about 28 percent, as compared with an increase of 19 percent for

Table 13.25. Duration of marriage to separation prior to divorce, separation to divorce, and marriage to divorce: Selected states, 1973

Number of years	Duration of marriage to separation	Duration of separation	Duration of marriage
	Prior to divorce[a]		
Percent[b]	100.0	100.0	100.0
1 year or less	24.3	71.1	13.1
2 years	10.2	12.0	9.0
3 years	8.8	6.1	9.2
4 years	6.9	3.2	8.1
5 years	5.7	1.9	6.9
6 years	4.8	1.3	5.8
7 years	4.1	0.9	5.1
8 years	3.5	0.6	4.4
9 years	3.1	0.5	3.8
10 years or more	28.6	2.4	34.6
Median years	5.0	0.7	6.6

Source: U.S. National Center for Health Statistics, Monthly Vital Statistics Report, Vol. 24, No. 4 Supplement, "Summary Report, Final Divorce Statistics, 1973," table 3, and unpublished tabulations.

[a]Basic data include reported annulments.

[b]First two columns based on data for California, Connecticut, Hawaii, Kansas, Missouri, Nebraska, New York, Vermont, Virginia, and Wisconsin. Third column based on data for the Divorce Registration Area (29 states).

the total population. During the 1960's, however, the contrast was far greater: the number of divorced men increased by 48 percent and divorced women by 62 percent, while the total population increased by only 13 percent. And during the 4 years between 1970 and 1974, the number of divorced persons increased by another 20 percent, with the number of divorced men reaching 2.3 million and the number of divorced women 3.6 million by 1974 (see the source of Table 13.8 above). In those 4 years, the total population increased by less than 4 percent. In round numbers, there were 15 divorced persons (who had not remarried) in 1974 for every 8 in 1960.

The rate of increase in the divorced population between 1960 and 1970 was much higher among young adults and the elderly than it was among those 35 to 44 years old — the age group born in the depression years of the 1930's and among whom the proportion married was most nearly universal (Table 13.26). The number of divorced persons under 25 years old, both men and women, doubled during the 1960's. Also, the number of divorced women 65 years old and over doubled during the decade, and divorced men of this age group increased by one-half. However, the corresponding increase for those 35 to 44 years old was only about one-third.

Statistics from a nationwide survey in 1971 show the tendency for persons who end their first marriage in divorce to do so at an earlier age in recent years. These data are from Table G of the source cited in Table 13.1. They show that women who were born in 1900 to 1914 and whose first marriages ended in divorce had a median age of 33

Table 13.26. Divorced persons, by age, relationship, and sex: United States, 1970 and 1960

(Numbers in thousands)

Age and relationship	Divorced men			Divorced women		
	1970	1960	$\frac{1970}{1960}$	1970	1960	$\frac{1970}{1960}$
Total	1,927	1,304	1.48	3,004	1,858	1.62
Age:						
Under 25 years	126	61	2.07	246	122	2.02
25-34 years	379	226	1.68	585	340	1.72
35-44 years	406	303	1.34	647	471	1.37
45-54 years	427	307	1.39	663	446	1.49
55-64 years	333	235	1.42	492	298	1.65
65 years and over	256	172	1.49	372	181	2.06
Relationship:						
In households	1,756	1,132	1.55	2,946	1,804	1.63
Head of household	1,125	603	1.87	2,275	1,236	1.84
Relatives present	224	128	1.75	1,312	692	1.90
No relatives	901	475	1.90	963	544	1.77
Child of head	304	219	1.39	307	250	1.23
Under 45 years	237	171	1.39	248	205	1.21
45 and over	67	48	1.40	59	45	1.31
Other relative	153	156	0.98	234	215	1.09
Under 45 years	55	54	1.02	51	58	0.88
45 and over	98	102	0.96	183	157	1.17
Nonrelative	174	154	1.13	130	103	1.26
In group quarters	170	172	0.99	59	53	1.11
Institution	106	93	1.14	42	32	1.31
Other group quarters	64	79	0.81	17	22	0.77

Source: U.S. Bureau of the Census, 1970 Census of Population, Vol. II-4B, Persons by Family Characteristics, table 2; Vol. II-4C, Marital Status, table 4; 1960 Census of Population, Vol. II-4B, Persons by Family Characteristics, table 2; and Vol. II-4E, Marital Status, table 4.

years at the time of that divorce. Corresponding medians for younger women were 31 for those born in 1915 to 1919; 30 for those born in 1920 to 1924; 29 for those born in 1925 to 1929; and 28 for those born in 1930 to 1934. The last group, however, was only 37 to 41 years old at the time of the 1971 survey and therefore may be expected eventually to have a slightly higher median age at the ending of their first marriage — perhaps 29 or 30 years, but in any case lower than 33 years.

A substantial majority of divorced persons maintain their own households in bachelor quarters. In 1970, 76 percent of the divorced women and 58 percent of the divorced men were classified as house-hold heads. However, divorced women were far more likely than divorced men to have relatives (usually children) sharing their living quarters, and this difference increased during the 1960's. With the sharp increase in the number of divorced mothers during the decade, the number of divorced women who were household heads with rela-tives present nearly doubled (up 90 percent). In the same period, the number of divorced men who were household heads with *no* relatives present also nearly doubled (up 90 percent). Information is not avail-able on how many of the divorced persons were sharing their living quarters with one or more unrelated adults.

Below-average increases occurred during the 1960's among di-vorced persons who lived in with their parents as "child of head." Far-below-average increases occurred among divorced persons who lived in with other relatives or with nonrelatives. Likewise, there was little absolute change in the number of divorced persons living in institutions or other group quarters. In fact, only one-tenth of the increase in the divorced population during the 1960's occurred among persons who were not heads of households.

By far the largest rate of increase in the number of separated per-sons during the 1960's (65 percent) occurred among young adults — those under 25 years of age (Table 13.27). However, part of this increase is attributable to the fact that those who were 18 to 24 years old in 1970 had been born during the period of high birth rates after World War II; the entire population in this age range increased by 51 percent between 1960 and 1970. Like the divorced population aged 35 to 44, the separated population in this range showed the smallest rate of increase.

Also, like divorced persons, separated persons generally maintained their own home and increased this tendency during the relatively af-

Table 13.27. Separated persons, by age, relationship, and sex: United States, 1970 and 1960

(Numbers in thousands)

Age and relationship	Separated men			Separated women		
	1970	1960	$\frac{1970}{1960}$	1970	1960	$\frac{1970}{1960}$
Total	1,046	878	1.19	1,740	1,316	1.32
Age:						
Under 25 years	116	69	1.68	271	167	1.62
25–34 years	228	179	1.27	430	329	1.31
35–44 years	213	203	1.05	394	330	1.19
45–54 years	209	184	1.14	324	251	1.29
55–64 years	155	134	1.16	200	150	1.33
65 years and over	125	109	1.15	122	89	1.37
Relationship:						
In households	958	775	1.24	1,705	1,278	1.33
Head of household	557	373	1.49	1,246	809	1.54
Relatives present	112	81	1.38	922	575	1.60
No relatives	445	292	1.52	324	234	1.38
Child of head	177	150	1.18	224	204	1.10
Under 45 years	151	128	1.18	201	187	1.07
45 and over	26	22	1.18	23	17	1.35
Other relative	103	123	.84	161	178	0.90
Under 45 years	66	58	1.14	64	78	0.82
45 and over	47	65	0.72	97	100	0.97
Nonrelative	121	127	0.95	74	72	1.03
In group quarters	88	103	0.85	35	38	0.92
Institution	54	57	0.95	22	24	0.92
Other group quarters	34	46	0.74	13	14	0.93

Source: U.S. Bureau of the Census, 1970 Census of Population, Vol. II-4B, Persons by Family Characteristics, table 2; Vol. II-4C, Marital Status, table 4; 1960 Census of Population, Vol. II-4B, Persons by Family Characteristics, table 2; and Vol. II-4E, Marital Status, table 4.

fluent period of the 1960's. Again, as for divorced persons, the most rapid increase occurred among sparated women who shared their homes with relatives (usually children) and separated men who maintained bachelor quarters with no relatives present. However, a larger proportion of separated persons than divorced persons in 1970 lived in with their parents or other relatives, partly because twice as large a proportion of the former were under 25 years of age.

Education and income of divorced persons by race. Tables 13.28 and 13.29 provide information on characteristics of the 3.6 million

Table 13.28. Percent known to have been divorced, for persons ever married 35 to 44 years old, by years of school completed, race, and sex: United States, 1970

Years of school completed and sex	Total	White	Black	Black White
Men ever married 35-44 years old	15.8	15.5	19.2	1.24
0-4 years of school	17.0	17.2	16.8	0.98
5-7 years	18.4	18.9	16.8	0.89
8 years	17.9	17.9	18.1	1.01
9-11 years	19.2	19.1	20.0	1.05
12 years	15.4	15.2	19.9	1.31
13-15 years	17.0	16.6	24.3	1.46
16 years	9.5	9.4	17.9	1.90
17 years or more	9.2	8.9	18.0	2.02
Median years completed	12.1	12.2	10.9	0.89
Women ever married 35-44 years old	17.5	16.9	22.8	1.35
0-4 years of school	17.2	16.4	20.9	1.27
5-7 years	20.1	20.4	19.5	0.96
8 years	20.4	20.3	21.0	1.03
9-11 years	23.0	23.0	23.4	1.02
12 years	15.2	14.6	23.3	1.60
13-15 years	16.5	15.7	28.6	1.82
16 years	9.4	8.7	20.1	2.31
17 years or more	16.7	16.1	25.7	1.60
Median years completed	12.1	12.1	11.3	0.93

Source: U.S. Bureau of the Census, 1970 Census of Population, Vol. II-4C, Marital Status, table 8.

persons 35 to 44 years old in 1970 who were known to have been divorced after their first marriage or after their most recent marriage.

In general, the proportion ever divorced is two to three times as large as the proportion currently separated or divorced; however, both sets of proportions in 1970 reached higher levels among those who started college but did not finish all 4 years than among those who terminated their education by graduating from high school (12 years) or from college (16 years). Moreover, "high school dropouts" (9 to 11 years) had the highest proportions known to have been divorced, exceeding the corresponding proportions who terminated their education after completing elementary school (8 years) or high school (12 years). As pointed out earlier, the type of personality and the experiences that cause a person to complete the broad level of school he or she starts must also tend to have a significant bearing on the chances that the marriage of such a person will last. One of the important experiences in this context is age at marriage; those who marry early are less likely to have completed the level of school that they entered.[22]

At nearly all levels of education, black persons 35 to 44 years old had a higher proportion ever divorced than did their white counterparts. Moreover, there was a definite tendency for this discrepancy to increase at the higher education levels. Evidently the mechanisms of social control that tend to inhibit divorce among better-educated whites must operate to a lesser degree among black persons with a similar amount of education.

Of special interest is the complex relation between money income and the extent of marital disruption in 1970 among different segments of the population 35 to 44 years old (Table 13.29). For white men, the percent ever divorced was consistently smaller at each successively higher level of income. Apparently families with relatively few worries about the provision of basic material necessities have more freedom to tackle the other problems they face.

For white women, the pattern is the reverse; the higher the woman's income, the larger the proportion who have been divorced. From the affluent woman's viewpoint a greater number of life-styles are available.

For black persons, the patterns are different from those for white persons. The range of variation in the percent known to have been divorced is smaller among the several income levels. Also, the relation between income and percent ever divorced is curvilinear for black men, with just as large a proportion ever divorced among high-income men as among low-income men. It may be that upper-level black men, on the economic scale as on the education scale, tend to experience less social pressure than upper-level white men to avoid ending a marriage in divorce. It is significant, however, that the pattern for black persons 35 to 44 is close to that of their white counterparts if the analysis of income data is limited to men with less than $10,000 per year (which includes approximately nine-tenths of the black men) and to women with less than $7,000 per year (which includes nine-tenths of the black women).

The last column of Table 13.29 brings out a strikingly consistent contrast between the proportion of blacks as compared with whites who were known to have been divorced: the higher the *man's* income,

Table 13.29. Percent known to have been divorced, for persons ever married 35 to 44 years old, by income in 1969, race, and sex: United States, 1970

Income in 1969 and sex	Total	White	Black	Black White
Men ever married 35-44 years old	15.8	15.5	19.2	1.24
Without income	30.6	32.8	25.9	0.79
With income:				
$1-$999 or loss	26.1	27.4	22.7	0.83
$1,000-$2,999	23.6	24.9	20.3	0.82
$3,000-$4,999	21.0	22.2	17.8	0.80
$5,000-$6,999	18.6	18.8	18.2	0.97
$7,000-$9,999	16.0	15.8	18.9	1.20
$10,000-$14,999	13.2	13.1	19.9	1.52
$15,000-$19,999	10.8	10.7	20.2	1.89
$20,000 and over	10.7	10.6	22.7	2.14
Median income	$8,409	$8,713	$6,127	0.70
Women ever married 35-44 years old	17.5	16.9	22.8	1.35
Without income	10.5	10.3	14.2	1.38
With income:				
$1-$999 or loss	15.6	14.7	22.5	1.53
$1,000-$2,999	19.9	19.1	24.0	1.26
$3,000-$4,999	22.6	22.1	26.5	1.20
$5,000-$6,999	27.2	27.0	29.4	1.09
$7,000-$9,999	30.2	30.5	29.1	0.95
$10,000-$14,999	31.6	32.2	29.5	0.92
$15,000 and over	30.0	30.9	25.5	0.83
Median income	$4,334	$4,103	$3,398	0.83

Source: U.S. Bureau of the Census, 1970 Census of Population, Vol. II-4C, Marital Status, tables 7 and 8.

the higher the ratio for *blacks* as compared with that for whites; however, the higher the *woman's* income, the higher the ratio for *whites* as compared with that for blacks. This is a remarkable demonstration of the extent to which the "rules of the game" may differ among socioeconomic groups with regard to how acceptable it is to enter into divorce sometime before the age of 45.

An interesting deviation from the overall pattern is the tendency for the proportion ever divorced among women 35 to 44 to taper off (or to fall slightly) at the upper part of the income distribution. This same pattern was also found among divorced women 14 and over in 1960 (Table 8.33). But the fact remains that the measure of divorce for *these* women in the upper-income groups remains well above the average for *all* women in their age group who have ever married.

Widows and Widowers

Age and living arrangements. One of every ten ever-married adults in the United States in 1970 had experienced widowhood — 4 percent of the men and 16 percent of the women. Of the 15.3 million persons 14 years old and over whose first or last marriage had ended in widowhood, 11.7 million, or three-fourths, were still widowed at the time of the census, according to data in the sources cited in Table 13.30. Although a majority of men in 1970 were "still married" by the time of their eighty-fifth birthday, one-fourth of these men had remarried. By contrast, a majority of women were still married shortly before their seventieth birthday, and one-fifth of these married women had remarried.

The number of widows rose substantially during the 1960's (by 22 percent), whereas the number of widowers changed very little. This is a reflection of the continuing increase in the gap between survival rates for men and women. The great majority of widowed persons are over 65 years old, but those who remarry usually have become widowed before they reach 65. Among widowed persons under 65, widows outnumber widowers by the lopsided ratio of 5 to 1 (5.1 widows per widower in 1970 and 4.8 in 1960). This situation results from a compounding of the effects of higher mortality and higher remarriage rates among widowers than widows.

Despite the great excess of widows as compared with widowers, only 13 percent more widows than widowers married in 1970. Moreover, only about one-half of the widowed persons who remarried were joined in marriage with another widowed person. Among the remaining remarriages of widowed persons, two-thirds were to divorced persons and one-third to single persons, for both men and women. Persons who remarry take into account many other characteristics of prospective partners than their previous marital status.

Among widowed persons, the type of living arrangement with the largest *volume* of increase during the 1960's was a home maintained apart from relatives. This growth is identified as the 2.0 million increase in widowed heads of households with no relatives present. Only 1 in 20 of the persons maintaining such homes had any nonrelatives living with them, and the other 19 out of 20 were living entirely alone

Table 13.30. Widowed persons, by age, relationship, and sex: United States, 1970 and 1960

(Numbers in thousands)

Age and relationship	Widowers			Widows		
	1970	1960	1970/1960	1970	1960	1970/1960
Total	2,131	2,082	1.02	9,615	7,862	1.22
Age:						
Under 55 years	323	296	1.09	1,540	1,425	1.08
55–64 years	365	380	0.96	1,988	1,808	1.10
65–74 years	595	656	0.91	2,946	2,529	1.16
75–84 years	615	573	1.07	2,402	1,674	1.43
85 years and over	233	177	1.32	739	426	1.73
Relationship:						
In households	1,951	1,916	1.02	9,057	7,536	1.20
Head of household	1,492	1,234	1.21	6,950	5,080	1.37
Relatives present	449	456	0.98	2,265	2,087	1.09
No relatives	1,043	778	1.34	4,685	2,993	1.57
Parent of head	256	378	0.68	1,471	1,613	0.91
Other relative	118	173	0.68	457	586	0.78
Nonrelative	86	131	0.66	179	258	0.69
In group quarters	180	166	1.08	559	326	1.71
Home for the aged	125	77	1.62	448	191	2.35
Nursing home[a]	40	33	1.21	144	87	1.66
Other	85	43	1.98	304	104	2.92
Other institution	30	44	0.68	58	67	0.87
Other group quarters	25	45	0.56	53	68	0.78

Source: U.S. Bureau of the Census, 1970 Census of Population, Vol. II-4C, Marital Status, table 1; Vol. II-4E, Persons in Institutions and Other Group Quarters, table 27; and 1960 data from the sources cited in Table 9.10.

[a]Persons in homes for the aged and dependent that were known to have nursing care.

as one-person households. Evidently more and more widowed persons are financially able and prefer, all factors considered, to make their home away from their sons and daughters or their siblings. (See the section above on living arrangements of children and adults.)

The largest *rate* of change in living arrangements of widowed persons was the doubling of the number living in nursing homes and other institutional facilities for elderly persons, from one-quarter of a million in 1960 to more than half a million in 1970. (No corresponding figures for the mid-1970's are available.) This development is apparently related to the increasing tendency for widowed persons to live alone; when they can no longer take care of themselves, they are more likely now than formerly to move to a rest home. This is corroborated by the one-quarter of a million decline during the 1960's in the number of widowed persons who were living with their children as parent of the head.

Comparison of widowed and divorced persons who do not remarry. In a cross-section of adults in 1970, the proportion of widowed persons who had remarried was only about one-half as large as that for divorced persons. This important difference is not simply a result of the older age of widowed persons. It is no doubt related to the fact that many persons obtain a divorce for the purpose of being free to marry someone else, whereas few persons become intentionally widowed in order to remarry! Documentation of the difference is presented in Table 13.31. This table features persons who were 45 to 54 years old in 1970, partly because this is the age range within which the number of widowed persons who remarry is at or near the peak, and partly because this age limitation reduces the possible bias that might result from differences between the ages of widowed and divorced persons.

The first number in the table shows that 1.7 percent of the men 45 to 54 in 1970 had become widowed and were still widowed when the census was taken. The second number shows that 4.2 percent had been widowed after their first or last marriage; these men are identified as "ever widowed." The third number shows that four-tenths (0.40) of those who were ever widowed (1.7 divided by 4.2) were still widowed. By reading across the first line of the table, it becomes apparent that only a little over one-half as large a proportion of the men who had ever been divorced, as compared with those who had ever been widowed, were still unmarried (0.22 versus 0.40). Likewise, for women 45 to 54 years of age the proportion of those who had remained unmarried was only about one-half as large for those who had ever been divorced (0.32) as for those who had ever been widowed (0.62). Although these overall findings are on a different level for men and women, they have a large measure of consistency. At the same time, some of the findings for persons in upper and lower socioeconomic groups vary widely, as is indicated below.

Among men, the proportion who are either widowed or divorced is much higher among those of low education or income than among those in the upper level. This observation is documented by the data on both current and previous experience with marital dissolution. The

Table 13.31. Remarriage of persons 45 to 54 years old known to have been widowed or divorced, by sex, years of school completed, and income in 1969: United States, 1970

Sex, years of school completed, and income	Percent currently widowed	Percent ever widowed	Currently Ever widowed	Percent currently divorced	Percent ever divorced	Currently Ever divorced
Men, 45-54 years	1.7	4.2	0.40	3.8	16.9	0.22
0-11 years of school	2.1	5.1	0.41	4.3	18.6	0.23
12 years	1.4	3.6	0.39	3.6	16.0	0.23
13-15 years	1.2	3.5	0.34	3.8	18.2	0.21
16 years	1.0	3.1	0.32	2.9	12.3	0.24
17 years or more	0.8	2.6	0.31	2.7	12.2	0.22
Under $3,000 or loss	4.0	8.4	0.48	9.1	26.3	0.35
$3,000-$4,999	2.5	6.0	0.42	5.8	21.1	0.27
$5,000-$6,999	1.9	4.7	0.40	4.3	18.3	0.23
$7,000-$9,999	1.4	3.8	0.37	3.2	16.5	0.19
$10,000-$14,999	1.0	3.1	0.32	2.4	14.6	0.16
$15,000 and over	0.8	2.7	0.30	1.8	12.4	0.15
Women, 45-54 years	7.9	12.7	0.62	5.5	17.4	0.32
0-11 years of school	9.7	15.2	0.64	5.4	19.3	0.28
12 years	6.4	10.6	0.60	5.3	15.9	0.33
13-15 years	6.6	10.9	0.61	6.7	17.3	0.39
16 years	5.4	8.9	0.61	5.1	11.7	0.44
17 years or more	6.5	11.1	0.59	7.6	17.4	0.44
Without income	1.8	5.8	0.31	1.0	11.5	0.09
$1-999 or loss	8.3	13.8	0.60	3.8	16.9	0.22
$1,000-$2,999	12.4	18.1	0.69	6.6	19.7	0.34
$3,000-$4,999	11.3	16.5	0.68	8.2	20.3	0.40
$5,000-$6,999	10.7	15.8	0.68	10.2	23.3	0.44
$7,000 and over	13.0	19.4	0.67	12.2	26.3	0.46

Source: U.S. Bureau of the Census, 1970 Census of Population, Vol. II-4C, Marital Status, tables 4 and 7.

lower widowhood rates among men in upper socioeconomic groups suggest, among other things, that these men and their wives tend to have superior health, and the lower divorce rates for upper-group men suggest that they have advantages in selecting a marital partner and in the promotion of stable adjustment after marriage.

Moreover, among men the extent to which remarriage occurs is more consistently related to income level than to educational level. The relatively small numbers of men in the upper income levels who become widowed or divorced are much more likely to remarry than those in the lower income levels. As a consequence, the proportion currently widowed or divorced is especially small for well-to-do men.

Among women, the results are in some key respects the reverse of those for men. For example, the tendency for divorced women to remarry decreases, rather than increases, with amount of income. Whether to remarry or not evidently tends to have very different connotations for divorced men than for divorced women with respect to such things as freedom of activity outside the home.

By contrast, the extent to which widowed women remarry bears little relation to their education or income level, except for a high remarriage rate among widows with little or no income. Although it is easy to understand the financial advantage for an impecunious widow to remarry, it is less easy to interpret the lack of relationship between the remarriage of widows and their socioeconomic status at the higher levels. Factors such as the possible reactions of relatives if a well-to-do widow should remarry may obscure variations in the *desire* for remarriage among widows of different socioeconomic levels.

Single Men and Women

Changes by age and race. As was pointed out in the section above on changes in marriage, divorce, and marital status, the marriage patterns of persons under 35 years old in the mid-1970's are quite different from those of persons 35 and older. Of special interest here is the fact that the younger generation has had a particularly strong tendency to postpone marriage (as well as to become separated or divorced at a relatively young age if they do marry). This tendency can be seen in the very large rate of increase in singleness among women in their twenties during the last decade and a half (Table 13.32). (The corresponding changes for men are not shown because they are obscured by differences between the coverage of men in the Armed Forces in 1960 and 1974, and for brevity of presentation.)

The proportion of women 20 to 24 years of age who had remained single was dramatically larger — about four-tenths larger — in 1974 than in 1960 (40 percent single in 1974 versus 28 percent in 1960). The corresponding increase was also large, one-fourth, for the next older group, 25 to 29 years old. Women in their twenties in 1960 had been born in the 1930's, whereas women in their twenties in 1974 had been born during the decade after the end of World War II — at the height of the baby boom. These two contrasting groups had experienced widely different social, economic, and political conditions during their formative years, and their marriage patterns evidently re-

Table 13.32. Percent never married, for women 14 years old and over by race and age: United States, 1974 and 1960

Age	All races			Races other than white		
	1974	1960	1974/1960	1974	1960	1974/1960
14 years and over	22.5	19.0	1.18	29.6	22.0	1.35
14-34 years	44.5	37.6	1.18	52.6	41.2	1.28
35 years and over	5.2	7.2	0.72	5.8	6.0	0.97
14-19 years	89.6	86.5	1.04	92.8	86.4	1.07
20-24 years	39.6	28.4	1.39	48.2	35.4	1.36
25-29 years	13.1	10.5	1.25	22.6	15.7	1.44
30-34 years	6.8	6.9	0.99	11.5	9.6	1.20
35-39 years	5.0	6.1	0.82	8.5	7.6	1.12
40-44 years	4.7	6.1	0.77	7.1	6.4	1.11
45-54 years	4.2	7.0	0.60	5.6	6.0	0.93
55-64 years	5.5	8.0	0.69	4.4	6.0	0.73
65 years and over	6.3	8.5	0.74	4.3	4.4	0.98

Source: U.S. Bureau of the Census, Current Population Reports, Series P-20, No. 271, "Marital Status and Living Arrangements: March 1974," table 1; and 1960 Census of Population, Vol. I, U.S. Summary, table 176.

flect these differences. One identifiable contributing factor was demographic: the "marriage squeeze" (page 81) was operating in opposite directions for these two groups; there was a scarcity of women of the most marriageable ages in the early 1950's and an excess of women of these ages in the late 1960's. No attempt will be made to assess the relative importance of this demographic factor as compared with that of such other factors as the delay in employment of young men because of more college attendance, more military service, and more competition for jobs among the large numbers of men and women who had been born soon after World War II.

Most of the women who were in their twenties in 1960 were 35 to 44 years old in 1974. The portion of these women who had remained single was smaller than that of women who had reached the same age by 1960. In fact, for each age group above 34 the percent single was significantly lower in 1974 than in 1960. Between these dates, many women who had appeared to be heading for a lifetime of singlehood decided to marry — in hopes of sharing the so-called "good life of married people."

Differences between white women and black women with respect to singlehood rates have increased since 1960. This inference can be made from the data in Table 13.32 for all women (88 percent of whom were white) as compared with data for women "other than white" (90 percent of whom were black). The percent single for women other than white was already higher in 1960 than that for women of all races combined, and between 1960 and 1974 the difference increased. To the extent that a high percent single tends to reflect a lack of confidence about future employment opportunities for prospective husbands and/or wives, the increasing singleness gap between black and white persons may be closely related to the high unemployment rates among blacks. According to the U.S. Bureau of Labor Statistics, the unemployment rate for black adults has been more than twice as high as that for white adults during most of the period since 1960.

Age and living arrangements of single adults. Tables 13.33 and 13.34 feature decennial census data for never-married adults under 35 and 35 years old and over, respectively, because their living arrangements are so different. The first table shows age detail in 5-year spans, the second in 10-year spans; therefore the number of single persons does not really reach a low point at ages 30 to 34, as a brief study of the two tables might suggest (for 1974 data, see Tables 13.8 and 13.9).

The combined effect of the baby boom after World War II and the sharp reduction in first-marriage rates after 1960 have caused the number of single women in their early twenties to nearly double (up 93 percent) between 1960 and 1974. The declining numbers of single persons between their mid-thirties and mid-fifties since 1960 reflect both past changes in birth rates and the much higher marriage rates during the 1950's than in the 1940's among those who were at the height of first marriage.

Overall changes during the 1960's in the living arrangements among single persons 14 to 34 years of age were dominated by the great majority living in their parental homes as "child of head." The rate of increase for this group was, therefore, about the same as that for the total. However, some very high rates of change occurred among the other 4.6 million.

More than twice as many single persons under 35 in 1970 as in 1960 were maintaining bachelor quarters in an apartment or house with no relatives present. Even more striking was the more than four

Table 13.33. Never-married persons 14 to 34 years old, by age, relationship, and sex: United States, 1970 and 1960

(Numbers in thousands)

Age and relationship	Never-married men			Never-married women		
	1970	1960	1970/1960	1970	1960	1970/1960
Total, 14-34 years old	17,625	12,426	1.42	14,673	9,435	1.56
Age:						
14-19 years	11,427	7,813	1.46	10,378	6,863	1.51
20-24 years	4,308	2,802	1.54	3,031	1,572	1.93
25-29 years	1,289	1,112	1.16	828	581	1.43
30-34 years	602	699	0.86	436	419	1.04
Relationship:						
In households	15,518	10,800	1.44	13,499	8,706	1.55
Head of household	1,151	548	2.10	972	387	2.51
Relatives present	147	110	1.34	272	104	2.62
No relatives	1,004	438	2.29	700	283	2.47
Child of head	12,991	9,027	1.44	11,302	7,369	1.53
Grandchild of head	283	236	1.20	242	183	1.32
Other relative	431	528	0.82	401	416	0.96
Unrelated partner	261	61	4.28	312	72	4.33
Other nonrelative	401	400	1.00	270	279	0.97
In group quarters	2,108	1,626	1.30	1,173	730	1.61
College dormitory	876	470	1.86	862	384	2.24
Military barracks	761	667	1.14	16	4	a
Correctional institution	125	124	1.01	5	4	a
Other institution	185	138	1.34	101	88	1.15
Other group quarters	161	227	0.71	189	250	0.76

Source: U.S. Bureau of the Census, 1970 Census of Population, Vol. II-4B, Persons by Family Characteristics, table 2; Vol. II-4C, Marital Status, table 1; 1960 Census of Population, Vol. II-4B, Persons by Family Characteristics, table 2; Vol. II-4E, Marital Status, table 1; and Vol. II-8A, Inmates of Institutions, table 26.

[a]Ratio not shown because base is very small.

times as many young adult single persons living in with someone else as an "unrelated partner." (Whether or not the partner was of the opposite sex is not ascertainable from published data for single persons. See the discussion in the section above on unrelated adults living together.) Other large rates of increase occurred among single residents of college housing quarters, which are typically quarters occupied by young adults not related to one another (even though they include many thousands of fraternity "brothers" and sorority "sisters"!).

The 2.6 times as many young single women in 1970 as in 1960 who were heads of households with relatives present are no doubt a direct

Table 13.34. Never-married persons 35 years old and over, by age, relationship, and sex: United States, 1970 and 1960

(Numbers in thousands)

Age and relationship	Never-married men			Never-married women		
	1970	1960	1970/1960	1970	1960	1970/1960
Total, 35 and over	2,801	2,877	0.97	2,952	2,892	1.02
Age:						
35-44 years	884	947	0.93	672	751	0.89
45-54 years	711	755	0.94	663	734	0.90
55-64 years	574	608	0.94	669	650	1.03
65 years and over	632	567	1.11	948	757	1.25
Relationship:						
In households	2,472	2,439	1.01	2,631	2,552	1.03
Head of household	1,338	1,141	1.17	1,398	1,169	1.20
Relatives present	334	338	0.99	419	373	1.12
No relatives	1,004	803	1.25	979	796	1.23
Child of head	582	547	1.06	530	533	0.99
Brother or sister[a]	271	332	0.82	428	496	0.86
Other relative	74	125	0.59	100	140	0.71
Nonrelative	207	294	0.70	175	214	0.82
In group quarters	330	438	0.75	321	339	0.95
Mental hospital	124	148	0.84	80	85	0.94
Home for the aged	82	56	1.46	105	57	1.84
Other institution	39	85	0.46	8	36	0.22
Other group quarters	85	149	0.57	128	161	0.80

Source: U.S. Bureau of the Census, 1970 Census of Population, Vol. II-4B, Persons by Family Characteristics, table 2; Vol. II-4C, Marital Status, table 1; 1960 Census of Population, Vol. II-4B, Persons by Family Characteristics, table 2; Vol. II-4E, Marital Status, table 1; and Vol. II-8A, Inmates of Institutions, tables 26 and 28.

[a]Includes natural and in-law brothers and sisters.

consequence of the increase in the proportion of children born out of wedlock, from 5 percent in 1960 to 11 percent in 1970 (and to 13 percent in 1973) according to reports of the U.S. National Center for Health Statistics. A sharply declining proportion of young single adults were living with their siblings, grandparents, or uncles and aunts as "other relatives."

Changes in the living arrangements of older single persons were in several respects like those of young singles, but the changes were much less striking. One reason was that the number of older singles remained virtually unchanged, while the number of younger singles increased approximately 50 percent during the 1960's. However, a noteworthy development was the substantial rate of increase among older single persons in homes for the aged. As noted above, persons without close family ties are more often spending their last few months or years in an institution.

Low incomes for single and separated men and high incomes for single and divorced women. In view of the large proportion of never-married adults under 25 years of age who are concentrated in their teens and are still enrolled in school, the income level of these persons is far below that for ever-married persons under 25, most of whom are concentrated in their early twenties. Accordingly, the analysis of income by marital status will feature the age range 25 to 64 years. As the lower part of Table 13.35 demonstrates, nearly all married men with wife present in 1970 had income, but nearly half of their wives did not. Married men and divorced men (most of whom will remarry soon) had the highest median incomes, whereas married women and separated women (many of whom were living with their husband during the income year, 1969) had the lowest incomes among those 25 to 64. The income figures discussed here include alimony and/or child support payments received from an absent or former spouse.

Single men shared with separated men the lowest median income level for each age group from 25 through 64. Moreover, the ratio of the median income of single or separated men to that of married men with wife present declined steadily within this age range. But the ratio of the median income of both divorced and widowed men to that of married men with wife present also declined with age. The conclusion appears to be that the selective factors that keep men married and living with a wife tend to be closely correlated with — and to include — a moderate-to-high income level. Stated otherwise, "a good income is like a cement that holds a solid marriage together." At the same time, it is obvious that many marriages end in divorce for reasons other than dire economic hardship, and the proportion that do so appears to be increasing.

Single women shared with divorced women the highest median income level among those 25 to 64 years old. However, the income level of single women was consistently above that of divorced women, probably as a consequence of several factors including more continuous work experience. Of special interest is the ratio of the median incomes of single men and single women. Among those approaching middle age (25 to 44 years old), the median income of single men was about

Table 13.35. Median income in 1969 by age, and percent without income in 1969, for persons 14 years old and over, by marital status and sex: United States, 1970

Age and sex	Total	Single	Married, spouse present	Sepa- rated	Divorced	Wid- owed
Median income for persons with income						
Men, 14 and over	$6,438	$2,093	$8,022	$4,826	$5,688	$2,653
14–24 years	2,151	1,433	5,344	3,753	4,077	2,645
25–34 years	8,016	5,844	8,460	5,990	6,924	6,202
35–44 years	9,167	6,116	9,556	6,129	7,307	6,825
45–54 years	8,876	5,511	9,277	5,479	6,542	6,515
55–64 years	7,361	4,212	7,851	4,106	4,860	5,205
65 years and over	2,794	2,224	3,230	2,148	2,287	2,211
Women, 14 and over	$2,474	$1,997	$2,649	$2,814	$4,048	$2,177
14–24 years	1,652	1,034	2,527	2,223	3,001	2,948
25–34 years	3,321	4,849	2,876	3,103	4,327	4,229
35–44 years	3,428	4,911	3,112	3,357	4,785	3,983
45–54 years	3,673	5,030	3,457	3,194	4,677	3,807
55–64 years	2,948	4,664	2,622	2,628	4,052	2,964
65 years and over	1,634	2,327	928	1,646	2,124	1,815
Percent with no income						
Men, 25–64 years	2.2	9.8	0.9	6.0	5.0	5.5
Women, 25–64 years	37.6	12.2	45.9	12.1	6.8	9.1

Source: U.S. Bureau of the Census, 1970 Census of Population, Vol. II-4C, Marital Status, table 7.

one-fifth higher than that of single women; but during middle age (45 to 64 years old), the relationship changed, with single women gaining ground and eventually surpassing single men in their income level at ages 55 to 64 years.

One conclusion from this set of findings is that attrition of men from singlehood into marriage tends to leave a residue of middle-aged single men with relatively little interest in earning very much money (or minimal ability to earn it), whereas the reverse seems to occur among single women. Moreover, in view of the fact that single women of mature age are more likely than other women to devote their energies to paid work, it might be said that women who have ever married but who devote much of their energy to paid work are conducting themselves more like traditional single women than traditional married women. This mode of behavior has been designated as "functional singlehood." [23]

Marital Status and Health

Health indicators by marital status. Recently collected information confirms the continuation of the generally more favorable health condition among married persons than among other ever-married persons (see Chapter 11). Within categories of race, sex, age, and family income, married persons (except separated) have distinctly fewer days of restricted activity per person per year than the other ever-marrieds (Table 13.36). Moreover, the average number of such days was smaller for white married persons than for married persons of other races; smaller for young married persons than for older ones; and

Table 13.36. Average number of days of restricted activity per person per year, for the civilian noninstitutional population 17 years old and over by marital status, race, sex, age, and family income: United States, 1971 and 1972

Race, sex, age, and family income	Total	Married, except separated	Widowed	Sepa-rated	Divorced	Single
Total, 17 and over	18.8	17.6	36.8	29.7	26.4	12.3
Race:						
White	18.1	17.2	34.5	25.5	24.8	11.8
All other	24.6	21.1	52.8	35.8	36.3	15.0
Sex and age:						
Male	16.6	16.9	32.1	27.3	25.7	11.4
17–24 years	9.4	9.2	a	20.7	18.9	9.2
25–34 years	10.9	10.2	46.3	19.0	13.2	12.3
35–44 years	12.7	11.9	16.8	25.5	23.5	12.5
45–64 years	20.7	19.6	30.4	33.6	31.2	23.7
65 years and over	32.0	31.8	33.6	36.1	41.6	25.1
Female	20.7	18.2	37.8	30.9	26.9	13.3
17–24 years	12.0	12.7	a	14.3	18.2	11.0
25–34 years	15.5	14.9	25.9	26.3	20.3	13.3
35–44 years	16.9	15.5	26.7	29.9	26.0	16.9
45–64 years	22.9	20.2	31.8	41.5	31.2	21.1
65 years and over	37.6	34.0	41.5	55.9	37.3	23.4
Family income:						
Under $7,000	27.9	27.1	40.6	36.5	33.9	16.6
$7,000 and over	13.4	13.5	27.9	13.8	16.5	9.5

Source: U.S. National Center for Health Statistics, <u>Vital and Health Statistics</u>, Series 10, No. 104, "Differentials in Health Characteristics by Marital Status, United States, 1971–1972."

[a]Figure does not meet standards of reliability or precision.

smaller for married persons with high family incomes than for those with lower incomes.

The largest number of days of restricted activity, as expected, was for widowed persons of all ages combined, because of the correlation of this indicator with age. However, within each age group above 35, widowed men fared better in this regard than separated and divorced men, and widowed women also fared as well as separated women but not divorced women. Single adults had the smallest number of restricted days, on the average, largely because of their concentration at the young adult ages — and because the information excludes persons in institutions, among whom single persons of middle age are disproportionately numerous.

Observed differences in restricted activity by marital status are substantial, but as Table 13.36 demonstrates, there are many other related variables (sex, age, and so forth) that help to determine the level of this type of activity. In addition, married women are most likely to report restricted activity associated with pregnancy, but they are probably least likely to report marginally restricted activity if they have an urgent need at the same time to care for other family members.

The relation between marital status and four other health indicators is shown in Table 13.37. In this table currently married persons have generally better health scores than other ever-married persons, but not so good as single adults on three of the four measures — chronic conditions, physician visits, and hospital episodes. However, on acute conditions, widowed persons have the best scores.

For conditions most closely related to age differences, the health measures show meaningful contrasts. Widowed persons are generally the oldest and consequently have the most limitation of activity because of chronic conditions, whereas the much younger single persons have few of these conditions. By contrast, single adults rank higher than either married or widowed persons on the incidence of acute conditions, which would include "downtime" because of accidents — to which young adults are especially prone. Separated and divorced persons also have relatively large frequencies of acute conditions, a fact that may result from tensions associated with the disruption of their marriages. Separated and divorced persons report conspicuously higher numbers of chronic conditions than any other group besides widowed persons. The available data do not indicate what proportion of these conditions was present before the marital disruption (and may

Table 13.37. Selected health conditions by marital status and sex, for the civilian noninstitutional population 17 years old and over: United States, 1971 and 1972

Health condition	Total	Married, except separated	Widowed	Separated	Divorced	Single
Percent limited in activity by chronic conditions						
Total	17.0	15.4	39.2	22.7	21.6	11.4
Male	18.1	18.0	44.9	25.9	25.4	12.6
Female	16.1	12.8	37.9	20.9	19.4	10.0
Number of acute conditions per person per year						
Total	1.7	1.7	1.4	2.3	2.2	2.0
Male	1.6	1.5	1.3	1.8	1.5	1.8
Female	1.9	1.9	1.4	2.6	2.5	2.2
Number of physician visits per person per year						
Total	5.4	5.4	6.8	6.7	6.3	4.2
Male	4.3	4.4	6.1	5.2	4.6	3.5
Female	6.3	6.4	7.0	7.5	7.3	4.9
Percent with one or more short-stay hospital episodes						
Total	13.0	13.8	15.1	18.1	14.0	7.9
Male	9.6	10.0	16.9	13.3	11.9	6.7
Female	15.9	17.5	14.7	20.6	15.2	9.4

Source: U.S. National Center for Health Statistics, Vital and Health Statistics, Series 10, No. 104, "Differentials in Health Characteristics by Marital Status, United States, 1971-1972."

have contributed to the parting of the husband and wife) and what proportion developed after the parting occurred.

Marital status of persons in institutions. The 2 million adults in institutions in 1970 were almost evenly divided between men and women. However, the age distributions for the two groups were very different and their marital status distributions therefore were also quite different. Nearly half of the men in institutions were under 45 years old, whereas more than half of the women in institutions were 75 or older; moreover, half of the men were single, and half of the women were widowed. This background helps to explain the differences among institutional inmates by type of institution and marital status, as shown in Table 13.38.

Over 95 percent of the 327,000 persons in correctional institutions in 1970 were men; and nearly half of those in custody (in prisons, reformatories, jails, workhouses, and homes for juvenile delinquents) were single. By contrast, two-thirds of the 926,000 persons in homes for the aged and needy were women; and 85 percent of these persons were widowed.

Table 13.38. Persons 14 years old and over in institutions, by type of institution, marital status, and sex: United States, 1970

Type of institution and sex	All inmates	Married, except sepa- rated	Wid- owed	Di- vorced	Sepa- rated	Single
Men in institutions (000's)	1,071	200	155	106	54	556
Percent by type of institution	100.0	100.0	100.0	100.0	100.0	100.0
Mental hospitals	22.1	22.5	8.2	22.1	24.6	25.7
Correctional institutions	29.2	42.5	4.8	44.2	46.9	26.7
Homes for the aged	28.3	27.6	80.9	23.2	18.9	15.7
Other institutions[a]	20.4	7.4	6.1	10.6	9.6	31.9
Percent by marital status	100.0	18.7	14.5	9.9	5.0	51.9
Mental hospitals	100.0	19.0	5.4	9.9	5.6	60.1
Correctional institutions	100.0	27.2	2.4	15.0	8.1	47.4
Homes for the aged	100.0	18.2	41.4	8.1	3.4	28.8
Other institutions	100.0	6.8	4.3	5.2	2.4	81.3
Women in institutions (000's)	974	106	506	42	23	297
Percent by type of institution	100.0	100.0	100.0	100.0	100.0	100.0
Mental hospitals	19.1	42.3	7.1	39.7	51.9	25.7
Correctional institutions	1.4	3.3	0.2	4.5	8.6	1.9
Homes for the aged	64.0	45.8	87.6	46.8	26.2	35.5
Other institutions[a]	15.5	8.6	5.1	9.0	13.3	36.8
Percent by marital status	100.0	10.9	51.9	4.3	2.3	30.5
Mental hospitals	100.0	24.2	19.2	8.9	6.4	41.3
Correctional institutions	100.0	24.8	8.5	13.3	13.8	39.6
Homes for the aged	100.0	7.8	71.1	3.1	1.0	17.0
Other institutions	100.0	6.0	17.0	2.5	2.0	72.5

Source: U.S. Bureau of the Census, 1970 Census of Population, Vol. II-4E, Persons in Institutions and Other Group Quarters, tables 16, 24, 25, and 27.

[a]Tuberculosis hospitals, other chronic disease hospitals, homes and schools for the mentally and physically handicapped, homes for dependent and neglected children, homes for unwed mothers, training schools for juvenile delinquents, and detention homes.

About 424,000 persons were in mental hospitals, about 55 percent of whom were men and half of whom were single. Mental hospital patients included a small proportion, but a substantial number (50,-000), of widowed persons. Whereas about 40 to 50 percent of the married, divorced, or separated men in institutions were in correctional institutions, similar large proportions of the institutionalized women who were in these same marital status categories were residing in mental hospitals. As pointed out in Chapter 11, this contrasting institutional pattern probably reflects not only different ways that men and women tend to behave under stress, but also the greater likelihood of a husband with a marginal emotional disturbance being cared for by his wife, whereas the wife under similar conditions might be cared for in a mental hospital.

Nearly four of every five persons 14 years old and over among the 369,000 residents of "other institutions" were single persons. The great majority of these persons were in their teens or early adulthood and were living in homes for the mentally handicapped, correctional homes or detention centers for juveniles, and homes for dependent and neglected children.

Changes in institutional rates by marital status. Table 13.39 updates the institutional-residence rates by type of institution and marital status that were shown for 1960 in Table 11.6. These rates per 10,000 population 45 to 64 years old amount to probabilities that middle-aged persons of a given marital status will be under care or custody in an institution. The categories of marital status are listed in the ascending order of the rates for women for 1970.

The overall institutional rates for both men and women were only about three-fourths as high in 1970 as in 1960, despite substantial proportional increases in the rather small rates for persons 45 to 64 in homes for the aged. For persons of each marital status, there was a particularly large decline in the rate of institutional care for mental disorders. Incarceration of men in correctional institutions also dropped sharply, the drop being by approximately the same proportion for men of each marital status. These findings do not necessarily mean that the incidence of mental problems or the frequency of crimes has diminished, but rather that more of the persons involved are being treated outside institutions.

Tremendous differences persist in institutional rates for middle-aged persons in the several marital status categories. Married persons (ex-

Table 13.39.   Institutional-residence rate per 10,000 population 45 to 64
years old, by type of institution, marital status, and sex:
United States, 1970 and 1960

Year, type of institution, and sex	All in- mates 45-64	Married, except sepa- rated	Wid- owed	Di- vorced	Sepa- rated	Single
1970						
Men in institutions	109	25	273	498	453	814
Mental hospitals	44	11	63	160	160	376
Correctional institutions	19	7	55	149	128	65
Homes for the aged	27	5	132	131	87	202
Other institutions	18	3	23	59	77	171
Women in institutions	67	18	98	143	178	468
Mental hospitals	32	12	32	73	98	207
Homes for the aged	23	5	58	56	37	133
Other institutions	12	2	7	14	43	128
1960						
Men in institutions	152	45	340	676	589	935
Mental hospitals	75	22	97	237	215	550
Correctional institutions	31	12	84	215	186	103
Homes for the aged	23	4	106	132	94	131
Other institutions	24	7	53	92	94	149
Women in institutions	90	37	99	193	247	475
Mental hospitals	62	31	51	150	193	297
Homes for the aged	14	2	37	27	22	64
Other institutions	13	3	9	11	23	111
1970/1960						
Men in institutions	0.72	0.56	0.80	0.74	0.77	0.87
Mental hospitals	0.59	0.50	0.65	0.68	0.74	0.68
Correctional institutions	0.61	0.58	0.65	0.69	0.69	0.63
Homes for the aged	1.17	1.25	1.25	0.99	0.93	1.54
Other institutions	0.75	0.43	0.43	0.64	0.82	1.15
Women in institutions	0.74	0.49	0.99	0.74	0.72	0.99
Mental hospitals	0.52	0.39	0.63	0.49	0.51	0.70
Homes for the aged	1.64	2.50	1.57	2.07	1.68	2.08
Other institutions	0.92	0.67	0.78	1.27	1.87	1.15

Source: U.S. Bureau of the Census, 1970 Census of Population, Vol. II-
4C, Marital Status, table 4; Vol. II-4E, Persons in Institutions and Other
Group Quarters, tables 16, 24, and 25; and 1960 rates from chapter 11, table
11.6.

cept separated) continue to have very low institutional-residence rates
compared with persons in each of the other categories, whereas those
who reach middle age without having married have by far the highest
rates. For example, only 0.25 percent of the married men, as compared with 8 percent of the single men, 45 to 64 years old were in

institutions in 1970. Nearly one-half of these men — both the married and the single — were residents of mental hospitals.

Separated, divorced, and single persons continued to have by far the highest rates of institutionalization among the middle aged. For each of these marital status categories, mental hospitalization was the most frequent cause for institutional residence. Moreover, two-thirds of the middle-aged married women in institutions were in mental hospitals. As a psychiatrist wryly observed to one of the authors, "It seems as if most of the women who receive psychiatric services (either in or outside mental hospitals) do so because they are *not* married — or because they *are* married!" The point, of course, is that emotional stress which is aggravated by such disturbing family situations as either the presence or the absence of close family ties is evidently a primary source of not only marital dissolution but also the need for help from specialists on mental problems.

Legal and Administrative Aspects of Marriage and Divorce

In recent years important changes have taken place in laws concerning marriage and divorce and in the thinking of members of the legal profession and others concerning the administration of these laws. Here, major changes in the laws are reviewed together with significant related events. The Uniform Marriage and Divorce Act, proposed in 1970, precipitated a major controversy between the Family Law Section of the American Bar Association and the Commission on Uniform State Laws. "No-fault divorce," which was advanced by the Uniform Act, and how it should be defined and implemented by the courts, were the major factors in the controversy. There has also been heightened interest in court procedures related to marital dissolution, especially efforts at conciliation and counseling through professional staffs attached to the courts.

Since 1970, stimulated by the proposed Uniform Act, much new state legislation has been enacted and tested in the state courts. Some early results of this state legislation and court action regarding it will be reviewed.

Marriage laws. The principal change in marriage laws in the past decade has been a marked reduction in the age at which persons may marry without parental consent. The right to vote was moved down from 21 years to 18 by constitutional amendment in 1971, and this doubtless stimulated changes in marriage laws. By early 1974 there were forty states that allowed both males and females to marry at age 18 without parental consent. For females, there were only three states that required an older age to marry; two states specified 19 years and one required 21 years. For males, more states specified an older age to marry without parental consent. Three states specified 19 years and eight plus the District of Columbia required 21 years for marriage without parental consent.

If the parents give consent, and frequently if approval is granted by a judicial authority (because of special circumstances such as the pregnancy of the girl), much younger ages at marriage are allowed by many states. A majority of states specified 16 years for the girl, but eleven states approved younger ages for the girl with judicial approval. Recently, state legislatures have not made a significant contribution to the problem of the young girl and boy who are involved in a pregnancy. Traditionally, marriage was considered the solution. Abortion is now approved by growing numbers with this problem, but on religious grounds abortion is disapproved by many. If neither abortion nor marriage takes place, the infant may be placed for adoption or the young mother may continue to care for her infant in her own home or in the home of her parents.

Minor changes in other marriage laws have occurred recently. Nearly all states now require some form of premarital examination. Unfortunately, the usual serological test, often cited as a test for venereal disease, is a more limited test for syphilis; it does not indicate the presence of the widespread venereal disease gonorrhea. A few states recently have added tests for sickle cell anemia, Tay-Sachs disease, and (for females) tests for immunity to German measles (rubella). Common-law marriages are still recognized in thirteen states (Alabama, Colorado, Georgia, Idaho, Iowa, Kansas, Montana, Ohio, Oklahoma, Pennsylvania, Rhode Island, South Carolina, and Texas) and the District of Columbia.[24] Most states specify a waiting period prior to issuance of a marriage license, most frequently three days. Enforcement of marriage laws has not significantly improved; it is still generally left to local, rather than state, officials.

A beginning has been made by some students of marriage to advance the idea of legal contracts between consenting partners in lieu of marriage. The conditions of the contract would conform to the needs and life-styles of the parties involved. They might include agreements with respect to the duration and terms of their relationship, as well as the conditions for its dissolution.[25] Issues that might be covered in such contracts range widely. Thus far this development is very much in the early stages of consideration, but the literature on the subject could have a desirable effect on those who study it in order to become more alert about the many facets of married life that must operate effectively to keep the relationship between husbands and wives in a healthy state of adjustment.

Divorce laws. Truly revolutionary changes in divorce laws have taken place during the past decade. No-fault divorce laws were urged during the early 1960's and were proposed by a state commission (California's) in 1966. Since 1970 they have been adopted by many states. The laws have appeared in a variety of forms and have sometimes been hailed as the answer to the divorce problem, but they have in turn led to a number of special problems.

Some of the changes wrought by the new no-fault divorce laws are purely cosmetic. "Plaintiff" and "defendant" become "petitioner" and "respondent"; "spousal support" replaces "alimony"; even "divorce" disappears and a decree "dissolves the marriage." Such changes are harmless as long as there is full awareness of the human problems and the tremendous emotions frequently involved in the termination of marriage.

The old legal grounds — cruelty, desertion, adultery, and the like (pages 365–369 and 374–378) — have become increasingly unsatisfactory as a basis for legal settlement of a marriage where the bonds of affection and trust between husband and wife have disappeared. The old approach assumed that there was an innocent and aggrieved party (in a majority of cases the wife) who was entitled to receive a divorce as well as other compensation from the guilty party (most frequently the husband) because he had committed a specific offense. This approach is obviously not in line with modern thinking about marital discord. While one may debate endlessly about who is to blame in a given marital dissolution, there is general agreement that in most cases the responsibility for the breakup rests with both husband and wife. Further than that, why explore *blame?* The essential fact is that a husband and a wife have come to the end of the road; there are irreconcilable differences. The old *fault* divorce laws were designed for a different society. A hundred years ago, the wife who was not affluent but who found herself in an intolerable marriage hesitated to seek divorce because her options were limited. She could hope to marry again, or she could return to the home of her parents or relatives, or she could seek employment for which she usually had limited skills.

Consequently, only in extreme cases did she seek divorce. In the same manner the husband of a hundred years ago, knowing how strongly public opinion would condemn him for seeking divorce from an "innocent" wife, was unlikely to sue for divorce unless there was clear evidence of wrongdoing by his wife. The "legal grounds" most frequently used a century ago reflect these facts.

No-fault divorce procedures avoid exploring and assessing blame and concentrate on dissolving the marriage and tidying up the inevitable problems — responsibility for the care of children (there still are children involved in a majority of divorce cases despite the decline in the birth rate), financial support for children, division of jointly owned property, and spousal support (alimony) if this seems indicated. The moment it is established that the question of blame is irrelevant to settlement of the case, some of the bitterness (but by no means all of it) goes out of the divorce proceedings.

Many states have modified their divorce laws either by adopting pure no-fault laws, or by adding no-fault provisions to their existing laws. Foster and Freed, two students of family law, have published a detailed tabulation of state divorce laws and have divided the states into five groups on the basis of their divorce laws in 1974 (in this classification the term "breakdown" refers, of course, to marriage):[26]

NO-FAULT AND FAULT GROUNDS

BREAKDOWN ONLY (except possibly "insanity"): Arizona, California, Colorado, Florida, Iowa, Kentucky, Michigan, Nebraska, Oregon, Washington

BREAKDOWN ADDED TO FAULT GROUNDS: Alabama, Connecticut, Georgia, Hawaii, Indiana, Maine, Montana, Missouri, New Hampshire, Texas, Vermont

INCOMPATIBILITY ADDED TO FAULT GROUNDS: Alaska, Delaware, Idaho, Kansas, Nevada, New Mexico, North Dakota, Oklahoma

SEPARATION ADDED TO FAULT GROUNDS: Arkansas, District of Columbia, Louisiana, Maryland, Minnesota, New Jersey, New York, North Carolina, Rhode Island, South Carolina, Tennessee, Utah, Virginia, West Virginia, Wisconsin, Wyoming (also Alabama, Connecticut, Delaware, Nevada, New Hampshire, North Dakota, Texas, and Vermont, listed supra)

FAULT ONLY GROUNDS: Illinois, Massachusetts, Mississippi, Montana (until new law becomes effective), Ohio, Pennsylvania (considering new law), South Dakota

This strange mixture of legal philosophies concerning divorce found in state laws is indicative of the present confused thinking on the subject. Only ten states fall into the *pure no-fault* (breakdown only) group, and, at the other extreme, only a shrinking group of six or seven states fall into the *fault only* group. All the other states have adopted some modifications or blending of the old and the new. A detailed listing of major provisions of all state divorce laws is given in the *Book of the States*.[27] The same source also lists the various provisions of the state marriage laws.

State legislators in large numbers seem to have found in "no-fault divorce" a magic phrase for solving a troublesome state problem. And, happily, it does not cost a lot of money. Clearly, a no-fault divorce law eliminates much of the hypocrisy and bitterness in the old fault divorce proceeding; still, it leaves many problems unresolved.

The 1966 commission appointed by the Governor of California that proposed no-fault divorce laws also made another major recommendation: that *all* divorce actions should be heard before a family court. The California legislature, unfortunately, adopted one provision but not the other (pages 378–381). There is no denying that properly staffed family courts are more expensive than traditional courts; the California state legislators were not convinced that such expenditures were justified.

In defense of family courts it should be pointed out that a reasonable and just unraveling of a marriage by divorce proceedings is rarely as simple as it might appear at first glance. There frequently are difficult human problems, and financial resources may be limited. After the divorce the wife may be planning to enter the labor market for the first time, or she may be planning to return to the job market after an absence of several years. In either case she may stand in urgent need of special training. How can this be financed? The husband may be planning to remarry, and this may involve expanding responsibilities for a new family. How can he provide for the old family and the new? Small children may be involved. How are they to be cared for?

The list of problems is long, and a first step toward a reasonable solution is a detailed listing of the financial resources of both the husband and the wife. This elementary move is sometimes surprisingly difficult, since concealment of assets may take place. Sometimes the laws are inadequate. A recent press dispatch reported enactment of a law in New York requiring full disclosure of all financial assets and income, as well as full information concerning the transfer of any assets during the preceding three years, before the start of a divorce trial (*New York Times,* August 10, 1975).

A divorce usually involves a grave crisis for one or more persons. The only way society can act wisely, through its courts, in such a situation is by a careful assembling of all the relevant facts. With these in hand the court is in a position to aid in finding solutions. Unfortunately, such procedures are expensive, since the aid of trained professionals is needed. And because of the expense most of the courts dealing with divorce cases probably lack adequate staffs.

Uniform Marriage and Divorce Act. A noteworthy development of the past decade has been the proposed Uniform Marriage and Divorce Act of the National Conference of Commissioners on Uniform State Laws. While attention was given primarily to changes in divorce laws, this group also made important proposals regarding state marriage laws. Although the conference of commissioners had been seeking uniformity in marriage and divorce laws since 1892, the current effort crystalized in 1965 with the presentation of a report by its committee on uniform divorce and marriage laws. The major recommendation was that the conference explore the possibility of *"nonfault"* *divorce laws.* The committee report was accepted, and a staff was assembled to proceed with the project.

The original version of the proposed Uniform Marriage and Divorce Act was approved by the National Conference of Commissioners on Uniform State Laws in August 1970. Some of its provisions immediately became controversial, especially to the lawyers most concerned with matrimonial problems, namely, the members of the Family Law Section of the American Bar Association. The section appointed a committee that met for two days in early 1971 with representatives of the National Conference of Commissioners, but the two groups failed to resolve their differences. A revised draft of the proposed Uniform Act was brought forward in 1971 and a third version in 1973. This last was approved in 1974 by the American Bar Association, but not before the Family Law Section had brought forth its own proposals for revision of the Uniform Act.[28] Some of the differences between the two will be reviewed in later pages.

Regarding the proposed uniform marriage laws, the work of the commission was marked by timidity. Noting that 13 states still recognize common-law marriage, the commission offered two alternatives: alternative A recognized the validity of common-law marriages, while alternative B found future common-law marriages in the state invalid. This is indeed a strange proposal for the model uniform law. In the same manner, the group could not bring itself to propose a minimum age for marriage. In the first (1970) draft of the proposed Uniform Act, after proposing 18 years as the minimum age to marry without parental consent, and 16 years as the approved age with parental consent or judicial approval, the group proposed that marriage below the age of 16, *but without any minimum age specified,* could take place if the parents gave their consent and the judicial authority approved. If these two conditions were met, child marriages of any age would be legal. However, in the final (1973) draft, this strange bow to child marriage was modified. The legality of marriages below 16 years was made optional, by placing this material in brackets.

Another weakness of the proposed marriage law, although a minor one, concerned the mechanics of application for a marriage license. The proposed law would allow *either* party to the proposed marriage to appear and submit the application. This would deny the necessity for a reasonable check by allowing the licensing authority to see both parties and to question them. The Uniform Marriage Act proposed to eliminate some of the existing prohibitions to marriage in certain state laws. Thus, for instance, the marriage of first or second cousins was to be approved.

The dissolution section of the proposed Uniform Marriage and Divorce Act is much longer than the marriage section. It is certainly not timid in its approach. It may be expected to have a profound effect on state legislatures during the next decade, as it has had already since 1970. It is clearly supportive of the no-fault approach to the termination of marriage. Some of its provisions will be noted below. Reference is to the 1973 draft unless otherwise indicated.

Any proceeding for the dissolution of marriage, legal separation, or declaration of invalidity of marriage must be entitled "in re the Marriage of _____ and _____," and a responsive pleading is to be called a response. Thus the adversary approach is taken out of the format of the legal procedures. The petition must set forth that the marriage is irretrievably broken. Either party, *or both parties,* may present the petition. Among the items of information to be presented to the court are age of children, whether the wife is pregnant, any financial arrangements for custody of children, and maintenance of a spouse.

The time-honored defenses to a divorce action (condonation, connivance, collusion, recrimination, insanity, and lapse of time) are swept away. After the petition has been presented, there may be temporary orders or injunctions related to maintenance, to assure that property and other financial assets are properly listed and utilized in fair manner, to assure that both parties are free from molestation, and to assure that one of the parties may be excluded from the family home.

The term "irretrievably broken" regarding the marriage is not defined in the 1970 draft of the model act, nor is it specified what evidence shall be produced to establish the fact. However, if there is disagreement between husband and wife regarding the fact of breakdown, then there may be court adjournment of 30 to 60 days, and, if the parties so desire, counseling services may be sought. Basically, the parties themselves decide whether the marriage is finished.

The dissolution decree is granted if one of the parties has been a resident of the state for 90 days and if the court concludes that all requirements have been met: breakdown of marriage, custody and support of children, spousal support, and division of property. If requested, a legal separation may be granted rather than a dissolution if both parties are agreeable to such a decree.

The Uniform Act provides for separation agreements and, unless the court found an existing agreement "unconscionable," it would enforce it. The act also makes specific provisions for disposition of property, maintenance of one spouse where appropriate, child support, and where reasonable, the payment of attorney's fees and costs by one of the parties. The Uniform Act also contains detailed provisions concerning the custody of any children coming within the jurisdiction of the court. The best interest of the child is to be the guiding principle for the judicial authority. A custody order may be modified if the evidence is clear that this is desirable for the child's physical or mental health.

Attorneys and no-fault divorce laws. The big change in the Uniform Marriage and Divorce Act put forward by the Conference of Commissioners on Uniform State Laws is the proposal for no-fault divorce proceedings. Some attorneys in the Washington area experienced in serving clients involved in divorce cases were asked in 1975 by one of the authors for their view on no-fault divorce. No great enthusiasm for the no-fault approach to divorce proceedings was encountered. While readily admitting that the old fault approach often engendered bitterness between husband and wife, the attorneys commented that frequently the bitterness was already there and the fault accusation simply served to bring it out into the open. One problem frequently encountered in divorce actions, it was stressed, is concealment of financial assets. There are many methods of concealment, and attorneys' efforts to obtain full information is often hampered by the wife's limited knowledge of her husband's business affairs. Removal of the adversary format in divorce proceedings does not change the fact that a genuine contest may be involved. A term frequently heard in such discussions is "leverage." In one case, the lawyer's client was the wife of a man believed to be quite wealthy but whose financial statements indicated only modest means. The wife was advised to sue on the ground of adultery — the proof of which was readily at hand — because this would give her more leverage; the husband's attorney would bargain more seriously regarding the financial settlement with the possibility of such a suit facing his client. If a financial settlement favorable to the wife was reached by means of this leverage, the wife would agree to a divorce on less pejorative grounds.

As a further complication, one attorney stressed that divorce looks quite different to a middle- or upper-class person than it does to one near the poverty level. The former may have many resources — family, relatives, and friends — to ease the transition; to the latter, the nature of the financial settlement — monthly payments for the wife, child support, and payment of all costs — is an immediate and overwhelming consideration. The middle-class woman may, and sometimes does, assert: "I don't want his money." Such sentiments are foreign to the woman near the poverty level. Her concern with her lawyer is to urge him to secure an adequate financial settlement; her husband, who probably found it difficult to maintain one household and may now be facing the prospect of trying to maintain two, is also deeply concerned with the money problem.

The cure for the concealment of financial assets in a divorce action would appear to be stronger laws governing the disclosure of all financial assets, together with severe penalties for failure to make an accurate statement. The family court system would be useful in bringing out all relevant facts.

Conciliation and counseling services. Recent changes in the divorce laws and the growing number of divorces have brought increased interest in conciliation and counseling services, available either in the courts or by referral. How good are such services, and what impact do they have on the divorce rate? This double-barreled query is frequently raised as if it were one question: actually, there are two distinct considerations and combining them into one question leads to endless confusion. A professional counseling service to troubled married couples might be excellent and yet result in higher, rather than lower, divorce rates (pages 381–382). Detailed analyses by social scientists of courts providing conciliation or counseling services are not numerous. One recent study[29] examined the Conciliation Court of Los Angeles County, but it was so narrowly focused that it leaves the major questions unanswered. It is reviewed here only briefly.

Maddi, the author, concentrated on the impact of court conciliation services on the rate of divorce decrees when a petition for dissolution of the marriage had previously been filed. Rigorously ruled out were all considerations of possible aid to petitioners by the actions of the staff of the conciliation court, including the 12 marriage counselors. Obviously, two people seeking a divorce (or *one* person seeking a divorce and opposed by the other spouse) have many possible problems. A skilled professional recognizes problems and stands ready to help; his caliber may be judged by his success in both aspects.

In Los Angeles County the number of persons seeking divorce each year is very large. In this particular study the author took as a sample for intensive study a 4-month intake of cases seeking divorce in 1970; the sample totaled over 6,500 cases. Of this larger group, a mere 330 cases requested conciliation services from the court. The bulk of the study is devoted to an exhaustive statistical analysis of the two groups: those who had applied for conciliation services and those who had not. Each case in the sample was followed for a minimum of 15 months, and during that period a majority of cases had received an interlocutory divorce decree. However, the group that had sought conciliation services had a substantially lower percentage divorced than was true of the group that had not sought such help. Why? Part of the answer, Maddi reported, was to be found in the varying characteristics of the two groups. Thus, the conciliation group had larger proportions of Catholics, of couples who had not separated prior to filing for divorce, and so on. Even after adjustment for these more obvious factors, there was still a lower divorce rate among the group that sought conciliation. However, because of the small proportion of the total number of cases seen by the court's marriage counselors, the overall effect on the total dissolution rate for Los Angeles County appeared to be negligible.

This study, unfortunately, asked the wrong questions. Counseling services are useful regardless of the effect on the divorce rate. Important questions that might be asked are along four lines:

(*a*) Why were steps not taken to increase the professional staff of the conciliation court? Maddi reported 47,000 family law petitions of various types filed each year in Los Angeles. The 12 marriage counselors had other duties, including premarital counseling, besides meeting with the applicants seeking divorce who requested their help.

(*b*) What so-called ancillary services did the conciliation court staff provide its clients? Was there credible evidence that the staff efforts significantly reduced bitterness over child custody, child support, alimony, and property division? Smoothing these final steps in a divorce proceeding is obviously important to the former wife, husband, and children.

(*c*) What of the referral services of the conciliation court; how extensive are they? Is there satisfactory cooperation between the court staff and reputable social agencies and private practitioners in the community?

(*d*) Finally, one should inquire about the conciliation court staff's effort to evaluate the effectiveness of its own work. Does it have a competent research staff, including social scientists, to prepare evaluative reports? What of its relation with interested research scientists in the community?

Questions along these lines posed by knowledgeable social scientists would add greatly to public understanding and evaluation of courts dealing with family problems.

Early evaluations of no-fault divorce laws. Although 1970 was the first year no-fault divorce laws became effective, several states hastened to modify their divorce laws; in 1974 Foster and Freed were able to examine results in 20 states that had recently changed their divorce laws.[30] They pointed out the limitations of "breakdown" as a ground for divorce if there is lacking a definition of the term and detailed guidelines for the court in administering the law. They concluded that legislative haste to humanize divorce laws had resulted in a lack of adequate safeguards. The authors reported that "in every case California courts have found 'irremediable breakdown' has been established." [31] They reached this conclusion after consulting local attorneys and examining the literature.

The authors present arguments for well-staffed family courts to hear divorce questions as well as all other family-related matters. They state that the movement toward family courts is as important as changing the divorce laws. However, they find that "the Uniform Act reflects hostility to, and a disdain for, family courts, counseling and conciliation services." [32]

In the opinion of Foster and Freed, the New York compulsory conciliation courts, established under the 1966 law and abolished in 1973, did a great deal of useful work on ancillary problems — alimony, child support, and the like — although the courts succeeded in preventing very few couples who desired divorce from continuing to the final decree. These authors oppose compulsory counseling, feeling that such services should be available if requested.

Under no-fault divorce, if the state also operates under the common law regarding property rights — as many states do — the loss to the wife may be substantial. The authors illustrate from the New York case of *Fischer* v. *Wirth*. In this strange case the earnings of husband and wife, in the early years of marriage, were pooled and the wife invested the excess funds. Later, in a new arrangement, the wife's earnings supported the family and the husband invested his income, in his own name, presumably for their later years. At divorce, after 40 years of marriage, the wife was awarded nothing from these investments made by the husband. The authors conclude that the pure common-law marital-property system lends itself to such outrageous results. What is desirable, they indicate, is that divorce should be treated as the dissolution of a partnership. [33]

Regarding the welfare of children, the authors conclude that no-fault divorce *increases* the risk that the interests of children will be overlooked because it may seem useless to struggle over custody if the divorce is to be granted on demand. [34]

The authors conclude, "In order to do an adequate job, the divorce court needs a professional staff to assist in conducting investigations . . . There should be a court officer . . . with responsibility for children . . . Instead of merely holding a mock inquest for allegedly dead marriages, courts should provide conciliation and counseling services and help the family to pick up the pieces and plan for the future." [35]

A somewhat different point of view from that of Foster and Freed was presented by Goddard,[36] who reviewed the early California experience with no-fault divorce law. The author, a third-year student at the University of California Law School, expressed his appreciation for guidance by Professor Herma H. Kay, one of the two principals in drafting the Uniform Act.

Goddard looked principally at the administration of the act in Alameda County. He found that spousal support (alimony) may be for shorter periods of time and for smaller amounts than was true under the old law. After interviewing judges, he concluded that the new law did not create divorce for the asking. He reported on a case in which the supreme court of the state had held that a certain procedure was legally impermissible and refused to grant a divorce. The wife had brought an action for divorce but had failed to appear and testify. Her defaulting husband was subpoenaed and testified to irreconcilable differences. A California judge is quoted to the effect that the law moves the state closer to divorce on unilateral request. Finally, Goddard concluded that the great weakness in the administration of the act was the lack of a family court to aid in implementation.

In the controversy over the proposed Uniform Marriage and Divorce Act the Family Law Section of the American Bar Association proposed the following clarification: "That the marriage is irretrievably broken in either that the parties have lived separate and apart for a period of more than one year . . . or that such serious marital misconduct has occurred which has so adversely affected the physical or mental health of the petitioning party as to make it impossible for the parties to continue the marital relation, and that reconciliation is improbable." [37]

The 1973 version of the proposed Uniform Act went part of the way toward meeting the wishes of the Family Law Section. The following language is used: "the court finds that the marriage is irretrievably broken, if the finding is supported by evidence that (1) the parties have lived separate and apart for a period of more than 180 days . . . or (2) there is serious marital discord adversely affecting the attitude of one or both of the parties toward the marriage; (3) the court finds that the conciliation provisions of Section 305 either do not apply or have been met." Although this language does define the irretrievably broken marriage, it is not specific except in the optional provision of separation for 180 days. The language "serious marital discord adversely affecting the attitude of one or both parties toward the marriage" does not give the court much guidance in deciding whether there has been a marital breakdown.

The nub of the controversy lies in the question of how difficult or how easy it should be for a couple, or for one of them, to secure a divorce. There was no difference between the two groups in cases where both marital partners want a divorce: it was agreed that it should be granted at once. But in cases where one partner wants a divorce and the other does not, the Family Law Section felt that the court should be given guidelines and definitions in processing the case. Traditionally, the states have gone their own way in enacting divorce laws, and these have varied from states where it was relatively simple to obtain a divorce to states where it was very difficult. For a time one state (South Carolina) did not grant divorce. Frequently, under the hodgepodge of laws, persons who very much wanted a divorce, and who could afford the expense, migrated temporarily to another state to obtain one (pages 369–374). And for over a century a national debate has gone forward regarding public policy on divorce. The trend to no-fault divorce marks a sharp turn toward easier divorce, but doubtless the old debate will be continued in a new setting.

NOTES / INDEX

NOTES

Chapter 1. Development of Statistics on Marriage and Divorce

1. George Elliott Howard, *A History of Matrimonial Institutions* (Chicago, Ill.: University of Chicago Press, 1904), vol. 2, pp. 121–327.

2. *Ibid.*, pp. 330–339.

3. *Ibid.*, pp. 366–368.

4. *Ibid.*, pp. 371–387.

5. National Center for Health Statistics, *Vital Statistics of the United States, 1950*, vol. 1, table 1.06. The following state files of marriage records were established before 1900: Connecticut, Hawaii, Iowa, Maine, Massachusetts, Michigan, New Hampshire, New Jersey, New York, Rhode Island, Vermont, Virginia, and the District of Columbia. The following were established between 1900 and 1950: Alabama, Alaska, Arkansas, California, Delaware, Florida, Idaho, Kansas, Louisiana, Maryland, Mississippi, Missouri, Montana, Nebraska, North Dakota, Ohio, Oregon, Pennsylvania, South Carolina, South Dakota, Tennessee, Utah, West Virginia, Wisconsin, Wyoming, and Puerto Rico.

6. *Ibid.* The following state files of divorce records were established before 1900: Maine, Michigan, New Hampshire, New Jersey, Vermont, and the District of Columbia. The following were established between 1900 and 1950: Alabama, Alaska, Arkansas, Connecticut, Delaware, Florida, Idaho, Iowa, Louisiana, Maryland, Mississippi, Missouri, Montana, Nebraska, North Dakota, Ohio, Oregon, Pennsylvania, South Dakota, Tennessee, Virginia, Wisconsin, Wyoming, and Puerto Rico.

7. Carroll D. Wright, *A Report on Marriage and Divorce in the United States, 1867 to 1886* (Washington, D.C.: Government Printing Office, 1889), pp. 1–14. This report includes an appendix relating to marriage and divorce in certain European countries.

8. U.S. Bureau of the Census, *Marriage and Divorce, 1867–1906*, pt. 1, Summary, Laws, Foreign Statistics, 1909, p. 4.

9. U.S. Bureau of the Census, *Marriage and Divorce 1916.*

10. U.S. Bureau of the Census, *Marriage and Divorce*, annual reports, 1922–1932 (1925–1934).

11. The Metropolitan Life Insurance Company made extensive collections of data. See *Statistical Bulletin* of that company for the December issues of 1940 through 1948; also, *Monthly Marriage Report,* Federal Security Agency, vol. 1, no. 13, March 1948. Marriage figures were also published in the Jeweler's Circular-Keystone. The Federal Home Loan Bank Board collected some marriage figures. Two sociologists prepared national estimates of marriages and divorces for the years 1933–1936: see S. A. Stouffer and L. M. Spencer, "Recent Increases in Marriages and Divorces," *American Journal of Sociology,* 44 (January 1939) 551–554. See also U.S. Bureau of the Census, *Estimated Number of Marriages by State: United States, 1937–1942*, 1942; and National Center for Health Statistics, *Marriage and Divorce in the United States, 1937*

to 1945, 1946. Beginning with 1946, final data have appeared in annual volumes: National Center for Health Statistics, *Vital Statistics of the United States,* and *Monthly Vital Statistics Report* (provisional data).

12. The agreement contains this statement: "The NOVS feels that the most essential statistical tabulations for the MRA must cover at least age, residence, previous marital status, and date and place of marriage." See *Implementation of the Marriage Registration Area (MRA)*, Public Health Conference on Records and Statistics, document no. 407-7/19/56, p. 3.

13. See the successive annual reports of the Committee on Marriage and Divorce Statistics in the *American Sociological Review* from 1955 to 1965. The successive chairmen of this committee for varying periods of time were: Robert F. Winch, Harold T. Christensen, P. K. Whelpton, William M. Kephart, Daniel O. Price, Charles E. Bowerman, C. Horace Hamilton, and Hugh Carter. See also Hugh Carter, "Plans for Improved Statistics on Family Formation and Dissolution in the United States," *Social Forces*, 39, no. 2 (1960), 163–169; Hugh Carter and Sarah Lewit, "Recent Developments in the Federal Marriage and Divorce Statistical Program," *Estadistica*, 15, no. 56 (1957), 617–630; and Hugh Carter, "The Federal Program for Statistics on Family Formation and Dissolution," *Marriage and Family Living*, 20, no. 3 (1958), 211–212.

14. The National Council on Family Relations at its annual meeting in August 1961 endorsed the program. The Rural Sociological Society gave its endorsement in 1961, as reported in *Rural Sociology*, 27 (1962), 247.

15. *Proceedings of the Board of Governors*, American Bar Association, October 19 and 20, 1961, p. 18 and exhibit H; and Hugh Carter, "The Program to Improve Registration and Statistics," *Proceedings of Section of Family Law*, American Bar Association, 1961.

16. See Hugh Carter, Carl E. Ortmeyer, and Alexander Plateris, "Statistics from the National Sample of Marriage and Divorce Transcripts," American Statistical Association, *Proceedings of Social Statistics Section*, 1962, pp. 24–33, esp. p. 28.

17. National Center for Health Statistics, *Vital Statistics of the United States, 1960*, vol. 3, "Marriage and Divorce," 1965.

18. *Ibid.*, tables 7–14 and 7–15.

19. National Center for Health Statistics, *Vital Statistics of the United States, 1950*, vol. 1, tables 1.03 and 1.04.

20. For a much fuller account of the subjects discussed in the balance of this chapter, see the following three chapters by Paul C. Glick: "Demographic Analysis of Family Data," in Harold T. Christensen, ed., *Handbook of Marriage and the Family* (Chicago, Ill.: Rand McNally & Co., 1964), pp. 300–334; "Family Statistics," in Philip M. Hauser and Otis Dudley Duncan, eds., *The Study of Population* (Chicago, Ill.: University of Chicago Press, 1959), pp. 576–603; and "Marital Characteristics and Family Groups," in Henry S. Shryock and Jacob S. Siegel, *Demographic Materials and Methods* (U.S. Bureau of the Census, 1971).

21. The census treatment of persons with consensual or common-law marriages deserves mention because the adult nonwhite population is more likely

than the white population to live in this type of (often unstable) union. In the collection process, enumerators are instructed to show such persons as married. In the editing process, instructions to coding clerks and computers likewise call for the treatment of such persons as married. Thus if a man and woman living together are recorded as head and wife of head of household, the computer automatically classifies them as "married." However, any study which might be designed to estimate the number of such unions from unedited census returns would very likely be far short of the actual number, partly because most persons living in consensual unions probably report themselves as married. The U.S. Bureau of the Census has not included marital status among the subjects covered in postcensal evaluation studies because of the possible effects on its public relations; the staff has reasoned that the required probing into this sensitive subject might create more problems than the statistical results would justify.

22. A detailed statement about the quality of data on marital status in the 1960 census is given in U.S. Bureau of the Census, *U.S. Census of Population: 1960, Subject Reports, Marital Status,* Final Report PC(2)-4E, pp. IX–XI. Among the findings in this statement that are relevant here is the fact that of all persons 14 years old and over, only 0.6 percent of the whites and 1.3 percent of the nonwhites *enumerated* did not report marital status. Of all white persons 14 and over, nonresponses were replaced with "allocated" entries of married for 0.1 percent, widowed for 1.2 percent, single for 1.6 percent, divorced for 2.2 percent, and separated for 2.9 percent; corresponding values for nonwhites were 0.5 percent, 2.0 percent, 2.7 percent, 3.1 percent, and 2.5 percent. The quality of the data on marital status may have been most seriously affected by the much larger proportion of nonwhite than white persons who were *not enumerated* in the census. This topic is effectively presented in David M. Heer, ed., *Social Statistics and the City* (Report of a Conference Held in Washington, D.C., June 22–23, 1967), (Cambridge, Mass.: Harvard University Press, 1968). On p. 4 of this report, estimates prepared by Jacob S. Siegel, of the Bureau of the Census, show the following proportions of under-enumeration in 1960: 2.2 percent for whites and 9.5 percent for nonwhites; 8.1 percent for nonwhite females and 10.9 percent for nonwhite males; and 17 percent, or one in every six, for nonwhite males 20 to 39 years old. Although this source provides no detail by marital status, a plausible hypothesis, based in part on the distribution of allocations for nonresponse given above, is that a disproportionately large part of the group missed in the census consisted of separated, divorced, widowed, and single persons. Yet for several reasons (including the relatively large proportion of young men with low incomes who have had trouble with legal authorities, and the procedures in many states in 1960 which made it easier for a mother to receive welfare assistance if she had no "man around the house"), a substantial proportion of the un-enumerated young adult males may have actually been married but simply not reported in the census.

Chapter 2. Comparative International Trends in Marriage and Divorce

1. John W. Moreland, *Keezer on the Law of Marriage and Divorce*, ed. 3 (Indianapolis, Ind.: Bobbs-Merrill Co., 1946), p. 298. See also Griselda Rowntree and Norman H. Carrier, "The Resort to Divorce in England and Wales, 1858–1957," *Population Studies*, 11, no. 3 (March 1958). The number of divorces in one year may be unusually high because of administrative changes. According to McGregor, England appointed special commissioners in 1947 and 1948 to hear divorce petitions, with the result that an accumulation of cases was cleared off quickly. Oliver Roass McGregor, *Divorce in England: A Centenary Study* (London: Heinemann, 1957), pp. 34–35.

2. In the United States by the mid-1960's, a contrary trend toward a smaller proportion of marriages in the teens was evident from current surveys. This change will be discussed further in Chapter 4.

Chapter 3. Trends and Variations in Marriage Rates, Divorce Rates, and Marital Status

1. See Mortimer Spiegelman, *Introduction to Demography*, rev. ed. (Cambridge, Mass.: Harvard University Press, 1968), table 8.5, p. 230. This table presents a meaningful summary of relationships between first-marriage rates and four social and economic characteristics: region, education, income, and occupation. For males and females in specified single and grouped years of age between 17 and 44, his table shows the category of each characteristic for which the first-marriage rate was highest (peak) and for which it was lowest (trough). The table is based on tables 16 and 17 of the report cited as the source of Table 3.7.

2. Hugh Carter and Gordon F. Sutton, "Factors Associated with Seasonal Variation in Marriage in the United States," *International Population Conference, Wien, 1959*, (Vienna: Christoph Reisser) pp. 161–172.

3. National Center for Health Statistics, *Vital Statistics of the United States, 1960*, vol. 3, "Marriage and Divorce," 1965.

4. *Ibid.*, 1960 and 1962.

5. *Ibid.*, 1960, table 1-R.

6. National Center for Health Statistics, *Vital Statistics — Special Report*, vol. 47, no. 7, table F.

7. The least reliable of these rates covers the years 1920–1921 and 1933–1939, when the national collection system for divorce statistics, as discussed in Chapter 1, was not functioning or was functioning inadequately. However, the overall trend is clear.

8. This measure was obtained by standardizing the proportions in each marital status on the basis of a stationary population; for both dates the L_x life-table values for 1959–1961 were used. This was done in order to eliminate the undue effects of the changing age composition of the actual populations on the distribution by marital status, and to permit summing the results meaningfully for all adult years combined.

Chapter 4. Group Variations in Age at Marriage

1. About 12.7 percent of white first births and 37.9 percent of nonwhite first births were reported as occurring within seven months after marriage, according to data for women married during the five years preceding a 1959 survey conducted by the U.S. Bureau of the Census. The results were reported in "Marriage, Fertility, and Childspacing: August 1959," *Current Population Reports*, series P-20, no. 108, tables 16 and 17.

2. Hugh Carter, Sarah Lewit, and William F. Pratt, "Socioeconomic Characteristics of Persons Who Married Between January 1947 and June 1954: United States," *Vital Statistics — Special Reports*, National Center for Health Statistics, vol. 45, no. 12, table 8.

3. U.S. Bureau of the Census, *U.S. Census of Population: 1960, Subject Reports, Marital Status*, Final Report PC(2)-4E, table 4.

4. Hugh Carter and Paul C. Glick, "Trends and Current Patterns of Marital Status Among Nonwhite Persons," *Demography*, 3, no. 1 (1966) 276–288, table 3.

5. Paul C. Glick and Robert Parke, Jr., "New Approaches in Studying the Life Cycle of the Family," *Demography*, vol. 2, (1965).

6. U.S. Bureau of the Census, "Marital Status and Household Characteristics: April 1949," *Current Population Reports*, series P-20, no. 26, table 10.

7. See Carter, Lewit, and Pratt, "Socioeconomic Characteristics," tables 15 and 16.

8. See especially Tables 3.4 and 3.5 in Chapter 3.

9. Clyde V. Kiser, "The Relation of Assortative Mating to Fertility," paper presented at the Fourth Princeton Conference on Population Genetics and Demography, November 9–11, 1967.

10. One of the advantages of completing a college education before marriage is the generally greater maturity of the person at the time of marriage. Such a person is likely to plan the number and spacing of children in a way that will permit the family to maintain its economic solvency. See Alvin L. Schorr, "The Family Cycle and Income Development," *Social Security Bulletin*, 29, no. 2 (February 1966), 14–25 and 47.

11. Nonwhite men's earnings overall were less than one-half the level for white men ($3,195 versus $6,563). This difference appears to have been largely a consequence of the greater concentration of nonwhites in occupations with low earnings. Actually, only nonwhite farm workers and managerial workers had mean earnings less than one-half the corresponding level for white men.

12. If data for Table 4.16 had been available on detailed occupations rather than on major occupation groups alone, the discriminating power of the occupational factor undoubtedly would have been greatly increased. For instance, separate data for professional workers in the relatively low income group of teachers at the elementary and high-school level and for those in the relatively high income group of lawyers, physicians, and engineers would have been enlightening. The data in Chapters 7, 8, 9, and 10 on marital status by detailed occupations demonstrate the usefulness of the finer classification of occupations for studying marriage patterns. This greater detail provides a basis for

checking hypotheses about the marriage patterns of men who tend to make occupational choices on the basis of probable income rather than intellectual satisfaction from their work.

13. Here, as elsewhere in the interpretation of the data on earnings during middle age by age at first marriage, the analysis undoubtedly would have been sharpened if the classification by age at marriage had been planned to include a fifth category comprising adjacent parts of the two intermediate age groups shown.

14. It should be noted that the earnings differentials, here, were the outgrowth of conditions that existed for many years prior to 1960. These men, 45 to 54 years old in 1960, began their education during or shortly after the end of World War I, and many of them started to work and married during the depression decade of the 1930's. At that time, educational and occupational opportunities differed markedly from those of today. The analysis was limited to one age group because of the complexities of the tabulation required, and the age group 45 to 54 years was chosen so that the results could be interpreted as representative of men at or near the peak of earning power.

15. A note of caution may be appropriate in interpreting the white-nonwhite differences in age at marriage by social and economic characteristics. Education, occupation, and income are not truly comparable even when identical levels were reported by white and nonwhite men. Especially at the time when the middle-aged men of today were attending school, the quality of education at each level tended to have been much poorer for nonwhites than whites. Moreover, the proportion of men in the lower-paying occupations in a given major occupation group still tends to be larger for the nonwhite men. Refinement of such measures of social and economic characteristics is obviously desirable.

Chapter 5. Intermarriage Among Educational, Ethnic, and Religious Groups

1. See Hyman Rodman, *Marriage, Family, and Society: A Reader* (New York: Random House, 1965), pt. 2, "Mate Selection," pp. 43–72.

2. The thesis of Robert F. Winch, *Mate-Selection: A Study of Complementary Needs* (New York: Harper & Row, 1958), is that many of the subtler needs of husbands and wives can be satisfied best if certain nondemographic characteristics of the husband and wife are complementary rather than identical.

3. Several types of statistics on intermarriage and other aspects of mate selection, which are discussed in the present chapter, became available for the first time on a nationwide basis from special tabulations of 1960 census data and from supplements to the Current Population Survey conducted during the 1950's. Therefore no attempt is made to infer historical trends in mate selection on the basis of data from successive censuses. Data are shown here for a cross-section of married couples at the time of the census or survey; variable portions of these data are affected by uneven losses from the total number of couples in first marriages through selective attrition by divorce or

the death of a spouse and uneven gains to the current number of married couples through selective increments by remarriage. In certain critical comparisons these disturbing factors are statistically controlled by such devices as limiting the detail to couples in primary marriages (that is, couples with both partners married only once) and by showing the detail for couples in cohorts according to period of first marriage of the husband.

4. U.S. Bureau of the Census, "School Enrollment, and Education of Young Adults and Their Fathers: October 1960." *Current Population Reports,* series P-20, no. 110, tables A, B, 9, and 10.

5. If occupation and income of the husband's father and of the wife's father had been available in relation to census data on the occupation and income of the husband, such information would have been quite useful.

6. The expected value is obtained by cross-multiplying a value in the total row with a value in the total column of Table 5.1. Thus, 1.5 percent (0.015) in the first row times 2.7 percent (0.027) in the first column equals the expected value 0.04 percent (0.000405); and the actual value 0.7 percent divided by the expected value 0.04 percent gives the quotient 17.5 shown in Table 5.2.

7. The values in Table 5.2 at or near the extremes of the diagonal tend to be relatively large. The corner values 17.5 and 9.1 are by far the highest, but they are based on the smallest numbers of cases on the diagonal, as Table 5.1 shows. They are large partially because the only possibilities are for the persons involved to marry a partner with the same amount of education or with a deviation in one direction only. Moreover, the value 9.1 is large in part because of the much greater supply of men than women with 5 or more years of college training; thus, 7 out of 8 married men with graduate-school training married women with less education than they had, whereas about one-half the wives with graduate training married men with no graduate training.

8. In prior censuses, the race item was generally recorded by the enumerator, without asking any questions, for all household members on the basis of the apparent race of the respondent. The enumerator in those censuses was asked to inquire about the race of resident employees or of other household members only where there was reason to believe that they might be of a race different from the respondent.

In the 1960 census, by contrast, replies to the race item were reported by self-enumeration, with follow-up by direct enumeration if the forms were not completed by a household member. At that time, however, an unknown proportion of couples with racially mixed marriages may have consciously misreported themselves as both of the same race in order to avoid the possible revelation that the facts were otherwise. Presumably the direction of the net bias in this situation would be to increase the proportion of couples with both husband and wife reported as white. In addition, if the self-enumeration forms were not completed by a household respondent before the enumerator called to pick them up, the enumerator obtained the required race information by direct interview as in previous censuses, and this probably led to the recording of less racial intermarriage than actually existed. Areas where this occurred may have had a larger proportion of mixed marriages than the average for the country as a whole. All the evidence, therefore, points to an undercount of unknown magnitude in the statistics on couples of unlike race.

9. The "total" columns for husbands classified by their race and wives classified by their race bring out the positive relationship between the size of racial group and the percent of married persons with a spouse of the same race. Of course, it would be physically possible for many (or all) of the members of a small racial group to marry a person of a different race; moreover, the geographic distribution of the members of such a race is often of sufficient breadth to permit few, if any, acceptable candidates of the same race to be considered as a marital partner. Hence the fact that there is a considerable amount of outmarriage among these groups should not be surprising, though the actual extent may exceed the level which most persons would expect.

10. A more adequate analysis of trends in racial mixture could be made if vital records of first marriages and remarriages by race of husband and wife for specified decades for the entire United States could be compared with subsequent census records tabulated in identical detail, to see what percent of the remarriages remained intact. In the absence of the desired historical series of vital data, some approximations of such series can be reconstructed from marital histories for persons in 30,000 households obtained by the Bureau of the Census in a survey conducted under contract with the Office of Economic Opportunity in the spring of 1967. The marital histories include information on when the first and last marriages were entered and when and how they were ended. Data from the 1967 survey appear in two publications: U.S. Bureau of the Census, *Current Population Reports,* Series P-20, no. 223, "Social and Economic Variations of Marriage, Divorce, and Remarriage, 1967"; and Paul C. Glick and Arthur J. Norton, "Frequency, Duration and Probability of Marriage and Divorce," *Journal of Marriage and the Family,* 33, no. 2 (May 1971), 307–317.

Still further valuable but unexplored items for a nationwide census or survey are date of birth, race, and education of each former spouse (or at least of the first and last spouses). Data on these items would permit a more definitive historical study than can be made from existing data of the proportion of couples in successive marriage cohorts who remain together for specified periods of time before obtaining a divorce.

For a description of new data of this type which were in preparation or being planned at the time of this writing, see Paul C. Glick, "Permanence of Marriage," *Population Index,* 33, no. 4 (October–December 1967), 517–526. The new data should be useful to marriage counselors; see the last two sections of Chapter 12.

11. See Rodman, *Marriage, Family, and Society.* Pages 56 and 57 contain a brief summary of theories of mate selection which have been presented by Robert K. Merton, Kingsley Davis, Milton L. Barron, Joseph Golden, Todd H. Pavella, and Marshall Sklare.

12. Of methodologic interest is the generally inverse relationship between the size of the diagonal value and the number of married persons in the national-origin group. For instance, those of Italian origin are the most numerous of all specific origin groups, and this group had one of the lowest diagonal values.

Yet persons of Italian origin could intermarry with non-Italians at a relatively restricted *rate* and still involve about as large a *number* of mixed-origin couples as a smaller origin group with a somewhat greater tendency to intermarry. Even with a small proportion of Italians marrying Irishmen, there were fully 37,000 Irish-and-Italian couples; at the same time, with a much larger proportion of Poles marrying Russians, there were nonetheless only about the same number (41,000) of Polish-and-Russian couples.

13. Median ages of males 14 and over in 1960 were as follows: native of native parentage, 40.7; native of foreign or mixed parentage, 43.8; and foreign born, 58.8.

14. Married couples or parent-child groups doubling up with relatives. See Chapter 6.

15. U.S. Bureau of the Census, *U.S. Census of Population: 1960, Subject Reports, Women by Number of Children Ever Born*, Final Report PC(2)-3A, table 9.

16. Among the numerous references which could be cited on substantive and methodologic aspects of intermarriage, only a few are given here: David M. Heer, "Negro-White Marriage in the United States," *Journal of Marriage and the Family*, 28, no. 3 (August 1966), 262–273; Jessie Bernard, "Note on Educational Homogamy in Negro-White and White-Negro Marriages, 1960," *Journal of Marriage and the Family*, 28, no. 3 (August 1966), 274–276; Rodman, *Marriage, Family, and Society* on pp. 61–65; Erich Rosenthal, "Studies of Jewish Intermarriage in the United States," *American Jewish Year Book*, 1963, vol. 64, pp. 3–53; William Petersen, "Religious Statistics in the United States," *Journal for the Scientific Study of Religion* (April 1962), 165–178; and Benson Y. Landis, "A Guide to the Literature on Statistics of Religious Affiliation with References to Related Social Studies," *Journal of the American Statistical Association*, 54 (June 1959), 335–357. Several hundred additional references on mate selection are listed in Joan Aldous and Reuben Hill, *International Bibliography of Research in Marriage and the Family, 1900–1964* (Minneapolis, Minn.: University of Minnesota Press, 1967).

Chapter 6. Family Composition and Living Arrangements of Married Persons

1. For a much more elaborate review of trends and differentials in childbearing and childspacing, see the monograph by Clyde V. Kiser, Wilson H. Grabill, and Arthur A. Campbell, *Trends and Variations in Fertility in the United States* (Cambridge, Mass.: Harvard University Press, 1968). One of the most comprehensive analyses of the family life cycle that has been made appears in the book by Evelyn Millis Duvall, *Family Development* (Chicago: J. B. Lippincott Co., 1971). The book was in process of revision in 1975.

2. As the number of children declined, the spacing intervals between the children tended to increase somewhat; then as the fertility rate rose after World War II and contracted again during the late 1950's and 1960's, additional changes (somewhat too complex to discuss here) occurred in the childspacing intervals. When a cohort of women is at the height of its reproductive period,

any tendency to postpone the timing of births or to advance it may not be fully compensated for later on. A very brief explanation is that women who postpone births tend to enjoy the personal advantages of having fewer children to rear, and those who advance births increase their period of exposure to having additional children.

3. Precise measurement of intervals between the later stages of married life is complicated by the increasing range of variation in the events (dates of birth of children, dates of marriage of children, dates of death of original spouses) which combine to determine the limits of these later stages. Consequently, although ages associated with the earlier phases are relatively well defined, those associated with the later phases are stated in terms of illustrative experience centering around the family behavior of those relatively few couples for whom the entire series of family-building and later "unbuilding" occurrences hovered near the average for all couples. In general, however, the deviations among married couples from the illustrative values shown should be about as large in one direction as the other.

4. The reasons why the median age at death of one spouse on this basis has changed very little during the century, despite the improvement in survival conditions, include the fact that this improvement is relatively small at the older ages and that it has been offset by a declining age at first marriage of the last child, so that exposure to death in the empty-nest period is now beginning at an earlier age.

5. These values are equivalent to the percentage of married couples "with their own household." The complement of such values is the proportion of married couples "without their own household," also referred to as "doubled couples" or "couples sharing the homes of others."

6. Of course, at least a minority of the couples had lived apart from their parents for a while and then moved in — or back in — with them.

7. Doubled couples living with the wife's grandparents are classified as living with an "other relative" of the husband.

8. The high proportion of "other families" with doubled couples must be interpreted in relation to the census definition of a family. This definition states that a family comprises two or more related persons who live together in the same housing unit (generally a one-family house or an apartment). Thus a family may consist of a head and a doubled couple. However, if the same three persons had been reported as a husband-wife family with an "adult relative" living in, there would have been no doubled couple present. The determination as to which person is reported as the head of the household is left to the respondent. Presumably the principal determining factors include who owns the home or in whose name it is rented, what patterns of dominance and subordination are recognized by the persons involved, and who is the chief breadwinner. The statistics show that the older generation is usually the host; this host generation probably also tends to dominate the guest generation largely because of long-standing role relationships, but also because the host generation is usually the main economic support of the family. Research to establish the rationale behind the designation of relationship by respondents might help to clarify this matter.

9. In addition, 6,500 families included three generations which were not consecutive; and at least 25,000 families included four generations. The detail shown in Table 6.9 on three-generation families by type of family composition is available only for white families.

10. For further discussion of "other families," see John Beresford and Alice M. Rivlin, "Characteristics of Other Families," *Demography*, 1, no. 1 (1964), 242–246.

11. The method of obtaining this index is as follows: The number of Japanese families in the United States in 1960 was 0.244 percent as large as the number of white families. Moreover, the number of Japanese families with three generations present comprising parent of head, HEAD, and child of head was 0.686 percent as large as the corresponding number of white families. Dividing 0.686 by 0.244 and multiplying the quotient by 100 gives the index 281. A parallel method was used to obtain the indexes of families comprising HEAD, child of head, and grandchild of head.

12. For a study of changes in social and economic characteristics of persons of second generation compared with those of first generation in the United States, see Charles B. Nam, "Nationality Groups and Social Stratification in America," *Social Forces,* 37, no. 4 (May 1959), 328–333.

13. According to the results of a survey of the aged conducted in 1963 for the Social Security Administration by the U.S. Bureau of the Census, nine out of ten persons 65 years old and over with living children but none in the same household live within a day's journey of at least one son or daughter. Seventeen percent of these aged persons live within a travel distance of over one hour but under one day to their nearest child, 12 percent over half an hour but under an hour, 24 percent over 10 but under 30 minutes, and 37 percent under 10 minutes. See U.S. Social Security Administration, *The Aged Population of the United States: The 1963 Social Security Survey of the Aged* (Research Report No. 19), 1967, pp. 163–165.

Chapter 7. Work Experience and Income of Married Persons

1. For a thorough examination of evidence on the difficulty which non-white husbands encounter in gaining and holding a position commensurate with their needs for income maintenance, see the 1960 census monograph by Daniel O. Price, *Changing Characteristics of the Negro Population* (Washington, D.C.: Government Printing Office, 1969).

2. U.S. Bureau of the Census, *U.S. Census of Population: 1960, Subject Reports, Families,* Final Report PC(2)-4A, table 38.

3. For a fuller exploration of this subject, see the monograph by Clyde V. Kiser, Wilson H. Grabill, and Arthur A. Campbell, *Trends and Variations in Fertility in the United States* (Cambridge, Mass.: Harvard University Press, 1968).

4. U.S. Bureau of the Census, *U.S. Census of Population: 1960, Subject Reports, Families.*

5. U.S. Bureau of the Census, *U.S. Census of Population: 1960, Subject*

Reports, Employment and Work Experience, Final Report PC(2)-6A, table 20.

6. U.S. Bureau of the Census, *Trends in the Income of Families and Persons in the United States: 1947 to 1960,* Technical Paper No. 8, 1963, tables A and D. See also note 10 below.

7. The extent to which men leave the teaching profession after a few years was among the subjects covered in a study of men college graduates initiated by the Bureau of the Census in 1967.

8. For current statistics on married persons enrolled in school, see U.S. Bureau of the Census, "School Enrollment: October 1965," *Current Population Reports,* series P-20, no. 162, March 24, 1967, table 7. This report shows that 21.9 percent of all college students in the fall of 1965 were married and living with their spouse. The corresponding figures for those attending college full time were only 6.2 percent married for women and 15.5 percent for men; but for those attending college part time the figures were 48.8 percent married for women and fully 61.5 percent for men.

9. U.S. Bureau of the Census, *U.S. Census of Population: 1960, Subject Reports, Educational Attainment,* Final Report PC(2)-5B, table 6.

10. U.S. Bureau of the Census, *U.S. Census of Population: 1960, Subject Reports, Occupational Characteristics,* Final Report PC(2)-7A, table 31.

11. U.S. Bureau of the Census, *Trends in the Income of Families and Persons in the United States: 1947 to 1964,* Technical Paper No. 17, 1967, table 3.

12. U.S. Bureau of the Census, *U.S. Census of Population: 1960, Subject Reports, Sources and Structure of Family Income,* Final Report PC(2)-4C, table 13.

13. A graphic presentation of the values in the last five columns of the upper section of Table 7.23 is shown in Paul C. Glick and Robert Parke, Jr., "New Approaches in Studying the Life Cycle of the Family," *Demography* (1965), 201.

14. The hypothesis concerning relatively permanent stratification of families by broad income levels throughout the family cycle is suggested by data from a cross-section of families at a given time rather than by a longitudinal study of cohorts of families passing through the cycle stages. Research currently in progress at the Bureau of the Census may provide corresponding data on a longitudinal basis for comparison.

15. After this monograph had been prepared, the following special report was published which throws further light on the subject matter discussed in this chapter: U.S. Bureau of the Census, *U.S. Census of Population: 1960, Subject Reports, Socioeconomic Status,* Final Report PC(2)-5C. This report gives "socioeconomic status scores" of adults classified by various subjects, including marital status, stage of the life cycle of the family, fertility, migration, race, nativity, ethnic origin, wife's contribution to family income, and housing characteristics. It also deals in a limited way with "status inconsistency," a frequent source of frustration and no doubt often a threat to marital stability.

Chapter 8. Group Variations Among Separated and Divorced Persons

1. For a summary of important research on this subject, see George Levinger, "Marital Cohesiveness and Dissolution: An Integrative Review," *Journal of Marriage and the Family,* 27, no. 1 (February 1965), 19–28.

2. The possibility that the increase in the number divorced is related to a rise in the proportion who leave the ranks of the separated to become divorced was raised by Calvin L. Beale in "Increased Divorce Rates Among Separated Persons as a Factor in Divorce Since 1940," *Social Forces,* 29, no. 1 (October 1950), 72–74.

3. Thomas P. Monahan, "When Married Couples Part: Statistical Trends and Relationships in Divorce," *American Sociological Review,* 27, no. 5 (October 1962), 625–633; and J. Richard Udry, "Marital Instability by Race, Sex, Education, and Occupation Using 1960 Census Data," *American Journal of Sociology,* 72, no. 2 (September 1960), 203–209.

4. The following partial explanation is offered for the older average age at divorce obtained from the Divorce-Census Match sample than from divorce records. In the former source, age was based on date of birth and related to April 1960, whereas in the latter source the age sometimes was related to the time when the divorce was applied for—a few days to several years before the divorce decree became final.

5. John D. Lillywhite, "Rural-Urban Differentials in Divorce," *Rural Sociology,* 17, no. 4 (December 1952), 348–355. In the fall of 1969 the first comprehensive set of *divorce rates* were published for the major cities of the United States. See *Divorce Statistics Analysis: United States, 1964 and 1965,* National Center for Health Statistics, U.S. Department of Health, Education, and Welfare, 1969, table 5. The combined rates in these 200 major city areas run in the expected direction: highest in central city counties, lowest in outlying metropolitan counties, and intermediate in the remainder of the country — the nonmetropolitan counties. About two-thirds of all 1965 divorces were granted in these 200 standard metropolitan statistical areas.

6. Analysis of the variance of separation ratios for native white and Negro women for 1960 shows that about twice as much of the variance can be explained by variation in residence by size of place as by variation in residence among the four regions of the United States:

Percent of variance accounted for by—	Separation ratio		Divorce ratio	
	Native white	Negro	Native white	Negro
Total	100.0	100.0	100.0	100.0
Size of place	63.1	69.2	82.5	49.7
Region	36.9	30.8	17.5	50.3

Variance of divorce ratios among native white women was even more readily explained by variation in residence by size of place, but that among Negro women was explained about equally by the two factors (size of place and region). This analysis is based on data from the same source as Tables 8.19 and 8.20. For a similar analysis based on white and nonwhite women for 1960 and an outline of the method of computation, see Paul C. Glick, "Marital Instability: Variations by Size of Place and Region," *Milbank Memorial Fund Quarterly*, 41, no. 1 (January 1963), 43–55.

7. National Center for Health Statistics, "Divorce Statistics, 1966," *Monthly Vital Statistics Report*, vol. 17, no. 10 supplement (January 6, 1969).

8. In 1960 an estimated 3.8 million of the 64 million (living) children under 18 years old were sons and daughters of persons who had ever been divorced. Of these, 2.1 million were living in the home of a divorced parent who had remarried, and most of the other 1.7 million were living with a parent who was still divorced; however, some of the parents had remarried and become widowed, and some of the children were living with neither parent. See Alvin L. Schorr, *Poor Kids: A Report on Children in Poverty* (New York: Basic Books, 1966), footnote on p. 118.

9. Another study of occupational concentrations of divorced persons in Philadelphia is given in William M. Kephart, "Occupational Level and Marital Disruption," *American Sociological Review*, 20, no. 4 (August 1955), 456–465.

10. Divorce records were adequate for matching only in five states and even in those states many records did not match, so that the results are far from definitive but are highly suggestive. To remove the distorting effect of age, the tabulations are limited to men 14 to 64 years old and women 14 to 54 years old, and both are standardized for age.

Chapter 9. Group Variations Among Widows and Widowers

1. National Center for Health Statistics, *Monthly Vital Statistics Report*, vol. 12, no. 13, table 7; and *Vital Statistics—Special Reports*, vol. 39, no. 7, table 1, and vol. 23, no. 2, table 1. See also the data presented in Tables 9.3 and 11.9.

2. Corresponding data were not collected in the 1960 census. Nor were data for men tabulated for 1950; the information was collected, but the punch cards containing the data were destroyed in the mid-1950's. Numerators for the rates shown here were based on a special tabulation of 1950 census data for women published in the report entitled *Duration of Current Marital Status*, and the bases were from the 1950 report entitled *Education*. The sample used as the source for the numerators did not extend into old age and did not include men. In computing the rates, one-half the widowed women in 1950 who reported themselves as having been widowed less than two years were divided by the number of married women in 1950 plus the number of widowed women just described, and the quotient was multiplied by 1,000. The rates have not been adjusted for any inaccuracies of reporting, and no means for doing so are readily available. Consequently, the absolute level of the rates may be subject to some error, yet it is believed that the approximate order of magnitude of the differences between social and demographic groups in widowhood rates can be properly gauged from the figures in the table.

3. Based on Current Population Survey data collected by the Bureau of

the Census for the period January 1950 to April 1953. See National Office of Vital Statistics, "Demographic Characteristics of Recently Married Persons: United States, April 1953," *Vital Statistics — Special Reports,* vol. 39, no. 3, table 4.

4. The first three columns of Table 9.3 were obtained directly from the report *Duration of Current Marital Status,* table 29. The absolute numbers used as the bases for the fourth column constitute one-half the widows in 1950 who reported that they had become widowed during the two years before the census. The fifth column was estimated by obtaining the percent of marriages in 1960 (when data for a larger number of states were available than in 1950) which were remarriages and applying the percent to the absolute number of marriages in 1950. The sixth column was derived from mortality data by marital status for 1949 to 1951 in the second report cited above in note 1. The seventh column was obtained by subtracting the fifth and sixth columns from the fourth.

5. Perhaps a majority of the women who become widowed at ages 22 to 24 years remarry after they become 25. This fact probably is one of the main reasons why the percentage of widows who remarry below the age of 25 is lower than that for women 25 to 34 years old.

6. The foregoing analysis of 1950 data on the occurrence of widowhood and departures from widowhood probably provides a better approximation to the relative importance of the several components than to the absolute sizes of the turnover rate for ages at which remarriage rates are the highest. Data collected in a survey of 30,000 households by the Bureau of the Census for the Office of Economic Opportunity in the spring of 1967 may provide a better source, in some respects, for studying annual additions of widowed persons (of all ages and of both sexes) and comparable data on their remarriages. Such data may be combined with vital statistics on deaths of widowed persons to make possible a thoroughgoing analysis of gross changes in widowerhood and widowhood. See also John P. Jones, "Remarriage Tables Based on Experience under OASDI and US Employees Compensation Systems," Actuarial Study No. 55, Social Security Administration, December, 1962.

7. As divorce has increased and as an increasing proportion of the population has survived to or beyond middle age as divorced persons, a correspondingly larger proportion of people in the United States is at risk of death as divorced rather than married persons. This is an additional factor in the declining proportion of middle-aged persons who are widowed.

8. There were actually more nonwhite (834,000) than white (782,000) children under 18 living with a parent who was reported as separated. Probably a majority of the separated parents of the white children involved were in the process of obtaining a divorce, and no doubt some of the separated parents were more or less permanently living apart with little prospect of obtaining a divorce; but many — possibly a majority — of the reportedly separated parents of the nonwhite children involved had really never been married. Among nonwhite children living with their mother only, 46 percent of the mothers were reported as separated and another 10 percent as single; among white children, the corresponding figures were only 21 and 1 percent.

9. The values on the total line of Table 9.15 for the last two columns are

larger than those for any age group, because the totals for nonwhites are more heavily weighted than those for whites by widowed persons at younger ages where labor-force-participation rates are relatively high.

10. See source of Table 9.18. This finding, interestingly, does not hold true for women of all ages combined because of the heavy weighting of widows 65 years old and over with incomes under $1,000. Except for age 65 and over, widows of every age group were more likely to have incomes between $1,000 and $2,999 than any other income group.

11. See U.S. Bureau of the Census, *U.S. Census of Population: 1960, Subject Reports, Sources and Structure of Family Income,* Final Report PC(2)-4C, table 7, data for female heads of families.

12. A longitudinal study initiated in 1966 by the Bureau of the Census for the Department of Labor should provide some data of the type mentioned here. Work and income history is to be traced for six years for a group of men 45 to 59 years old and a group of women 30 to 44 years old at the beginning of the study. The purpose of the study is to throw light on factors which determine the conditions under which men retire from the labor force and under which women re-enter the labor force when their children reach school age. Among the related items to be recorded and analyzed will be changes in marital status and changes in family composition.

Chapter 10. Group Variations Among Bachelors and Spinsters

1. U.S. Bureau of the Census, "Marital Status and Family Status: March 1967," *Current Population Reports,* series P-20, no. 170, table 1.

2. Walt Saveland and Paul C. Glick, "Nuptiality Tables for the United States: 1958–60 and Earlier Dates," paper presented at the annual meeting of the Population Association of America in Boston, April 19–20, 1968. The nuptiality tables for 1958–60 are based on 1960 census data and are for white and nonwhite men and women. They show for each year of age from 14 to 64 and 65 and over the probabilities of first marriage and (separately) death within one year, as well as various additional actuarial calculations. The 1958–60 tables prepared for this paper are compared with 1948 tables published by Jacobson and 1940 tables published by Grabill. See Paul H. Jacobson, *American Marriage and Divorce* (New York: Rinehart, 1959); and Wilson H. Grabill, "Attrition Life Tables for the Single Population," *Journal of the American Statistical Association,* 45, (1945), 364–375. See also note 9 below.

3. A classic study by Hollingshead in New Haven in 1949 provided evidence that the family tends to exert more pressure on daughters than on sons to marry a person in their own residential class or in an area of higher class. See August B. Hollingshead, "Cultural Factors in the Selection of Marriage Mates," *American Sociological Review,* 15, no. 5 (October 1950), 619–627.

4. Probably because of special circumstances, some of the cohort changes in percent single shown in Table 10.2 do not correspond to the expected patterns. Not even an abrupt decline in the marriage rate would lead one to expect that the percent single would rise between 1950 and 1960 for the following four cohorts, but it did: nonwhite men who were 45 to 49 years

old in 1950 and 55 to 59 years old in 1960; white women of the same age cohort; nonwhite women of the same cohort; and nonwhite women of the next younger cohort. (All other cohorts in the table show the expected decline in percent single from one census to the next.) The following are plausible explanations of the four unexpected changes. The increases for women may reflect errors of reporting marital status, with those of childrearing age in 1950 often reporting themselves incorrectly as separated while their children were present, but correctly as single a decade later after their children had left home. In addition, the coverage of the population in quarters difficult to enumerate — where many bachelors and spinsters reside — and the reporting of marital status under conditions of self-enumeration in 1960 may have been better than the corresponding coverage and reporting on marital status under conditions of direct enumeration in 1950.

5. See U.S. Bureau of the Census, *U.S. Census of Population: 1960, Detailed Characteristics, United States Summary,* Final Report PC(1)-1D, table 185.

6. In census classifications, "partners" are included in the category "lodgers." These are nonrelatives of the household head who usually share the cost of maintaining the home in the same manner in which two sisters might share. The same category includes "companions" and "friends," often of the opposite sex from that of the household head. In 1960, about 217,000 men 25 to 64 years old were living as primary individuals who shared their home with a nonrelative; about 93,000 of these men shared their home with a woman; about three-fourths of the women were reported as lodgers with the other fourth as resident employees. Nonwhite men were greatly overrepresented in this group. The vast majority (about 19 out of 20) of men 25 to 64 living as primary individuals, however, were enumerated as living entirely alone. See U.S. Bureau of the Census, *U.S. Census of Population: 1960, Subject Reports, Persons by Family Characteristics,* Final Report PC(2)-4B, table 15.

7. No doubt because of the difficulty of enumerating people in those parts of metropolitan centers where the unmarried tend to congregate, or of determining facts about them from neighbors, the nonresponse rate on the marital-status item was half again as large for central-city dwellers as for the population as a whole (0.9 percent versus 0.6 percent); nonresponse rates in both groups, however, were quite low.

8. For further discussion of aids in the location of an acceptable person to marry, including the use of computerized lists of potential dates, see Paul C. Glick, "Permanence of Marriage," *Population Index* (October–December 1967), pp. 517–526.

9. A similar conclusion is drawn by Walt Saveland and Paul C. Glick, "First-Marriage Decrement Tables by Color and Sex for the United States in 1958–60," *Demography,* 6, no. 3 (August 1969), pp. 243–260.

Chapter 11. Marital Status and Health

1. National Center for Health Statistics, *Vital and Health Statistics,* series 11, no. 10, "Coronary Heart Disease in Adults: United States, 1960–1962,"

table 17; and series 11, no. 13, "Hypertension and Hypertensive Heart Disease in Adults: United States, 1960–1962," table 15.

2. National Center for Health Statistics, *Vital and Health Statistics,* series 11, no. 9, "Findings on the Seriological Test for Syphilis in Adults: United States, 1960–1962," table 10.

3. Women 45 to 54 years old in private nursing homes in 1960 had 0.5 year more education, on the average, than those in public nursing homes; and those in private homes for the aged not known to have nursing care had 1.6 years more of education than those in public homes of the same type.

4. For evidence that single persons under 65 years old have the lowest discharge rates for patients in short-stay hospitals (except for boys and young men 14 to 24 years old) and that married and separated women under 45 have by far the highest short-stay discharge rates, see National Center for Health Statistics, *Vital and Health Statistics,* series 10, no. 30, "Hospital Discharges and Length of Stay: Short-Stay Hospitals, United States, July 1963– June 1964," p. 12 and table 27.

5. From tables 25 to 28 of the 1960 report on *Inmates of Institutions.* See source note in Table 11.6.

6. For a study of personal and family characteristics of persons admitted to mental hospitals in Louisiana and Maryland during the year between July 1, 1960, and July 1, 1961, see the American Public Health Association monograph by Morton Kramer, Earl S. Pollack, Richard W. Redick, and Ben Z. Locke, *Mental Disorders/Suicide* (Cambridge, Mass.: Harvard University Press, 1972).

7. For a discussion of problems involved in making reliable estimates of mortality differentials by marital status, see the American Public Health Association monograph by Evelyn M. Kitagawa and Philip M. Hauser, *Differential Mortality in the United States: A Study in Socioeconomic Epidemiology* (Cambridge, Mass.: Harvard University Press, 1973). Because of the substantial discrepancies in the reporting of marital status on death certificates and census records found by Kitagawa and Hauser, and because of other problems of measurement even for the young-to-middle-age group covered here (15 to 64), the author of this chapter intentionally has not attached analytical significance to variances of less than 25 percent between the death rates for persons in different marital-status categories.

8. Dewey Shurtleff, "Mortality among the Married," *Journal of the American Geriatrics Society,* 4, no. 7 (July 1956), 654–666, esp. 658.

9. Mindel C. Sheps, "Marriage and Mortality," *American Journal of Public Health,* 51, no. 4 (April 1961), 547–555, esp. 552.

10. Cancer of the respiratory system (essentially lung cancer) and tuberculosis deserve special comment. Between 1950 and 1960, the crude death rate from tuberculosis for the entire population of the United States fell precipitously — from 20.6 to 5.6 — while the death rate from lung cancer rose much less spectacularly — from 14.1 to 22.2. In other words, tuberculosis fell 15 points, whereas lung cancer rose 8 points, so that the net change for the two causes was a decrease of 7 points.

11. Shurtleff, "Mortality among the Married," p. 660.

12. William Haenszel, Michael B. Shimkin, and Herman P. Miller, *Tobacco*

Smoking Patterns in the United States, Public Health Monograph no. 45, Department of Health, Education, and Welfare, 1956, pp. 44–50 and 94. For widowed and divorced men 45 to 54 years old (mostly divorced), the proportion who smoked over one 20-cigarette pack per day was larger (18 percent of men and 8 percent of women) than corresponding figures for persons of the same age in other marital-status groups. Married men with wife absent had smoking patterns similar to those of divorced men but had an even higher proportion (40 versus 32 percent) who smoked moderately (10 to 20 cigarettes per day). By far the highest proportions of persons who had never smoked were spinsters (73 percent) and bachelors (32 percent). Married women with husband absent had a relatively small proportion of moderate smokers (14 percent), along with a quite small proportion for spinsters (10 percent). White and nonwhite persons had about equal proportions of smokers, but whites had double the nonwhite proportion of heavy smokers. Farm and professional workers had the highest proportions of nonsmokers.

13. *Ibid.*

14. In August 1967, the author of this chapter invited comment from Arthur E. Callin of the Atlanta office of the National Communicable Disease Center, Department of Health, Education, and Welfare, about the hypothesis that women are more likely than men to seek medical treatment for syphilitic infection. He stated an alternative hypothesis, as follows: "Most of the experts in the field seem to agree that syphilis runs a milder course in females. . . . In our studies of possible BFP (biologic false positive) reactors it is apparent that many females go through life with no knowledge of their infections."

15. See, for example, J. R. McDonough, G. E. Garrison, and C. G. Hames, "Blood Pressure and Hypertensive Disease among Negroes and Whites: Study in Evans County, Georgia," *Annals of Internal Medicine,* 61, no. 2 (August 1964), 208–228.

Chapter 12. Legal and Administrative Aspects of Marriage and Divorce

1. Frances Kuchler, *The Law of Marriage and Divorce Simplified* (Dobbs Ferry, N. Y.: Oceana Publications, Inc., 1963), pp. 16–22.

2. Harold T. Christensen, "Child Spacing Analysis Via Record Linkage: New Data Plus a Summing Up from Earlier Reports," *Marriage and Family Living,* 25, no. 3 (August 1963), 272–280.

3. William F. Pratt, "A Study of Marriages Involving Premarital Pregnancies," dissertation, Dept. of Sociology, University of Michigan, 1965.

4. Kuchler, *The Law of Marriage and Divorce Simplified,* table 4, pp. 27–31.

5. *Ibid.*

6. *Ibid.,* table 2, pp. 23–26.

7. U.S. Supreme Court no. 395, June 12, 1967; no. 87, 1817 (Richard Perry Loving *et ux.* vs Commonwealth of Virginia). This decision lists the following states, in addition to Virginia, as having laws which prohibit and punish marriages on the basis of racial classifications: Alabama, Arkansas, Delaware, Florida, Kentucky, Louisiana, Mississippi, Missouri, North Carolina, Oklahoma,

South Carolina, Tennessee, Texas, and West Virginia. The following states were listed as having repealed such laws during the preceding 15 years: Arizona, California, Colorado, Idaho, Indiana, Maryland, Montana, Nebraska, Nevada, North Dakota, Oregon, South Dakota, Utah, Wyoming.

8. Kuchler, *The Law of Marriage and Divorce Simplified*, table 3, p. 26.

9. Dale L. Womble, "Trends in Falsification of Age at Marriage in Ohio," *Journal of Marriage and the Family*, 28, no. 1 (February 1966), 54–56.

10. Christensen, "Child Spacing Analysis Via Record Linkage," pp. 272–280.

11. The list is based on a chart issued by the Women's Bureau of the U.S. Department of Labor, "Divorce Laws as of July 1, 1965," giving the grounds for absolute divorce. Numerous qualifying and limiting footnotes are omitted. This table does not agree in every detail with a chart prepared by the National Legal Aid and Defender Association, American Bar Center, Chicago, Illinois, "Divorce, Annulment and Separation in the United States" (1965). The author of this chapter prepared a detailed listing, too voluminous to reproduce here, of all legal grounds by states in 1964; this did not completely agree with either of the charts mentioned — possibly because of a year's difference in dates. These minor variations do not seriously affect the present purpose, which is to indicate major grievances widely held as sufficiently serious to entitle a spouse to divorce. No implication of error in the cited lists is intended, but only a recognition of the difficulty of summarizing complex legal provisions.

12. National Center for Health Statistics, *Vital and Health Statistics,* "Divorce Statistics Analysis: United States, 1963," Public Health Service Publication No. 1000, series 21, no. 13, table F.

13. National Legal Aid and Defender Association, American Bar Center, Chicago, Illinois, "Divorce, Annulment and Separation in the United States" (chart), 1965.

14. Nelson M. Blake, *The Road to Reno: A History of Divorce in the United States* (New York: MacMillan Co., 1962), pp. 116–129.

15. William L. O'Neill, *Divorce in the Progressive Era* (New Haven, Conn.: Yale University Press, 1967).

16. *Ibid.*, pp. 33–56.

17. Herbert J. O'Gorman, *Lawyers in Matrimonial Cases: A Study of Informal Pressures in Professional Practice* (New York: Free Press, 1963).

18. Richard C. Dinkelspiel and Aidan R. Gough, "The Case for the Family Court — A Summary of the Report of the California Governor's Commission on the Family," *Family Law Quarterly,* 1, no. 3 (September 1967), 70–82.

19. J. Richard Udry, *The Social Context of Marriage* (Philadelphia, Pa.: J. B. Lippincott Co., 1966), p. 543. Udry quotes a survey on the subject published in *Americans View Their Mental Health* by Gerald Gurin, Joseph Veroff, and Sheila Feld (New York: Basic Books, 1960), p. 309.

20. Gerald R. Leslie, "The Field of Marriage Counseling," in *Handbook of Marriage and the Family*, Harold T. Christensen, ed. (Chicago, Ill.: Rand McNally & Co., 1964), pp. 912–943.

Chapter 13. Recent Changes in Marriage and Divorce

1. Hugh Carter, "Sociologists and the Improvement of Marriage and Divorce Statistics in the United States," in Dhirendra Narin, ed., *Explorations in the Family and Other Essays* (Bombay, India: Thacker and Co., Ltd., 1975), pp. 428–434.

2. Sweden, National Central Bureau of Statistics, *Marriage and Divorce Since 1950,* no. 4 (Stockholm, 1974).

3. Her Majesty's Stationery Office, *Social Trends,* No. 5 (London: Government Statistical Services, 1974).

4. Statistics Canada, *Perspective Canada: A Compendium of Social Statistics* (Ottawa, July 1974), p. 18.

5. *Social Trends,* note 3, p. 11.

6. Paul C. Glick and Arthur J. Norton, "Perspective on the Recent Upturn in Divorce and Remarriage," *Demography,* 10, no. 3 (August 1973), 301–314.

7. George Levinger, "Marital Cohesiveness and Dissolution: An Interpretive Review," *Journal of Marriage and the Family,* 27, no. 1 (February 1965), 19–28.

8. Peter Uhlenberg, "Marital Instability Among Mexican Americans: Following the Pattern of Blacks?", *Social Problems,* 20 (summer 1972), 49–56.

9. Paul C. Glick, "Some Recent Changes in American Families," U.S. Bureau of the Census, *Current Population Reports,* Series P-23, no. 52 (July 1975), 1–17. This is a revised version of Paul C. Glick, "A Demographer Looks at American Families," *Journal of Marriage and the Family,* 37, no. 1 (February 1975), 15–26.

10. Jessie Bernard, "Marital Stability and Patterns of Status Variables," *Journal of Marriage and the Family,* 28, no. 4 (November 1966), 421–439.

11. Thomas P. Monahan, "Are Interracial Marriages Really Less Stable?", *Social Forces,* 48, no. 4 (June 1970), 461–473.

12. David M. Heer, "The Prevalence of Black-White Marriage in the United States, 1960 and 1970," *Journal of Marriage and the Family,* 36, no. 2 (May 1974), 246–258.

13. Paul C. Glick, "Living Arrangements of Children and Young Adults," *Journal of Contemporary Family Studies,* in press.

14. Paul C. Glick and Karen M. Mills, "Black Families: Marriage Patterns and Living Arrangements," in Everett S. Lee and John D. Reid, eds., *The Black Population of the United States* (Athens, Ga.: University of Georgia Press, forthcoming).

15. Elizabeth Herzog and Cecelia E. Sudia, *Boys in Fatherless Families,* U.S. Children's Bureau, 1970. Also F. Ivan Nye, "Child Adjustment in Broken and in Unhappy Unbroken Homes," in Marvin B. Sussman, ed., *Sourcebook in Marriage and the Family,* ed. 3 (Boston: Houghton Mifflin Co., 1968), pp. 434–440.

16. Findings reported to one of the authors by William F. Pratt, based on data obtained in connection with the preparation of his 1965 Ph.D. dissertation in sociology at the University of Michigan, "A Study of Marriages Involving

Premarital Pregnancies." See also Lolagene C. Coombs, Ronald Freedman, Judith Friedman, and William F. Pratt, "Premarital Pregnancy and Status before and after Marriage," *American Journal of Sociology,* 75, no. 5 (March 1970), 800–820.

17. Reynolds Farley, "Family Stability: A Comparison of Trends Between Blacks and Whites," *American Sociological Review,* 36, no. 1 (February 1971), 1–17.

18. Frances Kobrin, "The Fall in Household Size and the Rise of the Primary Individual in the United States," *Demography,* 13, no. 1 (February 1976), in press.

19. Angus Campbell, "The American Way of Mating: Marriage Sí, Children Only Maybe," *Psychology Today,* 8, no. 12 (May 1975), 37–43.

20. Glick and Mills, "Black Families," note 14.

21. Abbott L. Ferriss, *Indicators of Trends in the Status of American Women* (New York: Russell Sage Foundation, 1971).

22. Larry L. Bumpass and James A. Sweet, "Differentials in Marital Stability: 1970," *American Sociological Review,* 37, no. 6 (December 1972), 754–766.

23. Teresa Donati Marciano, "The Unmarriageability of Educated Women," paper presented at the Joint Groves Conference and International Workshop on the Changing Sex Roles in Family and Society, Dubrovnik, Yugoslavia, June 1975.

24. Beatrice Rosenberg and Ethel Mendelsohn, "Legal Status of Women," in Council of State Governments, *The Book of the States,* 1974–75 (available from U.S. Women's Bureau, 1975), pp. 402–411.

25. Lenore J. Weitzman, "Legal Regulation of Marriage: Tradition and Change," *California Law Review,* 62, no. 4 (July-September 1974), 1169–1288. Also Marvin B. Sussman, "Marriage Contracts: Social and Legal Consequences," paper presented at the Joint Groves Conference and International Workshop on the Changing Sex Roles in Family and Society, Dubrovnik, Yugoslavia, June 1975.

26. Henry H. Foster and Dorothy Jonas Freed, "Divorce Reform: Brakes on Breakdown?", *Journal of Family Law,* 13, no. 3 (1973–74), 443–493.

27. Rosenberg and Mendelsohn, "Status of Women," note 24, pp. 412, 413.

28. The Uniform Marriage and Divorce Act is printed in the *Family Law Quarterly,* 5, no. 2 (June 1971), 204–251. Detailed comments of the national conference are included. See also the report on the Uniform Marriage and Divorce Act of the Joint Meeting between the Representatives of the Section on Family Law and the Commissioners on Uniform State Laws held in New Orleans on April 3 and 4, 1971 (*Family Law Quarterly,* 5, no. 2, June 1971, 125 ff.). The text of the final version of the Uniform Act is available from the National Conference on Uniform State Laws, 645 North Michigan Avenue, Chicago, Illinois 60637. The version prepared by FLS-ABA was published as the Proposed Revised Uniform Marriage and Divorce Act, *Family Law Quarterly,* 7, no. 1 (January 1973), 135–168.

29. Dorothy Linder Maddi, "The Effect of Conciliation Court Proceedings on Petitions for Dissolution of Marriage," *Journal of Family Law,* 13, no. 3 (1974), 495–566.

30. Foster and Freed, "Divorce Reform," note 26.

31. *Ibid.,* p. 449.

32. *Ibid.,* p. 457.

33. *Ibid.,* p. 480.

34. *Ibid.,* p. 491.

35. *Ibid.*

36. Wendell H. Goddard, "A Report on California's New Divorce Law: Progress and Problems," *Family Law Quarterly,* 6 (1972), 405–421.

37. Proposed Revised Uniform Marriage and Divorce Act, *Family Law Quarterly,* 7, no. 1 (January 1973), 146.

INDEX

Abandonment, as grounds for divorce, 374

Abortion, for premarital pregnancy, 456

Accidental deaths, of unmarried persons, 349. *See also* Motor-vehicle accidents

Accountants, proportion divorced, 261

Actors, 317

Actresses, 317

Acute health conditions, and marital status, 450

Administrative mechanisms: for enforcing marriage laws, 362–365, 456; for enforcing divorce laws, 374–381, 467. *See also* Divorce laws; Marriage laws

Adult life, stages of related to marital status, 64–66

Adultery, as grounds for divorce, 27, 366, 374

Age: related to civil ceremony, 53; at divorce, 57–58, 226–234, 392, 432–433; and marital status, 59, 63–66, 397–400; at first marriage, 77–82, 388–392, 406–407, 442–443; at remarriage, 82–85, 408–409, 438; and relationships in shared home, 154–156; in three-generation families, 158–162; and residential movement, 163; and home ownership, 166–167; and employment, 170; and occupational choice, 190–191, 193; and income, 205–206, 214–215; residential patterns of divorced persons by, 251–252; of widowed persons, 275–278, 438; of bachelors and spinsters, 299–301; death rates by, 342–343

Age, marriage rate by, 20–26, 38; under twenty, 20–21; over sixty, 21; of women between twenty and twenty-nine, 21–26, 442–443; of men between twenty and thirty-four, 21–26, 285–286

Age at marriage, 77–110, 406–409; at first marriage, 77–82, 388–392, 406–407, 442–443; at remarriage, 82–85, 225–226, 408–409, 438; by type of residence, 85–87; by age of spouse, 87–90; by ethnic origin, 90–92; by educational level, 92–93, 107; by occupational groups, 93–97, 107; by income level, 98–110; marital dissolution by, 234–238; laws relating to, 358–360, 455–456, 461; enforcing of, 362–364; by marital status, 407–409; and marital stability, 409

Aged, homes for, 335

Alabama: divorce laws in, 367, 458; migratory divorce in, 373; common-law marriages recognized in, 456

Alameda County, divorce laws in, 467

Alaska, 68; proportion of remarriages in, 53; Orientals in, 70; divorce laws in, 367, 458; migratory divorce in, 371

Alcoholism, chronic, premarital tests for, 361, 414

Aldous, Joan, 479

Alimony, 378, 379

American Bar Association, 9, 455, 460

American Indian children, with parents of different race, 415–416

American Indian–white marriages, 119, 413–414

American Indians: marital status of, 68; subfamilies of, 158, 161; employment rates of married women among, 178, 180; percent divorced, 243; widowed among, 280; bachelors and spinsters among, 303; in interracial marriages, 362, 413–414

American Sociological Association, 384

Annulment of marriage, 54, 366; defined, 26

Argentina, divorce not granted in, 27, 392

Arkansas: residence requirements in, 373; divorces in, 373; divorce laws in, 458

Arizona: lack of state files in, 383; divorce laws in, 458

Armed Forces: proportion of married men in, 189; marriage data from, 399

Arthritis, incidence of by marital status, 328

Artists, 317

Auditors, proportion divorced, 261

Australia: marriage rates in, 17, 20, 388; divorce rates in, 30, 31, 32, 39; early marriage in, 389

Austria: divorce rates in, 30, 390; marriage rates in, 386–387

Baby boom, 81, 444

Bachelors: defined, 298; age distribution of, 299–301; ethnic origin of, 302–305; living arrangements of, 305–308; urban vs. rural residence for, 308–310; educational level of, 310–313; work experience of, 313–318; income of, 318–320; late marriage vs. nonmarriage of, 320–323; percent in institutions, 335; percent in mental hospitals, 336–337. *See also* Single persons